Current Topics in Microbiology 126 and Immunology

Editors

A. Clarke, Parkville/Victoria · R.W. Compans,
Birmingham/Alabama · M. Cooper, Birmingham/Alabama
H. Eisen, Paris · W. Goebel, Würzburg · H. Koprowski,
Philadelphia · F. Melchers, Basel · M. Oldstone,
La Jolla/California · R. Rott, Gießen · P.K. Vogt, Los Angeles
H. Wagner, Ulm · I. Wilson, La Jolla/California

Specificity and Function of Clonally Developing T Cells

Edited by B. Fleischer, J. Reimann, and H. Wagner

With 60 Figures

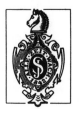

Springer-Verlag
Berlin Heidelberg New York Tokyo

BERNHARD FLEISCHER, M.D.
JÖRG REIMANN, M.D.
HERMANN WAGNER, M.D.
Department of Medical Microbiology and Immunology
University of Ulm
Oberer Eselsberg
D-7900 Ulm

ISBN-13:978-3-642-71154-1   e-ISBN-13:978-3-642-71152-7
DOI: 10.1007/978-3-642-71152-7

This work is subject to copyright. All rights are reserved, whether the whole
or part of the material is concerned, specifically those of translation, reprinting,
re-use of illustrations, broadcasting, reproduction by photocopying machine or
similar means, and storage in data banks. Under § 54 of the German Copyright
Law where copies are made for other than private use, a fee is payable to
"Verwertungsgesellschaft Wort", Munich

© by Springer-Verlag Berlin Heidelberg 1986
Softcover reprint of the hardcover 1st edition 1986

Library of Congress Catalog Card Number 15-12910

The use of registered names, trademarks, etc. in this publication does not imply,
even in the absence of a specific statement, that such names are exempt from
the relevant protective laws and regulations and therefore free for general use.

Product Liability: The publishers can give no guarantee for information about
drug dosage and application thereof contained in this book. In every individual
case the respective user must check its accuracy by consulting other pharmaceutical literature.

2123/3130-543210

Preface

The international workshop on "Specificity and Function of Clonally Developing T Cells" was held at Schloß Reisensburg (near Ulm, West Germany) on March 17–20, 1985. The meeting brought together immunologists studying clonal T-cell development in man and mouse in various in vitro systems at the cellular as well as molecular level. It was an attempt to provide an overview of the current research interests of groups working on (a) the developmental potential of in vitro expanding primary T-cell clones (investigated using limiting dilution analysis) and cloned T-cell lines established in long-term culture; (b) the signals required for the expression of particular patterns of (functional and antigen receptor) phenotypes by T cells which are either freshly explanted in vitro, or maintained in vitro as cloned long-term lines; and (c) the generation of an MHC-restricted T-cell repertoire.

In the study of thymocytes emphasis has shifted towards the presumably immature adult/embryonic subset(s) which is (are) devoid of subset-specific differentiation markers (L3T4, Lyt-2). Neither the signal requirement(s) for clonal expansion in vitro of these cells, nor their precursor role for any functional T-cell lineage are as yet unambiguously established. The multiple modes of human T-cell activation (e.g., via Tp44, T11, T3/Ti molecular complexes) were emphasized by a number of presentations and raised the question of whether these different modes of activation induce different functional activities in individual T-cell clones. The fact that two or more different functional phenotypes (e.g., helper and/or cytotoxic activity) can be activated in many human T-cell clones established in long-term culture raised the fundamental question of whether distinct T-cell lineages irreversibly committed to the expression of a particular pattern of functional phenotypes do exist, or alternatively whether every individual T-cell clone is multipotential with respect to the patterns of functional phenotypes it can express, with environmental influences deciding on the functional activity actually realized.

The sessions on the generation of T-cell receptor diversity addressed three topics central to the issue. (a) The role of somatic diversification in generating the T-cell receptor diversity was discussed. In contrast to the B-cell system, the available experimental evidence for a somatic diversification of the T-cell repertoire is preliminary. (b) The question of the self/nonself discrimination of the T-cell receptor repertoire has become more complex, as the difference between "physiologic self-reactivity" and "autoimmune reactivity" has become exceedingly difficult to define. The presence of self-reactive T-cell clones in the intact immune system was acknowledged, but its functional significance remains controversial. (c) The role of MHC determinants in "guiding" the generation of diversity of the T-cell repertoire was discussed with reference to the two previous topics. New data on allorestricted T-cell repertoire development in vitro raised basic questions on the role of MHC structures in directing the process of unfolding of the T-cell repertoire.

We are grateful for support from the Deutsche Forschungsgemeinschaft and indebted to Springer Verlag, for its interest in editing and publishing these proceedings.

Ulm, Spring 1986

HERMANN WAGNER
BERNHARD FLEISCHER
JÖRG REIMANN

Table of Contents

Part A: Development of T Lymphocytes in the Thymus

R. SCOLLAY: Introductory Remarks 3

K. SHORTMAN, R. SCOLLAY, P. ANDREWS, and R. BOYD: Development of T Lymphocytes Within the Thymus and Within Thymic Nurse Cells. With 3 Figures 5

H. VON BOEHMER: Thymus Development 19

R. CEREDIG: Major Histocompatibility-Restricted Cytolytic T-Lymphocyte Precursors from the Thymus of In Vivo Primed Mice: Increased Frequency and Resistance to Anti-Lyt-2 Antibody Inhibition. With 1 Figure 27

J.J.T. OWEN, E.J. JENKINSON, and R. KINGSTON: Thymic Stem Cells: Their Interaction with the Thymic Stroma and Tolerance Induction 35

Part B: Murine T-Cell Receptor Genes

M. STEINMETZ and Z. DEMBIĆ: Organization, Rearrangement, and Diversification of Mouse T-Cell Receptor Genes. With 1 Figure 45

L. ADORINI, G. PALMIERI, A. SETTE, E. APPELLA, and G. DORIA: Expression of T-Cell Receptor by a Mouse Monoclonal Antigen-Specific Suppressor T-Cell Line 53

H.U. WELTZIEN and K. EICHMANN: Somatic Variation of Antigen-Recognition Specificity in H-2^b-TNP-Specific Cytotoxic T-Cell Clones 63

J.T. EPPLEN, S. ALI, A. RINALDY, and M.M. SIMON: The Change of Specificity, Karyotype, and Antigen-Receptor Gene Expression is Correlated in Cytotoxic T-Cell Lines 69

VIII   Table of Contents

Part C: Phenotype and Functional Potential of T-Cell Clones

H. VON BOEHMER: Introductory Remarks 77

C.G. BROOKS: A Study of the Functional Potential of
Mouse T-Cell Clones 79

J.P. TITE, B. JONES, M.E. KATZ, and C.A. JANEWAY:
Generation, Propagation, and Variation in Cloned,
Antigen-Specific, I a-Restricted Cytolytic T-Cell
Lines 93

B. FLEISCHER and H. WAGNER: Significance of T4 or
T8 Phenotype of Human Cytotoxic T-Lymphocyte
Clones. With 1 Figure 101

K. SHORTMAN and A. WILSON: Natural and
Unnatural Killing by Cytolytic T Lymphocytes.
With 2 Figures 111

G. PAWELEC, F.-W. BUSCH, E.M. SCHNEIDER, A.
REHBEIN, I. BALKO, and P. WERNET: Acquisition of
Suppressive and Natural Killer-Like Activities
Associated with Loss of Alloreactivity in Human
"Helper" T-Lymphocyte Clones. With 3 Figures 121

J. HEUER, E. KÖLSCH, and K. RESKE: Expression and
Function of Class II I-A^k Antigens on an Antigen-
Specific T-Suppressor Cell Clone. With 2 Figures 131

Part D: Signal Requirements for T-Cell Activation

H. WAGNER: Introductory Remarks 141

H. WAGNER and C. HARDT: Heterogeneity of the
Signal Requirements During the Primary
Activation of Resting Lyt-2$^+$ Cytotoxic T-
Lymphocyte (CTL) Precursors into Clonally
Developing CTL. With 2 Figures 143

A.C. OCHOA, G. GROMO, S.-L. WEE, and F.H. BACH:
Regulation of Lytic Function by Recombinant IL2
and Antigen. With 4 Figures 155

T. HÜNIG: The Target Structure for T11: A Cell
Interaction Molecule Involved in T-Cell
Activation? With 3 Figures 165

M.M. SIMON, S. LANDOLFO, T. DIAMANTSTEIN, and
U. HOCHGESCHWENDER: Antigen- and Lectin-
Sensitized Murine Cytolytic T Lymphocyte-

Precursors Require Both Interleukin 2 and
Endogenously Produced Immune (γ) Interferon for
Their Growth and Differentiation. With 3 Figures   173

H.R. MacDonald and F. Erard: Activation
Requirements for Resting T Lymphocytes 187

**Part E: Self-Nonself Discrimination in the T-Cell
Compartment**

M. Feldmann: Introductory Remarks   197

G.J.V. Nossal, B.L. Pike, M.F. Good, J.F.A.P.
Miller, and J.R. Gamble: Functional Clonal
Deletion and Suppression as Complementary
Mechanisms in T Lymphocyte Tolerance   199

M. Feldmann, J.R. Lamb, and M. Londei: Human
T Cell Clones, Tolerance, and the Analysis of
Autoimmunity. With 1 Figure 207

M.H. Claësson and C. Röpke: Antiself Suppressive
(Veto) Activity of Responder Cells in Mixed
Lymphocyte Cultures. With 6 Figures   213

H.-D. Haubeck, O. Kloke, and E. Kölsch:
Analysis of T Suppressor Cell Mediated Tumor
Escape Mechanisms. With 2 Figures   225

M.K. Hoffmann, M. Chun, J.A. Hirst, and U.
Hämmerling: The T-Cell Receptor Recognizes
Nominal and Self Antigen Independently. A
Theoretical Alternative to the Modified Self
Concept. With 3 Figures   231

Part F: T-Cell-Mediated Autoreactivity

R.G. Miller: Introductory Remarks 241

J. Reimann, K. Heeg, D. Kabelitz, H. Wagner,
and R.G. Miller: T-Cell Reactivity to
Polymorphic MHC Determinants. I. MHC-Guided
T-Cell Reactivity   243

K. Heeg, D. Kabelitz, H. Wagner, and J.
Reimann: T-Cell Reactivity to Polymorphic MHC
Determinants. II. Self-Reactive and Self-Restricted
T Cells. With 6 Figures 259

D. Kabelitz, K. Heeg, H. Wagner, and J.
Reimann: T-Cell Reactivity to Polymorphic MHC

Determinants. III. Alloreactive and Allorestricted
T Cells. With 9 Figures 275

P. BENVENISTE and R.G. MILLER: Appearance of
New Specificities in Lectin-Induced T-Cell Clones
Obtained from Limiting Dilution T-Cell Cultures.
With 2 Figures 291

M.H. CLAËSSON and C. RÖPKE: Syngeneic
Cytotoxicity and Veto Activity in Thymic
Lymphoid Colonies and Their Expanded Progeny.
With 4 Figures 301

T. SAITO and K. RAJEWSKY: Functional Analysis of
a Self-I-A Reactive T-Cell Clone Which
Preferentially Stimulates Activated B Cells . . . 311

Indexed in Current Contents

List of Contributors

ADORINI, L., ENEA-Euratom Immunogenetics Group, Laboratory of Pathology, CRE Casaccia, CP 2400, I-00100 Rome AD

ALI, S., Max-Planck-Institut für Immunobiologie, Stübeweg 51, D-7800 Freiburg

ANDREWS, P., Walter and Eliza Hall Institute of Medical Research, Post Office, Royal Melbourne Hospital, Victoria 3050, Australia

APELLA, E., Laboratory of Cell Biology, NCI, NIH, Bethesda, MD 20205, USA

BACH, F.H., Immunobiology Research Center, Departments of Laboratory Medicine, Pathology, and Surgery, University of Minnesota, MN 55455, USA

BALKO, I., Immunology Laboratory, Medizinische Klinik, D-7400 Tübingen

BENVENISTE, P., Ontario Cancer Institute and Department of Immunology, University of Toronto, 500 Sherbourne St., Toronto, Ontario M4X 1K9, Canada

BOEHMER, H. VON, Basel Institute for Immunology, Grenzacher Str. 487, CH-4005 Basel

BOYD, R., Department of Pathology and Immunology, Monash University Medical School, Melbourne, Australia

BROOKS, C.G., Basic Immunology, Fred Hutchinson Cancer Research Center, 1124 Columbia Street, Seattle, WA 98104, USA

BUSCH, F.-W., Immunology Laboratory, Medizinische Klinik, D-7400 Tübingen

CEREDIG, R., Ludwig Institute for Cancer Research, Lausanne Branch, CH-1066 Epalinges

XII List of Contributors

CHUN, M., Memorial Sloan-Kettering Cancer Center, New York, NY 10021, USA

CLAËSSON, M.H., Institute of Medical Anatomy, Dept. A, University of Copenhagen, The Panum Institute, Blegdamsvej 3, DK-2200 Copenhagen N

DEMBIĆ, Z., Basel Institute for Immunology, Grenzacher Str. 487, CH-4005 Basel

DIAMANTSTEIN, T., Immunologische Forschungseinheit, Klinikum Steglitz, Freie Universität, D-1000 Berlin

DORIA, G., ENEA-Euratom Immunogenetics Group, Laboratory of Pathology, CRE Casaccia, CP 2400, I-00100 Rome AD

EICHMANN, K., Max-Planck-Institut für Immunbiologie, Stübeweg 51, D-7800 Freiburg

EPPLEN, J.T., Max-Planck-Institut für Immunbiologie, Stübeweg 51, D-7800 Freiburg

ERARD, F., Ludwig Institute for Cancer Research, Lausanne Branch, and Genetics Unit, Swiss Institute for Experimental Cancer Research, CH-1066 Epalinges

FELDMANN, M., ICRF Tumour Immunology Unit, Zoology Department, University Colege London, Gower Street, London WC1E 6BT, U.K.

FLEISCHER, B., Department of Medical Microbiology and Immunology, University of Ulm, D-7900 Ulm

GAMBLE, J.R., Walter and Eliza Hall Institute of Medical Research, Post Office, Royal Melbourne Hospital, Victoria 3050, Australia

GOOD, M.F., Walter and Eliza Hall Institute of Medical Research, Post Office, Royal Melbourne Hospital, Victoria 3050 Australia

GROMO, G., Immunobiology Research Center, Departments of Laboratory Medicine, Pathology, and Surgery, University of Minnesota, MN 55455, USA

HÄMMERLING, U., Memorial Sloan-Kettering Cancer Center, New York, NY 10021, USA

HARDT, C., Department of Medical Microbiology and Immunology, University of Ulm, D-7900 Ulm

HAUBECK, H.-D., Department of Immunology, University of Münster, Domagkstr. 3, D-4400 Münster

HEEG, K., Department of Medical Microbiology and Immunology, University of Ulm, D-7900 Ulm

HEUER, J., Department of Immunology, University of Münster, Domagkstr. 3, D-4400 Münster

HIRST, J.A., Memorial Sloan-Kettering Cancer Center, New York, NY 10021, USA

HOCHGESCHWENDER, U., Max-Planck-Institut für Immunbiologie, Stübeweg 51, D-7800 Freiburg

HOFFMANN, M.K., Memorial Sloan-Kettering Cancer Center, New York, NY 1021, USA

HÜNIG, T., Institute for Virology and Immunobiology, Versbacher Str. 7, D-8700 Würzburg

JANEWAY, C.A., Jr., Department of Pathology, Howard Hughes Medical Institute at Yale University School of Medicine, 310 Cedar Street, New Haven, CT 06510, USA

JENKINSON, E.J., Department of Anatomy, Medical School, University of Birmingham, Birmingham, U.K.

JONES, B., Department of Pathology, Howard Hughes Medical Institute at Yale University School of Medicine, 310 Cedar Street, New Haven, CT 06510, USA

KABELITZ, D., Department of Medical Microbiology and Immunology, University of Ulm, D-7900 Ulm

KATZ, E., Department of Pathology, Howard Hughes Medical Institute at Yale University School of Medicine, 310 Cedar Street, New Haven, CT 06510, USA

KINGSTON, R., Department of Anatomy, Medical School, University of Birmingham, Birmingham, U.K.

KLOKE, O., Department of Immunology, University of Münster, Domagkstr. 3, D-4400 Münster

KÖLSCH, E., Department of Immunology, University of Münster, Domagkstr. 3, D-4400 Münster

LAMB, J.R., ICRF Tumour Immunology Unit, Zoology Department, University College London, Gower Street, London WC1E 6BT, U.K.

LANDOLFO, S., Institute of Microbiology, University of Torino, I-Torino

LONDEI, M., ICRF Tumour Immunology Unit, Zoology Department, University College London, Cower Street, London WC1E 6BT, U.K.

MacDonald, H.R., Ludwig Institute for Cancer Research, Lausanne Branch, and Genetics Unit, Swiss Institute for Experimental Cancer Research, CH-1066 Epalinges

Miller, J.F.A.P., Walter and Eliza Hall Institute of Medical Research, Post Office, Royal Melbourne Hospital, Victoria 3050, Australia

Miller, R.G., Ontario Cancer Institute and Department of Immunology, University of Toronto, 5000 Sherbourne St., Toronto, Ontario M4X 1K9, Canada

Nossal, G.J.V., Walter and Eliza Hall Institute of Medical Research, Post Office, Royal Melbourne Hospital, Victoria 3050, Australia

Ochoa, A.C., Immunobiology Research Center, Departments of Laboratory Medicine, Pathology and Surgery, University of Minnesota, MN 55455, USA

Owen, J.J.T., Department of Anatomy, Medical School, University of Birmingham, Vincent Drive, Birmingham B15 2TJ, U.K.

Palmieri, G., ENEA-Euratom Immunogenetics Group, Laboratory of Pathology, CRE Casaccia, CP 2400, I-00100 Rome AD

Pawelec, G., Immunology Laboratory, Medizinische Universitätsklinik, D-7400 Tübingen

Pike, L., Walter and Eliza Hall Institute of Medical Research, Post Office, Royal Melbourne Hospital, Victoria 3050, Australia

Rajewski, K., Institute for Genetics, University of Cologne, D-5000 Cologne

Rehbein, A., Immunology Laboratory, Medizinische Klinik, D-7400 Tübingen

Reimann, J., Department of Medical Microbiology and Immunology, University of Ulm, D-7900 Ulm

Reske, K., Department of Immunology, University of Mainz, Hochhaus am Augustusplatz, D-6500 Mainz

Rinaldy, A., Max-Planck-Institut für Immunbiologie, Stübeweg 51, D-7800 Freiburg

Röpke, C., Institute of Medical Anatomy, Department A, University of Copenhagen, The Panum Institute, 3 Blegdamsvej, DK-2200 Copenhagen N

SAITO, T., Institute for Genetics, University of Cologne, D-5000 Cologne

SCHNEIDER, E.M., Immunology Laboratory, Medizinische Klinik, D-7400 Tübingen

SCOLLAY, R., Walter and Eliza Hall Institute of Medical Research, Post Office, Royal Melbourne Hospital, Victoria 3050, Australia

SETTE, A., ENEA-Euratom Immunogenetics Group, Laboratory of Pathology, CRE, Casaccia, CP 2400, I-00100 Rome AD

SHORTMAN, K., Walter and Eliza Hall Institute of Medical Research, Post Office, Royal Melbourne Hospital, Victoria 3050, Australia

SIMON, M.M., Max-Planck-Institut für Immunbiologie, Stübeweg 51, D-7800 Freiburg

STEINMETZ, M., Basel Institute for Immunology, Grenzacherstr. 487, CH-4005 Basel

TITE, J.P., Department of Pathology, Howard Hughes Medical Institute of Yale University School of Medicine, 310 Cedar Street, New Haven, CT 06510, USA

WAGNER, H., Department of Medical Microbiology and Immunology, University of Ulm, Oberer Eselsberg, D-7900 Ulm

WEE, S.-L., Immunobiology Research Center, Departments of Laboratory Medicine, Pathology, and Surgery, University of Minnesota, MN 55455, USA

WELTZIEN, H.U., Max-Planck-Institut für Immunbiologie, D-7800 Freiburg

WERNET, P., Immunology Laboratory, Medizinische Klinik, D-7400 Tübingen

WILSON, A., Walter and Eliza Hall Institute of Medical Research, Post Office, Royal Melbourne Hospital, Victoria 3050, Australia

Part A: Development of T Lymphocytes in the Thymus

Introductory Remarks

R. SCOLLAY

This section focuses mainly on the small population of thymocytes which expresses neither Ly-2 nor L3T4. These cells (3% – 5% of all thymocytes) represent the most easily identified precursor cells in the thymus, and for reasons made clear in the three following papers, are perhaps one of the most interesting in terms of the critical events of intrathymic T-cell differentiation. There was general agreement between speakers and discussers on most areas with the possible exception of the significance of cortical staining with the antibody MEL-14 (see below).

The Ly-2$^-$ L3T4$^-$ cells are by no means homogeneous. Ceredig (Lausanne) shows that they were heterogeneous for a number of markers including MEL-14 and IL-2 receptor expression. Shortman et al. (Melbourne) show that they could be subdivided into at least four further subpopulations on the basis of Ly-1 and Thy-1 staining but pointed out that there were differences between adult and embryonic Ly-2$^-$ L3T4$^-$ cells. Cross-correlations of all the various markers have not yet been performed, so how far this subdivision can reasonably go remains to be seen.

With regard to T-cell antigen-receptor expression on these cells, von Boehmer (Basel), using an ontogenetic approach, and Schwartz (Bethesda), using adult Ly-2$^-$ L3T4$^-$ cells and lines made from fusions of them with BW5147 (personal communication), both suggest that β-chain rearrangement was probably occurring among these cells, since some were rearranged and some were not. Data for the α-chain genes were not yet available. Full-length γ-chain and β-chain message is present in at least some of the cells (although not yet detectable in the day 15 embryo), but whether any protein is expressed and what form it takes (γ, β heterodimers?) remains entirely speculative. (More details are given in the von Boehmer paper.)

Attemps to induce differentiation of Ly-2$^-$ L3T4$^-$ cells in vitro have so far had limited success, but MacDonald (Lausanne) reports some adult derived Ly-2$^-$ L3T4$^-$ lines which could be induced with IL-2 and PMA to become Ly-2$^+$ L3T4$^-$ (personal communication), and von Boehmer (Basel) describes some fetal-derived Ly-2$^-$ L3T4$^-$ cells which would also become Ly-2$^+$ L3T4$^-$. However, the possibility of contamination by mature cells or filler cells remains to be excluded in these experiments. Conditions have not yet been described which will allow development of Ly-2$^-$ L3T4$^+$ cells or continuous production of Ly-2$^+$ L3T4$^+$ cells in vitro. This lack is a major stumbling block in the field. However, Schwartz (Bethesda) reports experiments from Fowlkes (Bethesda) which show that when

---

Walter and Eliza Hall Institute of Medical Research, Post Office, Royal Melbourne Hospital, Victoria 3050, Australia

used to reconstitute irradiated thymuses in vivo, the Ly-2$^-$ L3T4$^-$ population contains precursors of all other major subpopulations (personal communication) while Owen et al. (Birmingham) report that lymphocyte-depleted thymus organ cultures could be repopulated with a single fetal thymocyte (i.e., Ly-2$^-$ L3T4$^-$ cell), generating eventually all other major subpopulations (personal communication). Clearly then, as earlier experiments with organ cultured fetal thymus showed, Ly-2$^-$ L3T4$^-$ cells do contain all the precursor activity for the other subpopulations, and presumably conditions will eventually be found which allow expression of this potential in simplified culture systems.

Shortman et al. (Melbourne) discusses thymic nurse cells and shows that they seem to represent structures which are enclosed in vivo, and that they contain cells of both mature and immature phenotypes. Surprisingly, and in contrast to other reports, he did not find any CTL activity in cells isolated from within nurse cells. Whether this discrepancy is due to differences in purity of isolated nurse cell lymphocytes remains to be determined.

Finally, Reichert (Stanford) reports the data on MEL-14 staining of thymocyte suspensions and thymus frozen sections (personal communication). MEL-14 is the antibody which recognizes a receptor involved in lymphocyte migration into lymph nodes. Its strong expression on a small percentage of isolated cells in the thymic cortex, but not in the medulla (frozen sections), has led to speculation that these cortical cells are the ones about to migrate to the periphery. The predominantly cortical location of the brightest MEL-14 cells was clear on the sections, but in cell suspensions, the strongest MEL-14$^+$ cells included many Ly-2$^-$ L3T4$^-$ blasts. There is some disagreement between Reichert, Ceredig, and Scollay as to how many of the brightest MEL-14$^+$ cells were Ly-2$^-$ L3T4$^-$ and how many were of a more mature phenotype (Ly-2$^+$ L3T4$^-$ or Ly-2$^-$ L3T4$^+$), but all agree that single positives did exist among the strong MEL-14$^+$ cells. The absence of such cells in the medulla in the sections therefore suggests either a cortical location for some mature MEL-14$^+$ cells, or a discrepancy between the section and suspension staining. Again, further experiments are needed to resolve this issue.

In summary, a clearer picture is emerging of the early thymocytes as a heterogeneous population scattered through the cortex with various degrees of T-cell antigen receptor chain rearrangement probably in progress. However, the details of lineage determination and antigenic selection events remain as mysterious as ever.

Development of T Lymphocytes Within the Thymus and Within Thymic Nurse Cells

K. Shortman[1], R. Scollay[1], P. Andrews[1], and R. Boyd[2]

1 The Main Thymocyte Subpopulations   5
1.1 Medullary and Cortical Thymocytes   6
1.2 T-Cell Lineage Markers on Cortical and Medullary Thymocytes   6
1.3 Size and Division Rate   7
1.4 Immunocompetence   7
2 Developmental Steps Involving the Main Thymocyte Subpopulations   8
2.1 Development and Fate of Cortical Thymocytes   8
2.2 Development and Fate of Medullary Thymocytes   8
2.3 Conclusions   9
3 Definition of Putative Early Thymocytes   9
3.1 Ly-2$^-$ L3T4$^-$ Thymocytes   10
3.2 B2A2$^-$ Thymocytes   10
3.3 Overlap Between Ly-2$^-$ L3T4$^-$ and B2A2$^-$ Thymocytes   11
4 Division of Putative Early Thymocytes by Multiparameter Analysis   12
5 Intrathymic Location of Subsets of Putative Early Thymocytes   12
6 Possible Developmental Streams   12
7 Lymphocyte-Epithelial Cell Interactions and Thymic Nurse Cells   13
8 Phenotype of Intra-Nurse-Cell Lymphocytes   15
9 Functional Capacity of Intra-Nurse-Cell Lymphocytes   16
10 Conclusions   16
References   17

1 The Main Thymocyte Subpopulations

Any detailed study of T-cell development within the thymus requires, as a first step, the ability of distinguish the subpopulations of lymphoid cells which may be steps along a developmental pathway. About 95 % of adult murine thymic lymphocytes can be assigned to one of four discrete subpopulations as summarized in Table 1. These major subpopulations, and many of their surface markers, have been recognized for some time, and the recent application of multiparameter flow cytometric analysis (Scollay and Shortman 1983) has merely served to emphasize how clearcut this four-way division can be. This subdivision is obtained as follows.

---

[1] Walter and Eliza Hall Institute of Medical Research, Post Office, Royal Melbourne Hospital, Victoria 3050, Australia
[2] Department of Pathology and Immunology, Monash University Medical School, Melbourne, Australia

6   K. Shortman et al.

Table 1. The established murine thymocyte subpopulations

	Cortex		Medulla	
Antigenic phenotype	PNA^{++} Thy-1^{++} Ly-1$^+$ H-2K$^{\mp}$ B2A2^{++} Ly-2$^+$ L3T4$^+$		PNA$^{\mp}$ Thy-1$^+$ Ly-1^{++} H-2K^{++} B2A2$^+$ Ly-2$^+$ L3T4$^-$ and Ly-2$^-$ L3T4$^+$	
Size and division rate	Small (LS 100) nondividing	Large (LS 155) rapidly dividing	Medium (LS 128) | (LS 118) non- (or slowly) dividing	
Immuno- competence				Functional
	Nonfunctional		Cytolytic (Class I restricted)	Helper (Class II restricted
Percent of thymocytes	65	15	4	8

The data are summarized from SCOLLAY and SHORTMAN (1983), SCOLLAY et al. (1984a, b, c) and SHORTMAN et al. (1985), and are based on the analysis of 5-week-old male CBA mice. LS, relative low-angle light scatter

1.1 Medullary and Cortical Thymocytes

Some 12 % of all adult male CBA mouse thymocytes are found within the medullary region, and these cells differ in surface antigenic phenotype from the thymocytes in the cortex; very few (<1 %) of cells of medullary phenotype can be detected in the cortex, and vice versa (SHORTMAN et al. 1985). Medullary thymocytes are like peripheral T cells by most surface markers (PNA$\mp$ Thy-1$^+$ Ly-1^{++} H-2K^{++}) as well as by the lineage markers discussed below. However, they differ slightly from peripheral T cells in both physical properties and in expression of the antigenic marker B2A2, which is positive (but low) on medullary cells, and negative on peripheral T cells (SCOLLAY et al. 1984a, 1984b). According to all these markers, the two main groups of cortical thymocytes have a "thymus-unique" surface phenotype, opposite or quantitatively very different from medullary thymocytes and peripheral T cells.

1.2 T-Cell Lineage Markers on Cortical and Medullary Thymocytes

The development of monoclonal antibodies against the T-cell sublineage markers Ly-2 und L3T4 (the equivalent of T8 and T4 in the human) provided a further means of distinguishing cortical from medullary thymocytes (REINHERZ et al. 1980; DIALYNAS et al. 1983; CEREDIG et al. 1983a; SCOLLAY et al. 1984a). Medullary thymocytes, like peripheral T cells, express one or other of these antigens in a mutually exclusive way and are thus already divided into the separate functional lineages. By contrast, the typical cortical populations express both markers

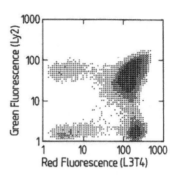

Fig. 1. Two-color fluorescent analysis of adult CBA mouse thymocytes for the expression of Ly-2 and L3T4. The figure is reproduced from SCOLLAY and SHORTMAN (1985). The major, "double-positive" population corresponds to cortical thymocytes (both small and large), the two single-positive populations to medullary thymocytes. The 4%–5% "double-negative" population represents the putative early blast cells

Table 2. The limited immunocompetence of nurse-cell lymphocytes

	Precursor frequency	
	PTL-P	CTL-P
Cortisone-resistant (medullary) thymocytes	0.88 ± 0.04	0.13 ± 0.03
PNA⁺ (cortical) thymocytes	0.003 ± 0.001	0.0008 ± 0.0002
Nurse-cell lymphocytes	0.030 ± 0.008	0.0000 ± 0.0000

The data are summarized from ANDREWS et al. (1985). PTL-P represents the total frequency of cells forming proliferating clones measured by ^{3}H-TdR uptake 9 days after Concanavalin A stimulation. CTL-P represents the total frequency of cells forming cytolytic clones measured by PHA-enhanced cytolysis of ^{111}In-labeled P815 8 days after Concanavalin A stimulation. Nurse-cell thymocytes were obtained as the cells released from individual nurse cells isolated by micromanipulation and incubated for 4–6 h in Terasaki tray wells. The control samples of cortical (PNA⁺) or medullary (cortisone-resistant) thymocytes were cultured and assayed side by side with the nurse-cell lymphocytes

simultaneously. The major, "double-positive cortical population and the two "single-positive" medullary populations can readily be distinguished by two-color immunofluorescent flow-cytometric analyses, as shown in Fig. 1.

1.3 Size and Division Rate

Amongst cortical thymocytes there is a clear division by size (or low-angle light scatter) into the large, medium-sized rapidly dividing blast cells and the uniformly small, nondividing product cells that constitute the most thymocyte subgroup (SCOLLAY and SHORTMAN 1983).

1.4 Immunocompetence

The earlier evidence that functional cells within the thymus are concentrated in the medullary subset has now been amply confirmed by limit-dilution precursor-frequency analysis (CEREDIG et al. 1982; CHEN et al. 1982, 1983a, b; KISIELOW et al. 1982). Examples are given in Table 2. Medullary thymocytes (such as the cortisone-resistant thymocytes of Table 2) give a very high frequency of cells responsive by proliferation to Concanavalin A (PTL-P) and a high frequency of precursors of cytolytic clones (CTL-P). The PTL-P are both Ly-2$^+$ L3T4$^-$ and Ly-2$^-$ L3T4$^+$, whereas CTL-P are almost entirely Ly-2$^+$ L3T4$^-$ (CHEN et al. 1983b). The majority of medullary thymocytes appear to be immunocompetent in such assays (CHEN et al. 1983a). In contrast PNA^{++} thymocytes (equivalent to small cortical thymocytes and cortical blasts combined) give a very low precursor frequency, sufficiently low to be attributed to medullary cross-contamination (up to 1%). Neither high levels of T-cell growth factors (CHEN et al. 1983a), nor various thymus hormone preparations (ANDREWS et al. 1985) are able to induce cortical thymocytes to become responsive cells. Cortical thymocytes therefore appear to be immunologically inert.

2 Developmental Steps Involving the Main Thymocyte Subpopulations

Given the information about the subsets in Table 1, the earliest interpretation was that cortical cells were "immature," and the immediate precursors of the "mature" medullary cells (OWEN and RAFF 1970; RAFF 1971). This very reasonable deduction appears to have been wrong. Kinetic studies using ^{3}H-TdR demonstrated that small cortical thymocytes behaved as if on a separate developmental stream and were not the immediate precursors of medullary cells (SHORTMAN and JACKSON 1974; FATHMAN et al. 1975), and there ist little to suggest that the cortical blasts with the same phenotype have any more potential. Although at one stage there appeared to be evidence that cortical thymocytes developed into functional cells of medullary phenotype under the influence of T-cell growth factors (IRLÉ et al. 1978), it seems likely that this result was due to expansion of preexistent contaminants, rather than differentiation (CHEN et al. 1982). What then is the developmental fate of cortical and medullary thymocytes?

2.1 Development and Fate of Cortical Thymocytes

It is clear that the large and medium-sized dividing cortical thymocytes produce the small, nondividing cells (METCALF 1966; BORUM 1973). This represents the only clear precursor-product relationship between the four populations of Table 1. However, it involves no functional development, and there is no change in the surface antigens expressed beyond such minor effects as the reduction of H-2K from low to undetectable levels. The fate of the majority, if not all, small cortical thymocytes then appears to be death within the thymus. This radical view first expressed by METCALF (1966), then vigorously disputed, now seems confirmed by a variety of different experimental approaches (JOEL et al. 1977; McPHEE et al. 1979; SCOLLAY et al. 1980a).

2.2 Development and Fate of Medullary Thymocytes

There is little direct evidence on the fate of medullary thymocytes, beyond the observation that their turnover is much slower than that of cortical cells (SHORT-

MAN and JACKSON 1974). This turnover rate is, however, in line with the rate of exit of cells from the thymus (SCOLLAY et al. 1980a). Although it was once argued that all medullary thymocytes constituted a sessile pool (ELLIOT 1973), a recent reexamination (SCOLLAY 1984) showed that "long-lived" thymocytes constitute only a small fraction of all medullary cells. We consider it likely that medullary thymocytes are the immediate source of the cells which emigrate from the thymus to populate peripheral lymphoid tissues. The main argument for this view is the extremely close resemblance between thymus migrants and medullary thymocytes; thus, recent thymus migrants are $Ly-2^+ L3T4^-$ or $Ly-2^- L3T4^+$; $PNA\mp$, $Thy-1^+$, $Ly-1^{++}$, and $H-2K^+$; immunocompetent; and, finally, in contrast to most peripheral T cells, readily killed by B2A2 and complement (SCOLLAY et al. 1978, 1980b, 1984a, b, c; SCOLLAY 1982).

The main argument *against* this view is the low expression of the homing receptor (the receptor mediating entry into peripheral lymph nodes) amongst medullary thymocytes, and its high expression on a small population of cells in the cortex (REICHERT et al. 1984). This suggests thymic emigrants may originate in this small cortical population. However, we have failed to find a significant population of "mature" cells in the cortex using other markers in multiparameter analysis, or using precursor frequency assays (SHORTMAN et al. 1985), and our own experiments on the distribution of the homing receptor (Scollay, unpublished) suggest, rather surprisingly, that the homing-receptor positive cells in the cortex may be amongst the putative early thymocytes discussed below.

2.3 Conclusions

From the foregoing it seems that the key developmental events within the thymus are all over by the time the four major populations in Table 1 are formed. Thus, the typical cortical thymocytes, both the blast forms and the small thymocytes, seem fated for cell death, for reasons that remain obscure, and the decisions which led to this must have been made at some earlier developmental stage. On the other hand medullary thymocytes are already almost fully mature and functional; if they do exit as thymic emigrants, their postthymic maturation involves becoming a little smaller and more dense, losing some of the already low B2A2 antigen, and gaining the homing receptor. The key decisions determining mature phenotype and function must have been made earlier. This suggests that the interesting stages of T-cell development (lineage commitment, acquisition of immune responsiveness, repertoire development and selection) are to be found amongst the subpopulations not represented in Table 1, and so amongst the 5 % of thymocytes not yet classified. The remainder of this review concerns this area.

3 Definition of Putative Early Thymocytes

As a preliminary step in detecting earlier developmental steps in the thymus, we looked for cells lacking some of the surface antigenic markers characterizing the more developed thymocyte populations in Table 1. The first approach was to isolate cells lacking either of the function-associated lineage markers Ly-2 and L3T4. The second was to isolate cells resistant to killing by the monoclonal antibody B2A2 and complement.

3.1 Ly-2⁻ L3T4⁻ Thymocytes

Two-color fluorescent analysis of adult mouse thymocytes, as shown in Fig. 1, readily demonstrates that 4%–5% of the population is lacking Ly-2 and L3T4 (SCOLLAY et al. 1984a; SCOLLAY and SHORTMAN 1985). These cells can also be isolated by killing most thymocytes with a mixture of the monoclonal antibodies against Ly-2 and L3T4 and complement, followed by removal of damaged cells. These Ly-2⁻ L3T4⁻ cells are all large dividing cells, similar in light scatter characteristics to the Ly-2⁺ L3T4⁺ cortical blasts. They are lymphoid in appearance, surface immunoglobulin negative and, as shown below, they express other T-cell markers. Similar cells had already been reported in the human thymus (REINHERZ et al. 1980). Three lines of evidence suggest these are early precursor cells: (a) They are much more prominent in the embryonic thymus (Scollay, in preparation); (b) some of them when cultured become Ly-2⁺ L3T4⁺ cortical-type thymocytes (CEREDIG et al. 1983b; Ceredig, personal communication); (c) they include cells able to repopulate the thymus of irradiated recipients (FOWLKES et al. 1985).

3.2 B2A2⁻ Thymocytes

The antigen recognized by the monoclonal antibody B2A2 developed by Bartlett (SCOLLAY et al. 1984a) is expressed on most hemopoietic elements, but its expression on T-lineage cells has unusual characteristics. Although about 95% of bone marrow cells are B2A2 positive, most stem cells and at least half the cells able to repopulate a thymus are B2A2 negative. Thymocytes (cortical and medullary) and recent migrants from the thymus are mainly B2A2 positive. However, most mature peripheral T cells are B2A2 negative, as judged by resistance to killing by B2A2 and complement. Thus, both the least and the most mature cells in the T-cell lineage are classed as B2A2⁻ (SCOLLAY et al. 1984a). We reasoned that a cell within the thymus resistant to B2A2 and complement would be likely to be an early, prothymocyte-like cell, rather than a mature cell, since B2A2 expression is lost only *after* exit. Note, however, that if some activated mature peripheral cells return to the thymus, as has been suggested (NAPARSTEK et al. 1982), these could also be B2A2⁻. Treatment of the thymus with B2A2 and complement, followed by removal of damaged cells, allows the isolation of a 1%–2% subpopulation of resistant cells. These have a unique size distribution, being larger than most medullary thymocytes, but on the average smaller (using light-scatter measurement) than most cortical blasts. They are lymphoid in appearance and surface immunoglobulin negative. Since most developed hemopoietic cells are B2A2⁺, they seem likely to be T-lineage cells and as shown below most express other T-cell markers (SCOLLAY et al. 1984a).

Development of T Lymphocytes Within the Thymus and Within Thymic Nurse Cells   11

Table 3. Subpopulations of B2A2⁻ and Ly-2⁻ L3T4⁻thymocytes and their likely intrathymic location

Group	Full antigenic phenotype	Probable Intra-thymic location	Percentage of all thymocytes
B2A2⁻	B2A2⁻ Thy-1⁻ Ly-1⁻ Ly-2⁻ L3T4⁻	Cortical	0.2
and	B2A2⁻ Thy-1⁻ Ly-1⁺⁺ Ly-2⁻ L3T4⁻	Intermediate	0.8
Ly-2⁻ L3T4⁻	B2A2⁻ Thy-1⁺ Ly-1⁺⁺ Ly-2⁻ L3T4⁻	Intermediate	0.8
B2A2⁻	B2A2⁻ Thy-1⁺ Ly-1⁺⁺ Ly-2⁺ L3T4⁻	Medullary	0.7
but			
Ly-2⁺ or L3T4⁺	B2A2⁻ Thy-1⁺ Ly-1⁺⁺ Ly-2⁻ L3T4⁺	Medullary	0.8
B2A2⁺	B2A2⁺⁺ Thy-1⁻ Ly-1⁻ Ly-2⁻ L3T4⁻		0.5
but	B2A2⁺⁺ Thy-1⁺ Ly-1⁻ Ly-2⁻ L3T4⁻	Cortical	1.8
Ly-2⁻ L3T4⁻	B2A2⁺⁺ Thy-1⁺⁺ Ly-1⁺ Ly-2⁻ L3T4⁻		1.7

The data are summarized from SCOLLAY et al. (1984 and 1985). The main groups were first isolated by a combination of killing with monoclonal antibody and complement, in combination with FACS separation. The complete antigenic subdivision was then obtained by subsequent two-parameter immunofluorescent (red and green) analysis. Probable intrathymic location was based on the degree of blue fluorescent labeling of the subsets after dipping the intact thymus in Hoechst 33342 dye; measurement of this involved three-color fluorescent analysis. The Hoechst 33342 labeling of B2A2⁺ Ly-2⁻ L3T4⁻ was calculated for the group as a whole, but has not yet been determined on the individual subsets with the group. Note that an "intermediate" Hoechst 33342 labeling index could indicate an inner-cortical or corticomedullary location, or alternatively a uniform distribution across both cortex and medulla

3.3   Overlap Between Ly-2⁻ L3T4⁻ and B2A2⁻ Thymocytes

Have these two different approaches arrived at the same early thymocyte population? Since around 5% of thymocytes are Ly-2⁻ L3T4⁻ and only around 2% are B2A2⁻, complete identity seems unlikely; the modal low-angle light scatter characteristics of the populations also pointed to basic differences, although there was considerable overlap. Direct experiments demonstrated that only about one third of isolated Ly-2⁻ L3T4⁻ thymocytes are B2A2⁻. Likewise only about one half of isolated B2A2⁻ thymocytes are Ly-2⁻ L3T4⁻. The remaining B2A2⁻ cells are either Ly-2⁺ L3T4⁻ or Ly-2⁻ L3T4⁺ (like medullary thymocytes) and none are Ly-2⁺ L3T4⁺ (SCOLLAY et al. 1984a; SCOLLAY and SHORTMAN 1985). These overlap and nonoverlap groups are shown in Table 3, first column.

4 Division of Putative Early Thymocytes by Multiparameter Analysis

Since it was clear that the putative early thymocytes were a heterogeneous group, a complete multiparameter analysis of the expression not only of B2A2, Ly-2, and L3T4, but of Thy-1 and Ly-1 as well, was carried out (SCOLLAY and SHORTMAN 1985). Despite the problems in characterizing such minor subpopulations, eight subsets could be discerned with reasonable confidence (Table 3).

One very minor population was negative for all these markers and might therefore be considered a candidate intrathymic stem cell.

The remaining members of the "overlap" population expressed rather high levels of Ly-1, similar to medullary thymocytes, suggesting they might be on a "medullary" pathway. Such cells are not apparent in the embryonic thymus (Scollay, in preparation).

The cells that were B2A2$^-$ but expressed either Ly-2 or L3T4 (like medullary cells) were also low Thy-1 high Ly-1 (like medullary cells). Thus, they could be committed blasts of the medullary lineage. However, they could also be activated peripheral T cells recycling through the thymus (NAPARSTEK et al. 1982). Again such cells are not evident in the embryonic thymus.

The cells which were B2A2$^+$ but Ly-2$^-$ L3T4$^-$ could be divided into three groups which had certain cortical characteristics, namely high B2A2 expression and a tendency to high Thy-1 and low Ly-1 expression. Cells of this type are readily observed in the embryonic thymus (Scollay, in preparation).

5 Intrathymic Location of Subsets of Putative Early Thymocytes

The location of these multiple subsets within the thymus should give some clues to their relationship to the more developed populations. However, cells such as those in Table 3 which are defined by the lack of certain markers, or by quantitative differences in marker expression, or by the use of several markers simultaneously, are difficult to identify using conventional immunofluorescence on frozen sections. To determine intrathymic location we used instead the technique of dipping the intact thymus in a fluorescent dye which diffuses across the capsule, labeling first the subcapsular outer cortex, then the cortex, then the medulla; the labeling index then serves as a rough guide to location. This technique is able to distinguish cells of known outer cortical, general cortical, or medullary location. It cannot distinguish cells of intermediate (say inner-cortical) location from cells having an even distribution throughout the thymus. Both fluorescein isothiocyanate and Hoechst 33342 dyes were employed, the latter being the most useful since its blue fluorescence allowed subsequent two-color (red and green) immunofluorescent analysis of the resulting stained and unstained cells. Conclusions from this study (SCOLLAY and SHORTMAN 1985) are summarized in Table 3.

The B2A2$^-$ but Ly-2$^+$ L3T4$^-$ or Ly-2$^-$ L3T4$^+$ cells are poorly stained by transcapsular diffusion of the dyes, and in this they behave much like medullary cells. We assume they are located in the medulla. In line with their phenotype the

B2A2$^+$ but Ly-2$^-$ L3T4$^-$ cells are rapidly labeled by dye diffusing across the capsule, to the same extent as cortical blasts in general, and we therefore assume they are of cortical location. It is of interest that the candidate for the "earliest" cell, negative for all markers, also seems to be of cortical location. The B2A2$^-$ Ly-2$^-$ L3T4$^-$ cells with Ly-1 levels show intermediate labeling characteristics, indicating either an "inner-cortical" location, a cortical-to-medullary transition, or a uniform distribution. All we can say is that they are neither clearly cortical nor clearly medullary.

6 Possible Developmental Streams

Given this array of phenotypically different "early" thymocyte subsets, and using the intrathymic localization as a guide, is it possible to deduce developmental pathways? The correct answer is no, since we lack evidence of precursor-product relationships between the subsets. However, it is instructive to attempt an arrangement of these cells into some sort of sequence, guided by related location and phenotypic similarities, since this can provide a framework for future experiments. Or, to be more honest and less rationalizing, the temptation is irresistible. A mixture of logic and guesswork leads to the developmental schemes in Figs. 2 and 3. The "cortical stream" of Fig. 2 is the one we consider most reasonable, because the order of cells in the pathway has since been found to be the same as the order of appearance of phenotypically similar subsets in embryonic thymic development (Scollay, in preparation). The only aspect of this scheme we currently question is whether the prethymocyte at the start is B2A2$^-$, or whether a separate and so far undetected B2A2$^+$ prethymocyte initiates this B2A2$^+$ lineage. The "medullary stream" of Fig. 3 is more of an exercise in incorporating all the remaining "medullary-like" cells into a single pathway, and is clearly incorrect if any of these elements are in fact recycled peripheral T cells. It does, however, offer the concept that both cortical and medullary streams might have a single common precursor located in the cortex, in line with the view of Weissman (WEISSMAN 1973; FATHMAN et al. 1975) of a developmental stream from cortex to medulla.

7 Lymphocyte-Epithelial Cell Interactions and Thymic Nurse Cells

The preceding studies focus on the lymphoid components of the thymus. However, both intrathymic differentiation and selection of the specificity repertoire is believed to involve interaction of thymocytes (and in particular of these putative early thymocytes) with nonlymphoid elements, such as epithelial cells. One interaction complex that might serve as a model for a special intrathymic microenvironment is the "nurse cell," first isolated by WEKERLE and KETELSEN (1980) from enzymic digests of mouse thymus. The nurse cell consists of an outer-cortical epithelial cell which encloses 20–200 lymphocytes. It had already been established that an association between these lymphocytes and the epithelial cell

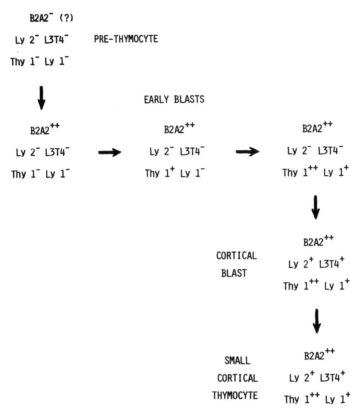

Fig. 2. A likely cortical pathway. The scheme is based on data of SCOLLAY and SHORTMAN (1985), and Scollay (in preparation). These subpopulations in this study isolated from the adult thymus also appear in this sequence during embryonic thymus development. Although we have never identified such a cell, we consider a B2A2$^+$ pre-thymocyte to be an alternative to the B2A2$^-$ pre-thymocyte at the beginning of this sequence

existed in the intact thymus prior to digestion (KYEWSKI and KAPLAN 1982), but it was not clear whether in vivo the lymphocytes were totally enfolded.

If the nurse cell lymphocytes are totally enclosed in situ, as in the digested and isolated structure, there should be two epithelial cell membranes separating the lymphocytes from the general thymic milieu. These membranes should constitute a barrier to certain dyes introduced by direct injection into the thymus. This postulate was tested by injecting substances such as the Hoechst 33342 nuclear stain, or the membrane carbohydrate stain alcian blue, or fluoresceinated anti-Thy-1 antibody, directly into the thymus, then afterwards isolating nurse cells. Although these substances stained most thymocytes, and although the epithelial cell outer membrane was stained with alcian blue and its nucleus with Hoechst 33342, lymphocytes within the nurse cell remained unstained (ANDREWS and BOYD 1985). This suggests the nurse cell could indeed represent a very specialized microenvironment, and we are examining the intranurse cell lymphocytes for clues to the biological function of the complex.

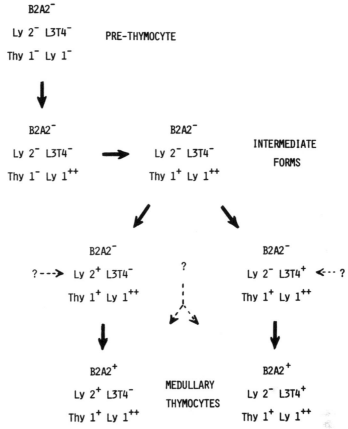

Fig. 3. One possible medullary pathway. The scheme is based on data from SCOLLAY et al. (1984a and SCOLLAY and SHORTMAN 1985). The prethymocyte, after seeding in the thymus, is located in the cortex, the first two "intermediate forms" are of indeterminate location, perhaps en route to the medulla, while the remainder of the subsets are in the medulla. There are many alternatives to this scheme. In particular the B2A2$^-$ but Ly-2$^+$ L3T4$^-$ or Ly-2$^-$ L3T4$^+$ forms may be activated peripheral T cells which have reseeded in the thymus, rather than being early developmental stages

8 Phenotype of Intra-Nurse-Cell Lymphocytes

The lymphoid cells released from purified nurse cells have been examined to see if they are especially enriched in any of the early thymocyte populations. The main result of our analysis to date is that the dominant cell type resembles the typical Ly-2$^+$ L3T4$^+$ small cortical thymocyte; this agrees with the results of KYEWSKI and KAPLAN (1982). However, it is clear that nurse cells also contain a small proportion of Ly-2$^-$ L3T4$^-$ blast cells, and as well some cells whose size, Thy-1, and PNA-receptor expression resemble medullary thymocytes. As yet we have not established the detailed phenotype or lineage commitment of these minority cells, since this will first require a complete elimination of all exogenous thymocyte contaminants. These studies are underway.

9 Functional Capacity of Intra-Nurse-Cell Lymphocytes

If most lymphocytes with nurse cells resemble small cortical thymocytes, they would not be expected to be immunocompetent. However, several groups have concluded that both cytotoxic and helper function may be generated from nurse cell lymphocytes, leading to the idea that they represent a special "intermediate" cell, in the process of developing from a cortical phenotype to a mature functional state (VAKHARIA 1983; VAKHARIA and MITCHISON 1984; FINK et al. 1984). Because of our concern that exogenous functional thymocytes might be contributing to the immune response observed in these experiments, we have determined the precursor frequency amongst nurse cell lymphocytes under very stringent conditions (ANDREWS et al. in preparation). Nurse cells were enriched, then individual nurse cells isolated by micromanipulation, placed in individual Terasaki tray wells, and checked for absence of any exogenous cells. The selected individual nurse cells were then incubated to release their contents, and the released lymphocytes then assayed at the one lymphoid cell per culture level in our high-cloning efficiency microculture systems. Their functional capacity was compared with other known thymus subpopulations in side-by-side assays. Some results are summarized in Table 2.

The majority of nurse cell thymocytes fail to proliferate and form clones in response to Concanavalin A in contrast to the high PTL-P frequency recorded for cortisone-resistant thymocytes. This is in agreement with the phenotypic data which suggest that most nurse-cell lymphocytes are like the inert small cortical thymocyte. However, around one in thirty nurse-cell lymphocytes (or two to six lymphocytes per nurse cell) is capable of forming a clone. Interestingly, not one of these clones (out of many hundreds tested) was cytolytic, and the CTL-P frequency was thus zero, in contrast to the results of FINK et al. (1984).

We conclude that nurse cells contain some cells capable of a proliferative response, but no mature precursors of the cytolytic lineage. An intriguing possibility, as yet untested, is that the proliferating cells are of the helper or Ly-2⁻ L3T4⁺ lineage, and that the nurse cell represents a selective environment for helper-cell development.

10 Conclusions

It seems likely that the key developmental steps within the thymus will be found, not amongst the 95 % of cells which constitute the better known and more developed subpopulations, but amongst the 5 % "early blast" group, or amongst the 1 % intra-nurse-cell lymphocytes. These minority populations are themselves heterogeneous and composed of subsets. This is to be expected if some complex developmental process is taking place at this level, but it poses a considerable technical challenge since the dominant populations tend to swamp the interesting minor subsets. Research at this level should nevertheless be more fruitful than the past investigations which assumed the main problems could be settled by a study of the already committed, dominant thymus subsets.

References

Andrews P, Boyd R (1985) The murine thymic nurse cell: an isolated thymic microenvironment. Eur J Immunol 15:36–42

Andrews P, Shortman K, Scollay R, Potworowski EF, Kruisbeek AM, Goldstein G, Trainin N, Bach J-F (1985) Thymic hormones do not induce proliferative ability or cytolytic function in PNA$^+$ cortical thymocytes. Cell Immunol 91:455–466

Borum K (1973) Cell kinetics in mouse thymus studied by simultaneous use of ^{3}H-thymidine and colchicine. Cell Tissue Kinet 6:545–552

Ceredig R, Glasebrook AL, MacDonald HR (1982) Phenotypic and functional properties of murine thymocytes. I. Precursors of cytolytic T lymphocytes and interleukin-2 producing cells are contained within a subpopulation of "mature" thymocytes as analysed by monoclonal antibodies and flow microfluorometry. J Exp Med 155:358–379

Ceredig R, Dialynas DP, Fitch FW, MacDonald HR (1983a) Precursors of T-cell growth factor producing cells in the thymus: ontogeny, frequency and quantitative recovery in a subpopulation of phenotypically mature thymocytes defined by monoclonal antibody GK–1.5. J Exp Med 158:1654–1671

Ceredig R, Sekaly RP, MacDonald HR (1983b) Differentiation in vitro of Lyt-2$^+$ thymocytes from embryonic Lyt-2$^-$ precursors. Nature 303:248–250

Chen W-F, Scollay R, Shortman K (1982) The functional capacity of thymus subpopulations: limit-dilution analysis of all precursors of cytotoxic lymphocytes and of all T cells capable of proliferation in subpopulations separated by the use of peanut agglutinin. J Immunol 129:18–24

Chen W-F, Scollay R, Clark-Lewis I, Shortman K (1983a) The size of functional T-lymphocyte pools within thymic medullary and cortical cell subsets. Thymus 5:179–195

Chen W-F, Scollay R, Shortman K (1983b) The Ly phenotype of functional medullary thymocytes. Thymus 5:197–207

Dialynas DP, Wilde DB, Marrack P, Pierres A, Wall KA, Havran W, Otten G, Loken MR, Pierres M, Kappler J (1983) Characterization of the murine antigenic determinant, designated L3T4a, recognized by monoclonal antibody GK1–5; expression on L3T4a by functional T cell clones appears to correlate primarily with class II MHC antigen-reactivity. Immunol Rev 74:29–56

Elliot EV (1973) A persistent lymphoid population in the thymus. Nature New Biol 242:150–152

Fathman CG, Small M, Herzenberg LA, Weissman IL (1975) Thymus cell maturation. II. Differentiation of three "mature" subclasses in vivo. Cell Immunol 15:109–128

Fink PJ, Weissman IL, Kaplan HS, Kyewski BA (1984) The immunocompetence of murine stromal cell-associated thymocytes. J Immunol 132:2266–2272

Fowlkes B-J, Edison L, Mathieson B, Chused TM (1985) In: U.C.L.A. Symposium, Regulation of the immune system. (to be published)

Irlé C, Piguet P-F, Vassalli P (1978) In vitro maturation of immature thymocytes into immunocompetent T cells in the absence of direct thymic influence. J Exp Med 148:32–45

Joel DD, Chanana AD, Cottier H, Cronkite EP, Laissue JA (1977) Fate of thymocytes: studies with ^{125}I-iododeoxyuridine and ^{3}H-thymidine in mice. Cell Tissue Kinet 10:57–69

Kisielow P, von Boehmer H, Haas W (1982) Functional and phenotypic properties of subpopulations of murine thymocytes. I. The bulk of peanut agglutinin-positive Lyt-1, 2, 3 thymocytes lacks precursors of cytotoxic T lymphocytes responsive to interleukin 2 (T cell growth factor). Eur J Immunol 12:463–467

Kyewski RA, Kaplan HS (1982) Lymphoepithelial interactions in the mouse thymus: phenotypic and kinetic studies on thymic nurse cells. J Immunol 128:2287–2294

McPhee D, Pye S, Shortman K (1979) The differentiation of T lymphocytes. V. Evidence for intrathymic death of most thymocytes. Thymus 1:151–161

Metcalf D (1966) The nature and regulation of lymphopoiesis in normal and neoplastic thymus. In: Wolstenholme GWE, Porter R (eds) The thymus: experimental and clinical studies, CIBA Foundation Symposium, Churchill, London, p. 242

Naparstek Y, Holoshitz J, Eisenstein S, Reshef T, Rappaport S, Chemke J, Ben-Nun A, Cohen IR (1982) Effector T lymphocyte line cells migrate to the thymus and persist there. Nature 300:262–264

Owen JJT, Raff MC (1980) Studies on the differentiation of thymus-derived lymphocytes. J Exp Med 132:1216–1232

18   K. Shortman et al.

Raff MC (1971) Evidence for a subpopulation of mature lymphocytes within the mouse thymus. Nature New Biol 229:182–183

Reichert RA, Gallatin WM, Butcher EC, Weissman IL (1984) A homing receptor-bearing cortical thymocyte subset: implications for thymus cell migration and the nature of cortisone-resistant thymocytes. Cell 38:89–99

Reinherz EL, Kung PC, Goldstein G, Levey RH, Schlossman SF (1980) Discrete stages of human intrathymic differentiation. Analysis of normal thymocytes and leukemic lymphoblasts of T cell lineage. Proc Natl Acad Sci USA 77:1588–1592

Scollay R (1982) Thymus cell migration: cells migrating from the thymus to peripheral lymphoid organs have a "mature" phenotype. J Immunol 128:1566–1570

Scollay R (1984) The long-lived medullary thymocyte re-visited: precise quantitation of a very small subset. J Immunol 132:1085–1089

Scollay R, Shortman K (1983) Thymocyte subpopulations: an experimental review, including flow cytometric cross-correlations between the major murine thymocyte markers. Thymus 5:245–295

Scollay R, Shortman K (1985) Identification of early stages of T lymphocyte development in the thymus cortex and medulla. J Immunol 134:3632–3642

Scollay R, Kocken M, Butcher E, Weissman I (1978) Lyt markers and thymus cell migrants. Nature 276:79–80

Scollay R, Butcher E, Weissman I (1980a) Thymus migration: quantitative studies on the rate of migration of cells from the thymus to the periphery in mice. Eur J Immunol 10:210–218

Scollay R, Jacobs S, Jerabek L, Butcher E, Weissman IL (1980b) T cell maturation: thymocyte and thymus migrant subpopulations defined with monoclonal antibodies to MHC region antigens. J Immunol 124:2845–2853

Scollay R, Bartlett P, Shortman K (1984a) T cell development in the adult murine thymus: Changes in the expression of the surface antigens Ly 2, L3T4 and B2A2 during development from early precursor cells to emigrants. Immunol Rev 82:79

Scollay R, Wilson A, Shortman K (1984b) Thymus cell migration: analysis of thymus emigrants with markers that distinguish medullary thymocytes from peripheral T cells. J Immunol 132:1089–1094

Scollay R, Chen W-F, Shortman K (1984c) The functional capabilities of cells leaving the thymus. J Immunol 132:25–30

Shortman K, Jackson H (1974) The differentiation of T-lymphocytes. I. Proliferation kinetics and interrelationships of subpopulations of mouse thymus cells. Cell Immunol 12:230–246

Shortman K, Mandel T, Andrews P, Scollay R (1985) Are any functionally mature cells of medullary phenotype located in the thymus cortex? Cell Immunol 93:350–363

Vakharia DD (1983) Demonstration of keratin filaments in thymic nurse cells (TNC) and alloreactivity of TNC-T cell population. Thymus 5:43–52

Vakharia DD, Mitchison NA (1984) Helper T cell activity demonstrated by thymic nurse cell T cells (TNC-T). Immunol 51:269–273

Weissman IL (1973) Thymus cell maturation. Studies on the origin of cortisone resistant thymic lymphocytes. J Exp Med 137:504–510

Wekerle H, Ketelsen UP (1980) Thymic nurse cells – Ia bearing epithelium involved in T-lymphocyte differentiation. Nature 283:402–404

Thymus Development

H. VON BOEHMER

1 Development of Thymocyte Subpopulations Defined by Surface Antigens 19
2 Growth Requirements of Immature T Cells 20
3 T-Cell Receptor-Gene Expression 21
3.1 DNA Rearrangement 21
3.2 T-Cell Receptor RNA 21
3.3 Expression of α, β Heterodimeric Proteins 23
4 Conclusion 24
References 24

It is generally believed that T lymphocytes develop from immature hemopoietic cells in the thymus. The thymus contains various subpopulations of lymphocytes, but little is known about their precursor-product relationship. Some of these connections have recently been studied in organ culture as well as in short-term culture of dissociated thymocytes and will be summarized below. In addition initial data on the ontogeny of T-cell receptor expression will be discussed.

1 Development of Thymocyte Subpopulations Defined by Surface Antigens

The murine thymus is colonized by hemopoietic cells at day 11–12 of gestation (MOORE and OWEN 1967). At day 14 one finds a population of large, dividing cells which are functionally incompetent and express Thy-1 and H-2 antigens, but neither Ly-2 nor MT4 antigens (Table 1). If the thymus is removed at this stage and put in organ culture, an exponential increase in cell numbers is observed during the next 6 days. During the same time period one observes differentiation of lymphocytes which is characterized (a) by the appearance of first large and then small cells expressing Ly-2 as well as MT4 antigens, and (b) the appearance of functional Ly-2$^+$, MT4$^-$ as well as Ly-2$^-$, MT4$^+$ cells (Table 1). It is also apparent from the data in Table 1 that on many cells Ly-2 is expressed before MT4. To verify this impression and to analyze the differentiation of early Ly-2$^+$, MT4$^-$ cells, the following experiments were conducted (Kisielow et al. unpublished): thymocytes from 16-day-old fetuses were stained with Ly-2 and MT4 antibodies after treatment with either Ly-2 or MT4 antibodies and complement or comple-

---

Basel Institute of Immunology, Grenzacher Strasse 487, CH-4005 Basel

Current Topics in Microbiology and Immunology, Vol. 126
© Springer-Verlag Berlin · Heidelberg 1986

20 H. von Boehmer

Table 1. Surface markers on embryonic thymocytes differentiating in vitro

Days in culture	Percent cells			
	Ly-2⁻, MT4⁻	Ly-2⁺, MT4⁺	Ly-2⁺, MT4⁻	Ly-2⁻, MT4⁺
0	100	0	0	0
2	79	6	13	1
4	23	51	14	12
6	10	70	10	10

ment alone. Treatment with Ly-2 antibodies plus complement removed all Ly-2 as well as MT4 positive cells, whereas treatment with MT4 antibodies plus complement removed all MT4, but not all Ly-2 positive cells. If the "early" Ly-2⁺, MT4⁻ cells are cultured for 24 h (survival, 40%) all cells acquire the expression of MT4. Thus, the sequence of differentiation may go from double-negative cells directly to double-positive cells (CEREDIG et al. 1983) or from double-negative cells to "early" Ly-2⁺, MT4⁻ cells and then to Ly-2⁺, MT4⁺ cells. The immediate precursors for the late Ly-2⁺, MT4⁻ as well as Ly-2⁻, MT4⁺ cells are, however, not known. While it is excluded that all double-positive thymocytes differentiate into single-positive cells (the turnover of the former populations is much faster than that of the latter (SCOLLAY and SHORTMAN 1983), it is uncertain whether a small proportion of double-positive cells contain the immediate precursors of single-positive cells. This differentiation step has not been observed in suspension culture of dissociated thymocytes (SCOLLAY and SHORTMAN 1983), but may nevertheless occur in situ. On the other hand, there is some evidence (discussed below) that some double-negative cells may produce single-positive cells in culture in the presence of certain growth factors. Whether or not this reflects physiological differentiation and whether or not there are a few intermediate double-positive cells is unknown. It is also unknown whether the thymus contains a common precursor for both Ly-2⁺, MT4⁻ and Ly-2⁻, MT4⁺ cells. Lineage experiments are being conducted using different methods, but conclusive data have not yet been obtained or published.

2 Growth Requirements of Immature T Cells

A significant proportion (> 50%) of 14-day-old fetal thymocytes expresses IL-2 receptors as observed by staining and precipitation of receptors with IL-2 receptor antibodies (TAKACS et al. 1984; RAULET 1985; CEREDIG et al. 1985; VON BOEHMER et al. 1985). The proportion of thymocytes expressing IL-2 receptors diminishes with age and is confined to the dividing population of double-negative blasts (Table 2) (VON BOEHMER et al. 1985; RAULET 1985). Even though not all dividing double-negative thymocytes express IL-2 receptors, the existence of these receptors on other cells raises the question of whether or not the growth of some early T cells requires only the interaction of IL-2 with their receptors. In

Table 2. The proportion of IL-2 receptor-positive thymocytes in embryonic life

Embryonic age (days)	IL-2 receptor positive (%)
14	90
15	72
16	20
20	4

Table 3. ^{3}H-thymidine incorporation by fetal thymocytes and activated T cells (CTL-L)

IL-2	15-day-old embryonic thymocytes	CTL-L
−	6700	9200
+	6900	115400

that case, one would expect that IL-2 receptor-positive cells would continue to divide in the presence of IL-2 in vitro. This is clearly not the case (Table 3) (VON BOEHMER et al. 1985). In addition, it has been reported that most IL-2 receptors on double-negative thymocytes have low affinity for IL-2 (CEREDIG et al. 1985). Finally, IL-2 cannot be induced by mitogens in fetal thymocytes expressing IL-2 receptors (KISIELOW et al. 1984). Thus it is unlikely that the division of double-negative thymocytes depends solely on the binding of IL-2 to receptors on fetal thymocytes.

Various attempts, however, were undertaken to grow IL-2 receptor expressing thymocytes in cultures containing IL-2. It has been claimed that addition of Concanavalin A (Con A) has some effect (RAULET 1985), but according to our experiment this effect is marginal. Other authors used phorbol myristic acid, which can increase growth of fetal thymocytes considerably (Ceredig et al. unpublished). The best growth is obtained by a combination of drugs leading to protein phosphorylation. It was shown by blocking with anti-IL-2 receptor antibodies that in this situation IL-2 was required for cell growth (PALACIOS and VON BOEHMER 1986). Single-positive cells have been observed in several of the cultures containing initially only double-negative cells, but these experiments need to confirmed with cloned double-negative cells. At present we have established several cell lines which are Thy-1$^+$, but not Ly-2 or MT4 antigen positive and their differentiation in vivo as well as in in vitro is being studied.

3 T-Cell Receptor-Gene Expression

3.1 DNA Rearrangement

Gene rearrangement is a prerequisite for the expression of T-cell receptors (HEDRICK et al. 1984), as it is for the expression of immunoglobulin. T-cell receptor-

22   H. von Boehmer

Table 4

Thymocyte subpopulations	Proportion of cells with β gene rearrangement (%)
Day 15 fetal thymocytes	< 30
Day 17 fetal thymocytes	75
Adult thymocytes	95
Ly-2$^+$, MT4$^+$ thymocytes	85

gene rearrangements can be detected by using cDNA probes and restriction enzyme digested DNA. Rearrangements of the β locus are easily detected on southern blots using a probe hybridizing to the constant Cβ_1 and Cβ_2 gene segments. The same does not apply to the α-chain locus: between Cα and some Jα there is a very large intron so that joining of V segments to some J segments is not detected by probes hybridizing to the Cα segment. For this reason, only β gene rearrangements have been analyzed in thymocyte subpopulations (SNOD-GRASS et al. 1985a). In 15-day-old fetal thymocytes there is relatively little rearrangement, whereas it is difficult to identify the β-germline bands in double-positive thymocytes or in thymocytes from adult mice. Table 4 shows a rough estimate of the extent of rearrangement in various cell populations using densitometric analysis. By use of appropriate restriction enzymes, one can show (SNOD-GRASS et al. 1985a) that rearrangements have occurred to J segments in front of both Cβ_1 and Cβ_2 gene segments. The experiments do not indicate whether the rearrangements represent VDJ or DJ joinings only. This question was analyzed by northern blot analysis probing for T-cell receptor-specific RNA.

3.2 T-Cell Receptor RNA

Hybridizing to α, β and γ RNA (the γ locus shores many structural and sequence characteristics with the α and β locus) cDNA probes detect larger (1.6, 1.3, and 1.5 kb for α, β, and γ respectively) and smaller (1.3, 1.0, and 1.2 kb for α, β, and γ respectively) transcripts in thymocytes. It has been shown for the β gene that the larger transcript represents a full-length RNA, while the smaller RNA represents a transcript from a DJ joining only. If only the larger transcripts are taken into consideration then 15-day-old fetal thymocytes express γ but not α or β transcripts; 17-day-old fetal thymocytes express γ and β, but few α transcripts; while adult thymocytes express α and β, but few γ transcripts (RAULET et al. 1985; SNODGRASS et al. 1985b). It is clear therefore that double-negative cells which enter the thymus and contain precursors for functional thymocytes do not express α, β heterodimers. Whether or not fetal thymocytes in the absence of an α transcript express a β, γ heterodimer is unknown, but it has been speculated that such a molecule may play a role in the selection of the T-cell receptor repertoire (RAULET et al. 1985; SNODGRASS et al. 1985b). The results obtained with probes for α and β transcripts together with those on the differentiation of 14-

day-old double-negative fetal thymocytes in organ culture (KISIELOW et al. 1984) indicate that precursors of T cells can enter the thymus prior to productive rearrangement of β- as well as α-gene segments and expression of full-length transcripts. Thus, there is little doubt that the thymus is one organ where T-cell diversity is generated. This does not exclude extrathymic differentiation of T cells, but makes the proposition unlikely that T-cell tolerance is exclusively acquired prethymically (MORISSEY et al. 1982).

The question of whether or not double-positive thymocytes express full-length transcripts of the α and β locus has been addressed using purified double-positive thymocytes as well as double-positive thymomas. Double-positive thymocytes were prepared by agglutination with peanut agglutinin and by killing of cells expressing high amounts of class I MHC antigens. Of these cells 98.5% express both Ly-2 and MT4 antigens and if RNA is isolated from this population one obtains only one sixth of that obtained from the same number of unfractionated thymocytes. Using northern blot analysis, full-length α and β transcripts are easily detected (SNODGRASS et al. 1985b). It can, however, not be excluded that these transcripts are derived from a few contaminating cells expressing high levels of RNA. This possibility has become more unlikely following recent experiments with Ly-2, MT4 double-positive, MEL14 negative thymomas. Two of two analyzed thymomas expressed high levels of full-length α and β transcripts.

3.3 Expression of α, β Heterodimeric Proteins

Whether or not the various thymocyte subpopulations which contain full-length α and β transcripts also express α and β dimers is at present difficult to analyze at the single-cell level since appropriate antibodies are not available. Nevertheless, receptor-like proteins can be analyzed using gel electrophoresis: disulfide-linked proteins can be separated by size in the first dimension under nonreducing conditions. In the second dimension they can be separated under reducing conditions. In this way receptors on T cells form a characteristic spot which is absent on B cells or fibroblasts. It cannot be excluded, however, that there exist other proteins with similar characteristics on T cells and it is for this reason that I refer to the proteins detected by this method as "receptor-like" proteins. Receptor-like proteins are not detected on 15-day-old fetal thymocytes, become apparent by day 17, and are also present on purified double-positive thymocytes (SNODGRASS et al. 1985a). While this parallels the appearance of full-length α and β transcripts in the various cell populations, further experiments were conducted to study the presence of α, β heterodimers, especially on double-positive thymocytes. For this purpose double-positive thymocytes, purified as described above, were stained with a recently developed monoclonal antibody F23 (STAERZ et al. 1985) which detects α, β heterodimers on 20% of peripheral T cells. We found, however, no significant staining on double-positive thymocytes. This result can be interpreted in at least three different ways: one, the receptor density on this population may be very low, two, receptors with the F23 marker may for some reason not be expressed in double-positive thymocytes, and, three, double-positive thymocytes may not express α, β heterodimers. These possibilities are pres-

24 H. von Boehmer

ently being addressed by further analysis and comparison of proteins from double-positive, MEL14 negative thymomas and proteins precipitated with F23 antibodies from functional T cells.

4 Conclusion

The Ly-2, MT4 negative lymphoblasts present in 14-day-old fetal thymus contain the precursors of nonfunctional double-positive as well as of single-positive Ly-2^+, MT4$^-$ and Ly-2$^-$, MT4$^+$ thymocytes. These cells enter the thymus prior to α and β gene rearrangement and expression of full-length transcripts coding the α and β chain of the T-cell receptor for antigen. These results leave little doubt that the thymus is one organ where T-cell diversity is generated. Since thymocytes are tolerant to a variety of antigens, prethymic tolerance (if it exists) cannot be a sufficient explanation for tolerance of thymocytes.

Double-negative cells are the immediate precursors of double-positive thymocytes which appear to express full-length α and β transcripts and whose expression of α, β heterodimers needs to be further analyzed. These double-negative precursor cells can, under certain conditions, be grown in media containing IL-2 and may occasionally differentiate into single-positive cells. Whether this differentiation bears any relationship to in situ differentiation is questionable, but may be tested by in vivo repopulation experiments.

References

Ceredig Rh, Sekaly RP, MacDonald HR (1983) Differentiation in vitro of Ly 2^+ thymocytes from Ly 2^- precursors. Nature 303:248

Ceredig Rh, Lowenthal JW, Nabholz M, MacDonald R (1985) Expression of interleukin 2 receptors as a differentiation marker on intrathymic stem cells. Nature 314:98

Hedrick SM, Cohen DI, Nielsen EA, Davis MM (1984) Isolation of c-DNA clones encoding T cell specific membrane associated proteins. Nature 308:149

Kisielow P, Leierson W, von Boehmer H (1984) Differentiation of thymocytes in fetal organ culture: analysis of phenotypic changes accompanying the appearance of cytolytic and interleukin 2-producing cells. J Immunol 133:1117

Moore MAS, Owen JJT (1967) Experimental studies on the development of the thymus. J Exp Med 126:715

Morissey PJ, Kruisbeck AM, Shanow SO, Singer A (1982) Tolerance of thymic cytotoxic T lymphocytes to allogeneic H-2 determinants encountered prethymically: evidence for expression of anti H-2 receptors prior to entry into the thymus. Proc Natl Acad Sci USA 79:2003

Palacios R, von Boehmer H (1986) Requirements for growth of immature thymocytes from fetal and adult mice in vitro. Eur J Immunol 16:12

Raulet D (1985) Embryonic and immature adult thymocytes express IL-2 receptors and respond to IL-2 in vitro. Nature 314:101

Raulet D, Gorman RD, Saito H, Tonegawa S (1985) Developmental regulation of T cell receptor gene expression. Nature 314:103

Scollay R, Shortman K (1983) Thymus subpopulations: an experimental review including flow cytometric cross-relations betwen the murine thymocyte markers. Thymus 5:245

Snodgrass HR, Kisielow P, Kiefer M, Steinmetz M, von Boehmer H (1985a) Ontogeny of the T cell antigen receptor within the thymus. Nature 313:592

Snodgrass R, Dembic Z, Steinmetz M, von Boehmer H (1985b) Expression of T cell antigen receptor gene during fetal development in the thymus. Nature 315:232

Staerz VD, Rammensee HG, Benedetto JD, Bevan MF (1985) Characterization of a murine monoclonal antibody specific for an allotypic determinant on the T cell antigen receptor. J Immunol 134:3994

Takacs L, Osawa H, Diamantstein T (1984) Detection and localization by the monoclonal anti-interleukin 2 receptor antibody AMT-13 of IL-2 receptor-bearing cells in the developing thymus of the mouse embryo and in the thymus of cortisone-treated mice. Eur J Immunol 14:1152

von Boehmer H, Crisanti A, Kisielow P, Haas W (1985) Absence of growth by most receptors expressing fetal thymocytes in the presence of interleukin 2. Nature 314:539

Major Histocompatibility-Restricted Cytolytic T-Lymphocyte Precursors from the Thymus of In Vivo Primed Mice: Increased Frequency and Resistance to Anti-Lyt-2 Antibody Inhibition

R. CEREDIG

1 Introduction 27
2 Results 28
3 Discussion 30
References 32

1 Introduction

The thymus is the primary site for the generation of immunocompetent T lymphocytes (MILLER and OSOBA 1967). It was generally assumed that there was an unidirectional flow of T cells from the thymus to peripheral lymphoid tissues, but recently evidence has accumulated suggesting that there may be recirculation of peripheral T lymphocytes back to the thymus (NAPARSTEK et al. 1982) and that the thymus may actively participate in an immune response. The functional participation of the thymus in an immune response was demonstrated by showing an increase in the frequency of thymic cytolytic T-lymphocyte precursors (CTL-P) responding to minor histocompatibility (minor-H) antigens following in vivo priming (FINK et al. 1984). Furthermore, in this study, it was suggested that the increased thymic content of CTL-P was the sum of three independent sources. Thus, prethymic and intrathymic T cells were primed within the thymus, but in addition there was evidence for recirculation back to the thymus of peripheral T cells.

In the studies reported herein, the responses of thymocytes from C57BL/6 female mice immunized with either the murine sarcoma virus-Moloney leukemia virus (MSV-MoLV) complex or syngeneic male spleen cells were determined by limiting dilution analysis of mixed leukocyte microcultures (micro-MLC). Responses to both MSV-MoLV (anti-MSV) (PLATA et al. 1976) and male spleen cells (anti-H-Y) (GORDON et al. 1975) are H-2 restricted and can usually only be detected among spleen cells following in vivo immunization with the corresponding antigen(s). For the thymus, it was demonstrated herein that there was a distinct increase in the frequency of CTL-P responding to either MSV-MoLV or male spleen cells following immunization. Furthermore, it could be shown that only a minority of anti-MSV cytolytic T lymphocytes (CTL) generated from the thymus of virus-immunized mice were inhibited in their effector function by anti-

---

Ludwig Institute for Cancer Research, Lausanne Branch, CH-1066 Épalinges

28   R. Ceredig

Lyt-2 monoclonal antibody (Mab). This lack of inhibition by anti-Lyt-2 has recently been shown to be a frequent property of CTL clones derived from in vivo immunized mice (MacDonald et al. 1982). Thus, functionally, most thymic anti-MSV CTL-P from MSV-immune mice gave rise to CTL progeny having a "primed" phenotype.

2 Results

Previous experiments had shown that cortisone-resistant thymocytes (CRT) were significantly enriched for CTL-P (Taswell et al. 1979; Ceredig and Cummings 1983). Therefore, in initial experiments, the responses of CRT from B/6 female mice, obtained at various times following injection with either the MSV-MoLV complex or male spleen cells, were tested in limit-dilution micro-MLC. This was done in order to determine the kinetics of increase in thymic CTL-P following immunization with two independent antigens. As shown in Table 1, by 14 days following immunization there had been a significant increase in the frequency of both anti-MSV and anti-male antigen (anti-H-Y) CTL-P. The specificity of the responses were shown by testing the same microwells against an irrelevant target cell. In the case of anti-MSV responses, the EL-4 thymoma, which does not express MSV antigens but is of the same H-2 haplotype ($H-2^b$) as the virus-expressing $H-2^b$ target cell MBL-2, was used as a control target cell. In the case of anti-H-Y responses, female B/6 blasts were used. As shown in Table 1, there was no significant increase in the frequency of wells lysing the irrelevant target cells, i.e., EL-4 for anti-MSV and female blasts for anti-male responses.

The responses of normal thymocytes and CRT from MSV-immune mice removed at 2–6 weeks following immunization were investigated further. In these experiments, the frequencies of B/6 thymic CTL-P responding to MSV antigens were always compared with the frequencies of the same pooled thymocytes responding to $H-2^d$ alloantigens as an internal control. An additional control group of mice was also included in these experiments, namely B/6 mice immunized with $H-2^d$ alloantigens. The results of these experiments are shown in Table 2.

When micro-MLC were tested for cytolytic activity, it was again clear that immunization with MSV resulted in a significant increase in CTL-P frequencies compared with the control $H-2^d$-immune mice. As expected, pretreatment of MSV-immune mice with hydrocortisone resulted in a further increase in CTL-P frequency. For anti-$H-2^d$ responses, immunization of B/6 mice with viable H-2-allogeneic tumor cells did not result in a significant increase in thymic anti-$H-2^d$ CTL-P frequencies above those found in normal nonimmune (not shown) or MSV-immune mice (Table 2).

Previous experiments had shown that immunization in vivo to H-2 alloantigens resulted in an increase in the frequency of splenic CTL-P whose clonal CTL progeny could not be inhibited in their cytolytic activity by anti-Lyt-2 antibodies (MacDonald et al. 1982). Therefore, micro-MLC wells were tested for their cytolytic activity in the presence or absence of anti-Lyt-2 antibody.

Major Histocompatibility-Restricted Cytolytic T-Lymphocyte Precursors   29

Table 1. CTL-P frequencies among C57BL/6 CRT: effect of in vivo priming

Thymus	Target	Days postimmunization[a]		
		0	7	14
MSV immune	MBL-2	1/7301	1/7830	1/403
		1/3186	1/2524	1/672
	EL-4	1/32162	1/15265	1/20554
H-Y immune	Blasts (Male)	1/23349	ND	1/2798
	Blasts (Female)	1/32763	–	1/40611

[a] CRT were obtained from mice injected 48 h previously with hydrocortisone acetate. Minimal estimates of CTL-P frequency were obtained according to TASWELL (1981)

ND, not done

Table 2. Inhibitability by anti-Lyt-2 Mab of thymic CTL-P

Thymus		Anti-MSV			Anti-H-2^d		
		Lyt-2$^-$	Lyt-2$^+$	Inhibited[a] (%)	Lyt-2$^-$	Lyt-2$^+$	Inhibited (%)
MSV immune	Total	1/4368	1/5934	27	1/7677	1/18477	60
	Total	1/9375	1/12055	33	1/2955	1/12774	77
	CRT	1/183	1/244	25	1/469	1/2492	81
	B2A2^{-b}	1/2933	1/2614	0	1/807	1/2194	64
H-2^d immune	Total	1/21169	1/65666	68	1/2275	1/7467	70
	Total	1/93987	1/234965	60	1/10648	1/85286	78
	CRT	ND	–	–	1/613	1/3242	81

Each line represents the results of an experiment with the same pooled thymocytes

[a] Calculated from the differences in CTL-P frequencies when micro-MLC wells were assayed either in the absence (Lyt-2$^-$) or presence (Lyt-2$^+$) of anti-Lyt-2 Mab

[b] Cells recovered following treatment of thymocytes with Mab B2A2+C'

ND, not done

Results of a typical experiment, where micro-MLC wells using thymocytes from H-2^d-alloimmune (panel A) or MSV-immune mice (panel B) as responder cells were tested for cytolytic activity in the absence (vertical axis) or presence (horizontal axis) of 500 ng anti-Lyt-2 Mab are shown in Fig. 1. The dose of responder cells (1000 and 3000) in the original wells was close to the CTL-P frequency (Table 2), and thus the probability of clonality was high (87%–98%). Whereas most CTL-positive microwells responding to H-2^d alloantigens could be inhibited in their lytic activity by the addition of anti-Lyt-2 Mab, those from MSV-immune thymuses could not.

Using data obtained in such a manner, the frequencies of CTL-P inhibited or not inhibited by anti-Lyt-2 Mab could be determined simultaneously and further-

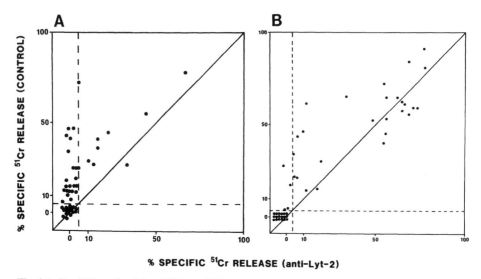

Fig. 1 A, B. Effect of anti-Lyt-2 Mab on CTL generated from in vivo primed mice. Each panel correlates the cytotoxicity data from individual micro-MLC wells tested either in the presence *(horizontal axis)* or absence *(vertical axis)* of 500 ng anti-Lyt-2 Mab. Panel **A** represents results from H-2^d-immune mice stimulated with H-2 alloantigens and tested on ^{51}Cr-labeled P815 target cells. The results of micro-MLC wells originally containing either 1000 or 3000 cells were pooled. Panel **B** is from MSV-immune mice stimulated with MSV antigens and tested on MBL-2. The original number of responder cells per micro-MLC well was similar to that in panel **A**

more, the percentage of CTL-P inhibited could be calculated. As shown in Table 2, upon immunization with MSV, there was a decrease (from 60%–68% to 25%–33%) in the percentage of wells inhibited by anti-Lyt-2 Mab. Immunization with H-2^d alloantigens did not appear to alter the proportion of wells inhibited by anti-Lyt-2 Mab (70%–81% vs 60%–81%).

Also shown in Table 2 is the response of B2A2$^-$ thymocytes from MSV-immune mice to either MSV or H-2^d. B2A2$^-$ thymocytes, which comprise about 1% of all cells are known to contain a subpopulation of mature thymocytes (SCOLLAY et al. 1984). However, from the results shown (Table 2) it appeared that B2A2$^-$ thymocytes generated CTL progeny that were as resistant as CRT to inhibition by anti-Lyt-2 Mab.

3 Discussion

In this report, the CTL-P frequencies of thymocytes from B/6 female mice immunized with either the MSV-MoLV complex, male spleen cells, or H-2 allogeneic tumor cells were determined by limit-dilution analysis of micro-MLC. Preliminary experiments where CRT were tested indicated that by 14 days after immunization there had been a significant (10- to 18-fold, Table 1) increase in specific anti-MSV or anti-H-Y CTL-P. Since the frequencies of anti-MSV CTL-P among

CRT from MSV-immune mice were relatively high (Table 1) in subsequent experiments, thymuses were also removed from mice without prior hydrocortisone injection.

As shown in Table 2, where normal thymocytes were tested, there was a significant (5- to 10-fold) increase in anti-MSV CTL-P following immunization. However, in contrast, there was no significant increase in alloreactive anti-H-2^d CTL-P frequencies among thymocytes from mice immunized with viable H-2-allogeneic P815 tumor cells. One reason for the failure to detect any increase in anti-H-2^d CTL-P frequencies may be that the frequency in normal unimmunized animals is already high and that any slight increase in frequency among thymocytes could not be determined by this method of analysis. Previous experiments from this laboratory indicated that in H-2-alloimmune mice there was only a 3- to 4-fold increase in the frequency of splenic CTL-P responding to the corresponding H-2 alloantigens (RYSER and MACDONALD 1979). Changes of this magnitude were not observed among thymocytes tested herein.

One difference that has been observed among CTL generated from normal or immune mice is their ability to be inhibited at the effector stage by anti-Lyt-2 Mab (MACDONALD et al. 1982). When analyzed at the clonal level, about 80% of CTL-P from normal mice gave rise to CTL progeny which could be inhibited by anti-Lyt-2 Mab. However, following in vivo immunization with H-2 alloantigens only about 20% of memory CTL-P gave rise to CTL progeny which could be inhibited in this way. Thus, one of the characteristic features of the CTL response from a primed animal is the relative decrease in the frequency of CTL clones susceptible to inhibition by anti-Lyt-2 Mab.

When micro-MLC wells were tested for CTL activity in the presence or absence of anti-Lyt-2 Mab, a clear difference was observed between those generated in response to H-2 alloantigens or MSV. The majority of thymic anti-H-2^d-immune CTL (Fig. 1A) were inhibited by anti-Lyt-2 Mab. This result with thymocytes differs from the results obtained with splenic CTL-P from primed mice, were immunization resulted in a decrease in anti-Lyt-2-inhibitable CTL (MACDONALD et al. 1982). The apparent failure of H-2 alloimmunization to change detectably the anti-Lyt-2 inhibitability of thymic CTL-P may be linked to the fact that following immunization, no changes in thymic anti-H-2^d CTL-P frequencies were detected (Table 2).

When mice were immunized with MSV-MoLV, there was a detectable change in both the frequency (Table 2) and anti-Lyt-2 inhibitability (Fig. 1B) of thymic CTL-P. Thus, the majority of CTL-P detected in this culture system had a "primed" phenotype, namely they were not inhibited in their effector function by anti-Lyt-2 Mab.

With these results an important question to be addressed is where, anatomically, in the mouse does this priming take place? Is it solely intrathymic or extrathymic or both? It is known that immunization with MSV-MoLV results in systemic dissemination of virus (COLLAVO et al. 1980) and even intrathymic injection of virus has been shown to immunize the peripheral lymphoid tissues (ZANOVELLO et al. 1984). Furthermore, the thymus does contain cells capable of presenting antigen to immunocompetent T cells (LONGO and SCHWARTZ 1980; KYEWSKI et al. 1984). Whether these cells become infected by MSV and conse-

32   R. Ceredig

quently present antigen to precursor T cells during the immune response is unclear at the present time.

Several independent observations have shown that peripheral T cells may recirculate back to the thymus and hence contribute to the increased frequencies of CTL-P detected following immunization (GALTON and REED 1966; NAPARSTEK et al. 1982; ZANOVELLO et al. 1984). In a recent study (FINK et al. 1984) it was shown that the thymic CTL response of C57BL/Ka mice primed to minor-H histocompatibility antigens was the sum of intrathymically and extrathymically generated responses. The kinetics of the thymic response to minor-H was similar to that reported herein for anti-MSV and anti-H-Y responses. As pointed out by FINK et al. (1984), the biology of the thymic response to immunization by foreign antigens needs to be further investigated. The results obtained with $B2A2^-$ thymocytes suggest that this subpopulation may contain cells recirculating back to the thymus.

One important direction for future work would include a study of the relative anatomical localization within the thymus of injected antigen and responding T cells. With monoclonal antibodies to a defined immunogenic protein antigen, the anatomical localization of injected antigen within the thymus could be investigated. However, there is as yet no phenotypic marker that allows one to readily distinguish activated recirculating peripheral T cells from thymocytes with a "mature" (or peripheral T-cell) phenotype.

Acknowledgments. I sincerely thank Françoise Besençon for excellent technical assistance, Dr. H. Robson MacDonald for helpful discussions, and P. Brunet for typing the manuscript.

References

Ceredig Rh, Cumming DE (1983) Phenotypic and functional properties of murine thymocytes. III. Kinetic analysis of the recovery of intrathymic cytolytic T lymphocyte precursors after in vivo administration of hydrocortisone acetate. J Immunol 130:33

Collavo D, Zanovello P, Leuchars E, Davies AJS, Chieco-Bianchi L, Biasi G (1980) Moloney murine sarcoma virus oncogenesis in T-lymphocyte-deprived mice: biologic and immunologic studies. J Nat Cancer Inst 64:97

Fink P, Bevan MJ, Weissman IL (1984) Thymic cytotoxic T lymphocytes are primed in vivo to minor histocompatibility antigens. J Exp Med 159:436

Galton M, Reed RB (1966) Entry of lymphoid cells into the normal thymus. Transplantation 4:168

Gordon RD, Simpson E, Samelson LE (1975) In vitro cell-mediated immune responses to the male specific (HY) antigen in mice. J Exp Med 142:1108

Kyewski BA, Fathman CG, Kaplan HS (1984) Intrathymic presentation of circulating non-major histocompatibility complex antigens. Nature 308:196

Longo DL, Schwartz RH (1980) T-cell specificity for H-2 and Ir gene phenotype correlates with the phenotype of thymic antigen-presenting cells. Nature 287:44

MacDonald HR, Glasebrook AL, Bron C, Kelso A, Cerottini J-C (1982) Clonal heterogeneity in the functional requirement for Lyt-2/3 molecules on cytolytic T lymphocytes (CTL): possible implications for the affinity of CTL antigen receptors. Immunol Rev 68:89

Miller JFAP, Osoba D (1967) Current concepts of the immunological function of the thymus. Physiol Rev 47:437

Naparstek Y, Holoshitz J, Eisenstein S, Reshef T, Rappaport S, Chemke J, Ben-Nun A, Cohen IR (1982) Effector T lymphocyte line cells migrate to the thymus and persist there. Nature 300:262

Plata F, Jongeneel V, Cerottini J-C, Brunner KT (1976) Antigenic specificity of the cytolytic T lymphocyte (CTL) response to murine sarcoma virus (MSV)-induced tumors. I. Preferential reactivity of in vitro generated secondary CTL with syngeneic tumor cells. Eur J Immunol 6:823

Ryser J-E, MacDonald HR (1979) Limiting dilution analysis of alloantigen-reactive T lymphocytes. III. Effect of priming on precursor frequencies. J Immunol 123:128

Scollay R, Shortman KD, Bartlett PF (1984) T cell development in the adult mouse thymus: change in the surface antigens Lyt-2, L3T4 and B2A2 during development from early precursors to emigrants. Immunol Rev 82:79

Taswell C (1981) Limiting dilution assays for the determination of immunocompetent cell frequencies. I. Data analysis. J Immunol 126:1614

Taswell C, MacDonald HR, Cerottini J-C (1979) Limiting dilution analysis of alloantigen-reactive T lymphocytes. II. Effect of cortisone and cyclophosphamide on cytolytic T lymphocyte precursor frequencies in the thymus. Thymus 1:119

Zanovello P, Collavo D, Ronchese F, de Rossi A, Biasi G, Chieco-Bianchi L (1984) Virus-specific T cell response prevents lymphoma development in mice infected by intrathymic inoculation of Moloney leukemia virus (M-MuLV). Immunology 51:9

Thymic Stem Cells:
Their Interaction with the Thymic Stroma and Tolerance Induction

J. J. T. Owen, E. J. Jenkinson, and R. Kingston

1 The Proliferative Capacity of Thymic Stem Cells: Implications for the Site of Diversification of
   T-Cell Receptors   35
1.1 Recolonization of Thymic Lobes by a Single Micromanipulated Stem Cell   36
2 Influence of the Thymic Stroma on the Development of the T-Cell Repertoire   37
2.1 Studies on Tolerance Induction In Vitro   37
2.2 Studies on Tolerance Induction In Vivo   38
References   40

1 The Proliferative Capacity of Thymic Stem Cells: Implications for the Site of Diversification of T-Cell Receptors

There are a number of lines of indirect evidence which suggest that lymphoid stem cells which migrate into the thymus have considerable proliferative potential. The first indication that this is the case was provided by Wallis et al. (1975) who derived estimates of the number of syngeneic bone marrow stem cells which repopulate the thymus of mice given a potentially lethal dose of irradiation. By injecting various mixtures of two syngeneic but chromosomally distinguishable bone marrow suspensions, they were able using probability analysis to estimate that fewer than 10 stem cells colonize a single thymus lobe. More recently, Ezine et al. (1984), using irradiated mice reconstituted with limited numbers of mixed bone marrow cells from congeneic donors differing at the Thy-1 locus, have demonstrated in frozen sections that patterns of lymphoid repopulation suggest that distinct cell clones develop within the thymus.

In order to provide a direct approach to the study of thymic stem cells we have tested the proliferative potential of "blast" cells derived by "teasing" 14-day mouse embryo thymus. Large "blast" cells first migrate into the mouse thymic primordium at 11 days' gestation but at 14 days, although more numerous, "blast" cells are still the predominant lymphoid cell type (Moore and Owen 1967). These immature cells will not proliferate in vitro when they are removed from the thymic environment. Although they express IL-2 receptors, addition of IL-2 to cultures does not prevent their rapid death (von Boehmer et al. 1985). Presumably, thymic stromal cells produce unique growth signals which may oper-

---

Department of Anatomy, Medical School, University of Birmingham, Birmingham, United Kingdom

The work of J. J. T. O. and E. J. J. described in this paper was supported by an MRC grant

36   J.J.T. Owen et al.

ate over a short range. We have adopted, therefore, an experimental approach in which thymic stem cells can be grown within an embryonic thymus which has been emptied of its own lymphoid cells by a period of organ culture in the presence of deoxyguanosine which is toxic to lymphoid cells, but spares the epithelial stroma (JENKINSON et al. 1982). When 14-day thymus "blast" cells or fetal liver cells are cocultured with deoxyguanosine-treated thymus in 20 μl hanging drops made by inverting Terasaki plates, the lobes are colonized by stem cells which associate with them at the tip of the drop. In order to allow optimal expansion of the stem cells that have migrated into the lobes, after 24–48 h each lobe is returned to organ culture for a further 10–14 days.

We have found that the frequency with which lobes are colonized is related to the number of thymus or fetal liver cells added to each hanging drop. About 20 % of lobes are colonized when 20000 14-day fetal liver cells are added, whereas over 66 % of lobes are colonized by as few as 2000 14-day thymus "blasts," presumably reflecting the difference in stem cell content in these two sources. Fetal liver cells can be enriched for stem cell activity by buoyant density fractionation over Percoll. Low density cells banding over 1.066 g/ml Percoll will colonize 80 % of lobes when 20000 cells are added and 33 % of lobes when 2500 cells are added.

1.1 Recolonization of Thymic Lobes by a Single Micromanipulated Stem Cell

In some cases we have found that as few as ten 14-day thymic "blasts" will colonize a deoxyguanosine-treated thymus. Encouraged by these results, we have examined over 300 deoxyguanosine-treated lobes to each of which a single 14-day thymic "blast" has been added using a micropipette. In 2 %–3 % of cases, the lobes have been recolonized by a single precursor giving yields of 2 to 11 $\times$ 10^4 lymphocytes for individual lobes over a 12-day culture period. By using allelic markers for Ly antigens, we have shown that all lymphocytes of repopulated deoxyguanosine-treated lobes are derived from donor stem cells.

Although the majority of lymphocytes derived from a single stem cell express an "immature" phenotype (Lyt-1$^+$, L3T4$^+$, Lyt-2$^+$), we have detected a small proportion of lymphocytes with "helper" (Lyt-1$^+$, L3T4$^+$, Lyt-2$^-$) and "cytotoxic" (Lyt-1$^-$, L3T4$^-$, Lyt-2$^+$) phenotypes. These results suggest that all subsets can be derived from a single thymic stem cell, a point much debated in the past. However, functional data is required to confirm this conclusion.

Perhaps equally important, these results suggest that diversification of the T-cell receptor repertoire by gene rearrangement is likely to occur mainly within the thymus. Extensive rearrangement prethymically is not compatible with the notion that a broad repertoire can be derived from a few stem cells migrating into the thymus. Recent evidence that T-cell receptor α and β chain rearrangement and expression progresses within the thymus as ontogeny proceeds (SNODGRASS et al. 1985) is also in line with a predominant thymic role in rearrangement. Although some level of extrathymic diversification is not excluded by these results and, indeed, is supported by the limited T-cell development found in nude mice, it is difficult to reconcile the reports on expression of antigen recognition receptors on prethymic precursors (MORRISSEY et al. 1982; CHERVENAK et al. 1985) with the results outlined above.

2 Influence of the Thymic Stroma on the Development of the T-Cell Repertoire

2.1 Studies on Tolerance Induction In Vitro

The experiments of Billingham, Brent, and Medawar (BILLINGHAM et al. 1956) showed that specific immunological tolerance to histocompatibility antigens can be induced in neonatal mice by injection of foreign cells. These observations (a) suggest that tolerance is most readily achieved when the immune system is immature and (b) are central to theories of tolerance in which it is postulated that interaction of immature lymphocytes with "self" antigens results in destruction or inactivation of autoreactive cells (BURNET 1962). However, recent studies have indicated that T-cell tolerance induction is not limited to the earliest phases of T-cell differentiation (FELDMAN et al. 1985), although these phases are likely to be crucial for tolerance induction to "self" during T-cell ontogeny.

The thymus as the primary site of T-cell production and diversification of the repertoire (see Sect. 1) is likely to be important in this respect. Both class I and class II MHC antigens are expressed by thymic epithelial cells from the earliest stages of thymus ontogeny (JENKINSON et al. 1981) and it has been suggested that tolerance to self-MHC antigens results from contact between these antigens and developing thymocytes (BURNET 1962; JERNE 1971). In order to test this proposition, we have constructed chimeric thymuses in vitro in which "empty" deoxyguanosine-treated thymic lobes are colonized by thymic or fetal liver stem cells of a different MHC haplotype (JENKINSON et al. 1985). We have asked the question: Do MHC antigens expressed on thymic epithelial cells induce tolerance in the lymphoid population as assessed by their proliferative responses to a panel of stimulators in a micro-MLC assay? The results demonstrate that lymphocytes maturing in a chimeric thymus are as responsive to MHC antigens of the thymic epithelial haplotype as they are to third-party antigens. However, they do not respond to MHC antigens of their own genotype.

How can these results be explained? Tolerance might be acquired at a prethymic level so that precursors entering the thymus are already tolerant. However, evidence presented in Sect. 1 that repertoire diversification is primarily intrathymic argues against this view. Another possibility is that tolerance is acquired within the thymus, but depends either upon interaction between thymus lymphocytes or upon interaction with a stromal cell type other than the epithelial component. The former seems unlikely in view of the low levels of MHC antigens expressed by thymocytes. With regard to the latter, the thymus contains a major population of class I and class II MHC antigen expressing cells – medullary dendritic cells, which are of hematogenous origin (BARCLAY and MAYROHOFER 1981). We have found that deoxyguanosine treatment of embryonic thymus not only eliminates lymphocytes, but also reduces and perhaps eliminates dendritic cells (OWEN and JENKINSON 1984). Furthermore, recolonized deoxyguanosine-treated thymic lobes are populated by dendritic cells of donor origin. Hence, these cells might direct the pattern of tolerance induction as outlined above.

In order to test the proposition that tolerance can be induced intrathymically, we have colonized deoxyguanosine-treated lobes with stem cells derived from two different mouse strains. We find that the lymphoid progeny of the two stem cell types are mutually unresponsive to stimulators of either haplotype in an MLC, but are fully responsive to third-party stimulators (JENKINSON et al. 1985). Furthermore, mixing of responder cells derived from separately organ-cultured thymus lobes of two different mouse strains does not suppress responsiveness to stimulator cells of either haplotype. Hence, we have concluded that tolerance to MHC antigens can be aquired within the thymus and this is not due simply to mutual suppression between MHC different lymphoid populations. The notion that dendritic cells colonizing the thymus together with lymphoid precursors are involved in tolerance induction is an attractive one, although direct evidence for it is lacking. In conclusion, tolerance to MHC antigens, as measured by MLC assays, can be induced within the thymus in vitro, but it is directed to the MHC haplotype of the colonizing stem cells rather than that of the thymic epithelium.

2.2 Studies on Tolerance Induction In Vivo

There is now a considerable amount of literature on the induction of tolerance in neonates by injection of allogeneic cells (reviewed in WOOD and STREILEIN 1984). However, the mechanisms of tolerance induction remain uncertain and the role of the thymus, in particular, is obscure. Another approach to the problem is provided by experiments in which tolerance induction is examined in nude mice grafted with allogeneic thymus. BESEDOVSKY et al. (1979) showed that these animals are tolerant to "self" and to MHC antigens of the allogeneic thymus haplotype. Tolerance to host "self" in these circumstances cannot depend upon MHC expression by the thymic epithelium (which is allogeneic) and the authors suggested that it was due to pre-T cell tolerance. However, thymus grafts are populated by host dendritic cells as well as lymphoid stem cells and intrathymic interaction with the former might be responsible for the tolerance noted.

Further, support for the notion that tolerance in thymus grafted nude mice does not depend on thymic epithelial antigen expression is provided by VON BOEHMER and SCHUBIGER (1984), who have shown that in nude mice grafted with allogeneic deoxyguanosine-treated embryonic thymus, cytolytic T-cell precursors for class I MHC antigens expressed on the epithelial thymus are present in normal numbers. This result is in line with the observations outlined in Sect. 1, where it was shown that in chimeric thymuses produced in vitro, differentiating lymphocytes are fully responsive to MHC antigens of the epithelial haplotype. Hence these studies are compatible with the idea that the thymic epithelium is not involved in tolerance induction, but that tolerance is imposed by some other element within the thymus, perhaps dendritic cells.

Of course dendritic cells are known to be potent stimulators of immunity in some situations (STEINMAN et al. 1983). Also dendritic cells are thought to be important immunogenic components of tissue grafts and their removal by in vitro treatments has been associated with prolonged graft survival (FAUSTMAN et al. 1981). Interestingly, deoxyguanosine-treated embryonic thymus lobes can be transplanted to normal mouse recipients across major or minor histocompatibility barriers without rejection (READY et al. 1984) and we have suggested that this is due to elimination of dendritic cells by deoxyguanosine, leaving an epithelial stroma which is neither immunogenic nor tolerogenic. How can this evidence for the potent lymphocyte activating function of dendritic cells be reconciled with the view that they may have a tolerogenic function within the thymus? The difference might depend upon the level of maturity of the lymphocytes involved with the least mature cells of the thymus receiving negative signals from dendritic cells, whilst the mature cells of peripheral organs receive activating signals.

Although the evidence outlined above supports the view that thymic epithelial MHC antigen expression does not play a direct role in the induction of tolerance in differentiating thymus lymphocytes, a recent study in nude mice grafted with allogeneic thymus lobes that had been subjected to a period of organ culture at 24° C has produced evidence that in this situation host-derived lymphocytes maturing within the graft are unresponsive to MHC antigens of the thymic epithelial haplotype (JORDAN et al. 1985). Culture at 24° C selectively depletes lymphocytes from the embryonic thymus and is known to reduce the immunogenicity of tissue grafts, suggesting that it might have an influence on dendritic cells also. Hence, it seems that it might have a comparable effect on the thymus to that of deoxyguanosine, but whether it eliminates the lymphoid component as reliably as deoxyguanosine is unclear. Perhaps this explains the different results obtained by VON BOEHMER and SCHUBIGER (1984) using deguanosine-treated grafts to nudes and JORDAN et al. (1985) using low-temperature cultured material, the former showing a lack of effect of thymic epithelium on cytotytic T-cell precursors, but the latter showing a tolerizing effect on proliferative T-cell responses.

However, neither group have reported on the status of the thymus grafted animals in terms of the survival of test allografts of other tissues. We have grafted nude mice reconstituted by deoxyguanosine-treated thymus with embryonic pancreas in order to test their tolerance status. BALB/c nude mice were grafted with four deoxyguanosine-treated lobes under the renal capsule. We limited the lobes transplanted to this number because we have found that when larger numbers of lobes are transplanted to normal mice, they are rejected, suggesting that a few residual immunogenic dendritic cells persist in these lobes and that a threshold activating number may be exceeded when multiple lobes are grafted. Such a number might also influence the tolerance pattern of nudes. Three months after reconstitution with four allogeneic (CBA/Ca) deoxyguanosine-treated lobes, the mice were grafted to either pole of the kidney with a single CBA/Ca and C57 B1 10 pancreas from 14-day embryos. Thus H-2^d nude mice given an H-2^k epithelial thymus were tested with H-2^k and H-2^b pancreas grafts. In a group of six mice, 6 weeks after pancreas transplantation, all mice were found to have an excellent H-2^k pancreas graft containing numerous islets, but only a fibrous scar was found at the site of the H-2^b pancreas graft.

Hence these results indicate that nude mice given allogeneic deoxyguanosine-treated grafts are immunocompetent and capable of rejecting third-party grafts, but are tolerant to the MHC haplotype of the thymic epithelial cells, suggesting a role for the epithelium in tolerance induction. However, the mechanism of nonresponsiveness here may be different, but perhaps complementary, to that operating in normal mice and this result may not be in such apparent conflict with the conclusions outlined in Sect. 2.1. We have found that these nude mice contain substantial numbers of lymph node, spleen, and thymus cells bearing Ia^k and K^k antigens presumably shed from the $H-2^k$ thymus grafts. For example, over 30% of lymph node cells, 20% of thymus cells, and 50% of spleen cells are positive for Ia^k with comparable figures for K^k of 75%, 20%, and 75%, respectively. We have found no trace of persisting donor lymphocytes or their precursors in deoxyguanosine-treated grafts and so these antigens must be acquired by host cells from the donor epithelium. Passive acquisition of MHC antigens by T cells has previously been reported (SHARROW et al. 1981), but its functional significance is obscure. Perhaps the high level of donor antigen on peripheral cells of thymus grafted nudes might provide an explanation for the nonresponsiveness to donor antigens found. If so, thymic epithelial MHC antigen expression might have a role in tolerance, but it is unclear whether this is unique to nudes. Certainly, such a mechanism would not exclude a role for dendritic cells (as described previously) and could not be the means by which T cells in these animals are tolerant to genetic "self."

In conclusion, although it is not easy to reconcile all of the experimental data discussed, it is likely that differentiating T cells acquire tolerance to "self"-MHC antigens at an intrathymic level, perhaps by interaction with MHC-expressing dendritic cells. The evidence provided by allogeneic thymus grafted nudes suggests that an additional mechanism, namely, shedding of thymic epithelial MHC antigens followed by extensive acquisition of these antigens by host lymphocytes, may play a part.

Acknowledgements. We thank Jackie Lidstone for help in the preparation of the manuscript.

References

Barclay NA, Mayrohofer G (1981) Bone marrow origin of Ia-positive cells in the medulla of rat thymus. J Exp Med 153:1660–1671

Besedovsky HO, Del Rey A, Sorkin E (1979) Role of prethymic cells in acquisition of self-tolerance. J Exp Med 150:1351–1358

Billingham RF, Brent L, Medawar PB (1956) Quantitative studies on tissue transplantation immunity. III. Actively acquired tolerance. Philos Trans R Soc Lond [Biol] 239:357–414

Burnet FM (1962) Role of the thymus and related organs in immunity. Br Med J 2:807–811

Chervenak R, Moorhead JW, Cohen JJ (1985) Prethymic T cell precursors express receptors for antigen. J Immunol 134:695–698

Ezine S, Weissman IL, Rouse RV (1984) Bone marrow cells give rise to distinct cell clones within the thymus. Nature 309:629–631

Faustman D, Hauptfeld V, Lacy P, Davie J (1981) Prolongation of murine islet allograft survival by pretreatment of islets with antibody directed to Ia determinants. Proc Natl Acad Sci USA 78:5156–5159

Feldmann M, Zanders ED, Lamb JR (1985) Tolerance in T-cell clones. Immunol Today 6:58–62

Jenkinson EJ, van Ewijk W, Owen JJT (1981) Major histocompatibility complex antigen expression on the epithelium of the developing thymus in normal and nude mice. J Exp Med 153:280–293

Jenkinson EJ, Franchi LL, Kingston R, Owen JJT (1982) Effect of deoxyguanosine on lymphopoiesis in the developing thymus in vitro: application in the construction of chimeric thymus rudiments. Eur J Immunol 12:583–587

Thymic Stem Cells: Their Interaction with the Thymic Stroma and Tolerance Induction 41

Jenkinson EJ, Jhittay P, Kingston R, Owen JJT (1985) Studies on the role of the thymic environment in the induction of tolerance to MHC antigens. Transplantation 39:331–333

Jerne NK (1971) The somatic generation of immune recognition. Eur J Immunol 1:1–9

Jordan RK, Robinson JH, Hopkinson NA, House KC, Bentley AL (1985) Thymic epithelium and the induction of transplantation tolerance in nude mice. Nature 314:454–456

Moore MAS, Owen JJT (1967) Experimental studies on the development of the thymus. J Exp Med 126:715–726

Morrissey PJ, Kruisbeek AM, Sharrow SO, Singer A (1982) Tolerance of thymic cytotoxic T lymphocytes to allogeneic H-2 determinants encountered pre-thymically: evidence of expression of anti-H2 receptors prior to entry to the thymus. Proc Natl Acad Sci USA 79:2003–2007

Owen JJT, Jenkinson EJ (1984) Early events in T lymphocyte genesis in fetal thymus. Am J Anat 170:301–310

Ready AR, Jenkinson EJ, Kingston R, Owen JJT (1984) Deoxyguanosine treatment of embryonic thymus allows successful transplantation across a major histocompatibility barrier despite continued class II antigen expression on donor thymic epithelium. Nature 310:231–233

Sharrow SO, Mathieson BJ, Singer A (1981) Cell surface appearance of unexpected host MHC determinants on thymocytes from radiation bone marrow chimerias. J Immunol 4:1327–1335

Snodgrass HR, Kisielow P, Kiefer M, Steinmetz M, von Boehmer H (1985) Ontogeny of the T-cell antigen receptor within the thymus. Nature 313:592–594

Steinman RM, Gutchinov B, Witmer MD, Nussenzweig MC (1983) Dendritic cells are the principal stimulators of the primary mixed leukocyte reaction in mice. J Exp Med 157:613–627

von Boehmer H, Schubiger K (1984) Thymocytes appear to ignore class I major histocompatibility complex antigens expressed on thymus epithelial cells. Eur J Immunol 14:1048–1052

von Boehmer H, Crisani A, Kisielow P, Haas W (1985) Absence of growth by most receptor-expressing fetal thymocytes in the presence of interleukin-2. Nature 314:539–520

Wallis VJ, Leuchars E, Chwalinski S, Davies AJS (1975) On the sparse seeding of bone marrow and thymus in radiation chimaeras. Transplantation 19:2–11

Wood PJ, Streilein JW (1984) Immunogenetic basis of acquired transplantation tolerance. Transplantation 37:223–226

Part B: Murine T-Cell Receptor Genes

Organization, Rearrangement, and Diversification of Mouse T-Cell Receptor Genes

M. STEINMETZ and Z. DEMBIĆ

1 Organization, Rearrangement, and Expression   45
2 Use of Specific V_β Gene Segments Does Not Correlate with Recognition of Certain MHC Alleles   47
3 Generation of Diversity   48
References   49

With the isolation of specific antibodies and cDNA clones it has recently become possible to study the molecular nature of the T-cell receptor that had for an unusually long time resisted characterization (for a review see, MÖLLER 1984). It has by now been firmly established that the T-cell receptor genes are members of the so-called immunoglobulin superfamily which includes the immunoglobulin, T-cell receptor, MHC class I and class II, T4, T8, Thy-1, Ox-2 and poly(Ig)receptor genes (HOOD et al. 1985; WILLIAMS 1985). The T-cell receptor genes use the same strategies as the immunoglobulin genes to generate diversity – namely, splitting of the coding information into a number of small gene segments and diversification of these segments by various somatic mechanisms (reviewed in STEINMETZ 1986). In the following, we will briefly review the organization and rearrangement of the T-cell receptor gene segments and compare somatic diversification mechanisms of immunoglobulin and T-cell receptor genes.

1 Organization, Rearrangement, and Expression

The T-cell receptor is a glycoprotein molecule, composed of two distinct, disulfide-linked polypeptide chains, called α and β, each about 40000 to 50000 daltons in molecular weight. The α and β chains both consist of a variable and a constant region domain which are linked to a segment that resembles a hinge region followed by a transmembrane region and a short cytoplasmic tail.

The organization of the β-chain gene segments, which are located on chromosome 6 in the mouse (CACCIA et al. 1984; LEE et al. 1984), is shown in Fig. 1. The variable region domain is encoded by three distinct gene segments, V, D, and J, which are present in several copies in the mouse genome. Seven V gene segments, out of a total of perhaps 15 to 30 (MARX 1985), have been described (PAT-

---

Basel Institute for Immunology, Grenzacher Strasse 487, CH-4005 Basel

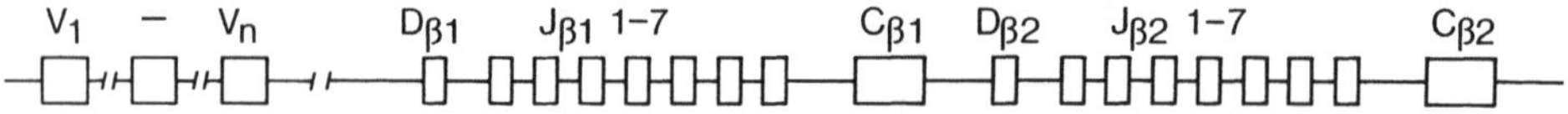

Fig. 1. Organization of mouse T-cell receptor β-chain gene segments (GASCOIGNE et al. 1984; MALISSEN et al. 1984; KAVALER et al. 1984; SIU et al. 1984). Gene segments, indicated by *boxes*, are not drawn to scale. The two D-J-C clusters are spread over approx. 15 kb. Both C_β gene segments are split into four exons and V gene segments consist of two exons. The number, orientation, and distance (with respect to the two D-J-C gene clusters) are not known for the V_β gene segments. All D, J, and C gene segments have the same 5' to 3' orientation

TEN et al. 1984), and two D gene segments (KAVALER et al. 1984; SIU et al. 1984), and 14 J gene segments, 12 of which appear to be functional (GASCOIGNE et al. 1984; MALISSEN et al. 1984), have been identified. The D and J gene segments are arranged into two clusters upstream of two C_β genes, respectively. The two C_β genes which code for the constant region domain of two distinct β chains are almost identical in their coding region, but differ extensively in the 3' untranslated region (GASCOIGNE et al. 1984, MALISSEN et al. 1984).

Expression of β-chain genes is preceded by a rearrangement of the β-chain gene segments to form a complete β-chain variable region gene. Two types of rearrangements of variable region gene segments have been found: joining of D and J gene segments only, leading to the production of a D-J-C mRNA molecule, 1.0 kb in size, and complete V, D, and J joining, giving rise to 1.3 kb mRNA transcripts, containing V, D, J, and C gene sequences (CHIEN et al. 1984a; SIU et al. 1984). Obviously, complete β chains can only be synthesized from the 1.3 kb mRNA transcripts. Some of the 1.0 kb mRNA transcripts might also be translated, although such a protein has not yet been identified (SIU et al. 1984). The $D_{\beta1}$ gene segment can combine with J gene segments of the first or the second cluster. V gene segments also use both clusters of D, J, and C gene segments (CHIEN et al. 1984a; KRONENBERG et al. 1985).

Conserved sequences have been identified immediately downstream of V gene segments, upstream of J gene segments, and on both sides of D gene segments (GASCOIGNE et al. 1984; SIU et al. 1984). These sequences are closely related to their immunoglobulin counterparts and are believed to be important for the rearrangement of the gene segments. The homology indicates that the same or very similar enzymes rearrange immunoglobulin and T-cell receptor genes. Whereas direct V-J joining, skipping the D gene segment, has never been observed for immunoglobulin heavy chain genes, such a rearrangement appears to be possible for β-chain genes. Indeed, some evidence for direct V-J joining has been obtained for human β-chain genes (YOSHIKAI et al. 1984).

The genomic organization of the T-cell receptor α-chain genes has not yet been worked out to a detail similar to that for the β-chain genes. It is known that a single C_α gene is present in the mouse genome on chromosome 14, closely linked to the gene coding for nucleoside phosphorylase (DEMBIĆ et al. 1985). The sequence organization of α-chain cDNA clones indicates that V, J, and possibly D gene segments will also be found (CHIEN et al. 1984b; SAITO et al. 1984b).

A third gene family, called γ, has ben described, which is closely related to α- and β-chain genes, and undergoes specific rearrangements in T cells (SAITO et al.

1984a). The function of the γ genes, however, is unknown and a protein product has not yet been identified. The γ gene family is composed of at least three V, three J, and three C gene segments. It appears that only one V, J, and C combination yields the productive rearrangement (HAYDAY et al. 1985). In the mouse, the γ gene family maps to chromosome 13 (KRANZ et al. 1985b).

The γ gene appears to be almost exclusively transcribed in cytotoxic T cells (KRANZ et al. 1984a) and its expression shows an interesting inverse correlationship with α gene expression during T-cell ontogeny (RAULET et al. 1985; SNODGRASS et al. 1985b). The γ genes are the first to be transcribed during ontogeny and their level of transcription declines when the α gene is activated. Transcription of β genes starts at an intermediate timepoint and appears to switch from primarily D-J-C transcripts to complete V-D-J-C transcripts (SNODGRASS et al. 1985a).

T-cell receptor β-chain genes have been found to be expressed in every helper and cytotoxic T cell tested. In contrast, most mouse suppressor hybridomas appear to lose the β-chain genes derived from the functional T cells, indicating that suppressor T cells might use a different gene family to code for one chain of the T-cell receptor (KRONENBERG et al. 1985; HEDRICK et al. 1985). Adorini et al. (this volume), however, describe a cloned suppressor T-cell line which appears to contain a functional β-chain gene. In addition they show that antibodies, directed against the β chain, bind soluble suppressor factor. At least some suppressor cells, therefore, might use the same β-chain genes as helper and killer T cells. This is in agreement with apparently functional β-chain gene rearrangements in human suppressor T-cell clones (ROYER et al. 1984; TOYONAGA et al. 1984).

2 Use of Specific V_β Gene Segments Does Not Correlate with Recognition of Certain MHC Alleles

Both the $C_{\beta1}$ and $C_{\beta2}$ constant region genes have been found to be expressed in cytotoxic and helper T cells, recognizing foreign antigen in the context of class I and class II MHC molecules, respectively (CHIEN et al. 1984a; SAITO et al. 1984a; KRONENBERG et al. 1985). Thus, usage of the two β-chain constant regions does not correlate with function or MHC specificity. Also V_β gene segments do not determine MHC specificity. The same V_β gene segment has been found to be expressed in two different helper T cells, one specific for hen egg lysozyme together with I-A^b as a restriction element and the other specific for pigeon cytochrome c with I-E^k (CHIEN et al. 1984a; GOVERMAN et al. 1985). Furthermore, it has been shown that the same V_β gene segment is used in a cytotoxic and a helper T cell, which differ in antigen and MHC specificity (Dembić et al., unpublished results). It also follows from these findings that recognition of a particular foreign antigen does not depend solely on the V_β gene segment used.

In contrast to the V_β gene segment, the sequences of the D_β and J_β gene segments differ between the two helper T cells, and between the cytotoxic and the helper T cell discussed above (CHIEN et al. 1984a; GOVERMAN et al. 1985; Dembić et al. unpublished results). One might therefore anticipate that the specificity of

48 M. Steinmetz and Z. Dembić

T-cell receptor combining sites, like those of antibody molecules, will be determined by residues encoded by all three variable region gene segments as well by variable residues located on the α chain.

3 Generation of Diversity

The mechanisms by which T cells diversify the germline repertoire of β-chain gene segments are fundamentally similar to those used by B cells to diversify immunoglobulin genes, although some differences exist. Table 1 compares the different mechanisms that have been found to diversify immunoglobulin (TONEGAWA 1983) and T-cell receptor β-chain genes (KAVALER et al. 1984; SIU et al. 1984; MALISSEN et al. 1984; PATTEN et al. 1984; HAYDAY et al. 1985; GOVERMAN et al. 1985).

Combinatorial joining of multiple germline gene segments obviously is an important somatic diversification mechanism used by both gene families. Clearly, differences in the numbers of various gene segments exist for immunoglobulin and T-cell receptor β-chain genes. However, the importance of this variation is not clear at all, since large variations in gene numbers are also found when immunoglobulin genes of different species are compared (REYNAUD et al. 1985). It is very well possible that the extent to which these various mechanisms contribute to the diversity of immunoglobulin and T-cell receptor molecules can vary without being directly related to the size of the functional repertoire.

Table 1. Generation of diversity in mouse immunoglobulin and T-cell receptor β-chain variable region genes in vivo

	Immunoglobulin genes	T-cell receptor β-chain genes
Multiplicity of germline encoded V region gene segments:	Light chain 90–300 V_κ 4 J_κ 2 V_λ 3 J_λ Heavy chain 100–200 V_H 12 D_H 4 J_H	15–30 V_β 2 D_β 12 J_β
Somatic diversification mechanisms:		
Combinatorial joining	yes	yes
Junctional flexibility	yes	yes
N-region diversity	yes	yes
Translational flexibility	some	yes
Combinatorial chain association	yes	likely
Somatic mutation	yes	unlikely

Organization, Rearrangement, and Diversification of Mouse T-Cell Receptor Genes 49

Junctional flexibility describes the inaccuracy that occurs when gene segments are joined. Individual amino acid residues at the junction site might either be encoded separately by V, D, and J gene segments or partly by V and D, D and J, or V and J gene segments.

N-region insertion has been observed in immunoglobulin heavy chain and T-cell receptor β-chain genes. It refers to the apparently random insertion of nucleotides at both ends of D gene segments.

Translational flexibility appears to be a special mechanism used by D gene segments of T-cell receptor β-chain genes. The two D_β gene segments lack translational stop codons in all three reading frames, in contrast to immunoglobulin D gene segments. Thus, a single D_β gene segment can be translated into three different protein sequences. By this means, β-chain genes may partly compensate for their apparently smaller numbers of D gene segments compared with mouse immunoglobulin heavy chain genes.

Combinatorial association is an important mechanism that contributes to the diversity of antibody molecules because the antigen-combining site is formed by residues from heavy and light chain variable regions. Random or almost random association of several thousand heavy chains with several hundred light chains can give rise to several million antibody molecules. It is very likely that T-cell receptor molecules will also show combinatorial association of α and β chains.

Finally, somatic mutation will further diversify immunoglobulin variable region genes. It is presently unclear to what extent somatic mutational mechanisms contribute to the diversity of T-cell receptor genes. Base changes that have been observed between V_β germline genes and their expressed counterparts might be due to strain polymorphism or sequencing errors (CHIEN et al. 1984a; GOVERMAN et al. 1985). On the other hand, clear evidence for the accumulation of mutations has been found in V region genes in cloned helper T-cell hybridomas during propagation in culture (AUGUSTIN and SIM 1984). Similarly, cytotoxic T-cell clones when propagated in culture change their specificity (Weltzien and Eichmann this volume). Some apparently change specificity by expressing new V_β gene segments (Epplen et al. this volune). Future experiments will show whether these recent findings reflect mechanisms which also operate on T-cell receptor genes in vivo.

Acknowledgements. We thank L. Hood for preprints and S. Ryser and R. Snodgrass for comments. The Basel Institute for Immunology was founded and is supported by Hoffmann-La Roche, Basel, Switzerland.

References

Augustin AA, Sim KG (1984) T cell receptors generated via mutations are specific for various major histocompatibility antigens. Cell 39:5–12

Caccia N, Kronenberg M, Saxe D, Haars R, Bruns GAP, Goverman J, Malissen M, Willard H, Yoshikai Y, Simon M, Hood L, Mak TW (1984) The T cell receptor β chain genes are located on chromosome 6 in mice and chromosome 7 in humans. Cell 37:1091–1099

Chien YH, Gascoigne NRJ, Kavaler J, Lee NE, Davis MM (1984a) Somatic recombination in a murine T-cell receptor gene. Nature 309:322–326

Chien YH, Becker DM, Lindsten T, Okamura M, Cohen DI, Davis MM (1984b) A third type of murine T-cell receptor gene. Nature 312:31–35

Dembić Z, Bannwarth W, Taylor BA, Steinmetz M (1985) The gene encoding the T-cell receptor α-chain maps close to the Np-2 locus on mouse chromosome 14. Nature 314:271–273

Gascoigne NRJ, Chien YH, Becker DM, Kavaler J, Davis MM (1984) Genomic organization and sequence of T-cell receptor β-chain constant- and joining-region genes. Nature 310:387–391

Goverman J, Minard K, Shastri N, Hunkapiller T, Hansburg D, Sercarz E, Hood L (1985) Rearranged β T-cell receptor genes in a helper T-cell clone specific for lysozyme: no correlation between V_β and MHC restriction. Cell 40:859–867

Hayday AC, Saito H, Gillies SD, Kranz DM, Tangigawa G, Eisen HN, Tonegawa S (1985) Structure, organization and somatic rearrangement of T cell gamma genes. Cell 40:259–269

Hedrick SM, Germain RN, Bevan MJ, Dorf M, Engel I, Fink P, Gascoigne N, Heber-Katz E, Kapp J, Kaufman Y, Kaye J, Melchers F, Pierce C, Schwartz RH, Sorensen C, Taniguchi M, Davis MM (1985) Rearrangement and transcription of a T-cell receptor β-chain gene in different T-cell subsets. Proc Natl Acad Sci USA 82:531–555

Hood L, Kronenberg M, Hunkapiller T (1985) T cell antigen receptors and the immunoglobulin supergene family. Cell 40:225–229

Kavaler J, Davis MM, Chien YH (1984) Localization of a T-cell receptor diversity-region element. Nature 310:421–423

Kranz DM, Saito H, Heller M, Takagaki Y, Haas W, Eisen HN, Tonegawa S (1985a) Limited diversity of the rearranged T-cell γ gene. Nature 313:752–755

Kranz DM, Saito H, Disteche CM, Swisshelm K, Pravtcheva D, Ruddle FH, Eisen HN, Tonegawa S (1985b) Chromosomal locations of the murine T-cell receptor alpha-chain gene and the T-cell gamma gene. Science 227:941–945

Kronenberg M, Goverman J, Haars R, Malissen M, Kraig E, Phillips L, Delovitch T, Suciu-Foca N, Hood L (1985) Rearrangement and transcription of the β-chain genes of the T-cell antigen receptor in different types of murine lymphocytes. Nature 313:647–653

Lee NE, D'Euchstachio P, Pravtcheva D, Ruddle FH, Hedrick SM, Davis MM (1984) Murine T cell receptor beta chain is encoded on chromosome 6. J Exp Med 160:905–913

Malissen M, Minard K, Mjolsness S, Kronenberg M, Goverman J, Hunkapiller T, Prystowsky MB, Yoshikai Y, Fitch F, Mak TW, Hood L (1984) Mouse T cell antigen receptor: structure and organization of constant and joining gene segments encoding the β polypeptide. Cell 37:1101–1110

Marx JL (1985) The T-cell receptor – the genes and beyond. Science 227:733–735

Möller G (ed) (1984) T cell receptors and genes. Immunol Rev 81

Patten P, Yokota T, Rothbard J, Chien YH, Arai KI, Davis MM (1984) Structure, expression and divergence of T-cell receptor β-chain variable regions. Nature 312:40–46

Raulet DH, Garman RD, Saito H, Tonegawa S (1985) Developmental regulation of T-cell receptor gene expression. Nature 314:103–107

Reynaud CA, Anquez V, Dahan A, Weill JC (1985) A single rearrangement event generates most of the chicken immunoglobulin light chain diversity. Cell 40:283–291

Royer HD, Bensussan A, Acuto O, Reinherz EL (1984) Functional isotypes are not encoded by the constant region genes of the β subunit of the T cell receptor for antigen/major histocompatibility complex. J Exp Med 160:947–952

Saito H, Kranz DM, Takagaki Y, Hayday AC, Eisen HN, Tonegawa S (1984a) Complete primary structure of a heterodimeric T-cell receptor deduced from cDNA sequences. Nature 309:757–762

Saito H, Kranz DM, Takagaki Y, Hayday AC, Eisen H, Tonegawa S (1984b) A third rearranged and expressed gene in a clone of cytotoxic T lymphocytes. Nature 312:36–40

Siu G, Kronenberg M, Strauss E, Haars R, Mak TW, Hood L (1984) The structure, rearrangement and expression of D_β gene segments of the murine T-cell antigen receptor. Nature 311:344–350

Snodgrass HR, Kieselow P, Kiefer M, Steinmetz M, von Boehmer H (1985a) Ontogeny of the T-cell antigen receptor within the thymus. Nature 313:592–595

Snodgrass HR, Dembić Z, Steinmetz M, von Boehmer H (1985b) Expression of T cell antigen receptor genes during fetal development in the thymus. Nature 315:232–233

Steinmetz M (1986) Genes of the immune system. In: Rigby PWJ (ed) Genetic engineering, vol 5. Academic, London, pp 117–158

Tonegawa S (1983) Somatic generation of antibody diversity. Nature 302:575–581

Toyonaga B, Yanagi Y, Suciu-Foca N, Minden M, Mak TW (1984) Rearrangement of T-cell receptor gene YT35 in human DNA from thymic leukaemia T-cell lines and functional T-cell clones. Nature 311:385–387

Williams AF (1985) Immunoglobulin-related domains for cell surface recognition. Nature 314:579–580

Yoshikai Y, Anatoniou D, Clark SP, Yanagi Y, Sangster R, van der Elsen P, Terhorst C, Mak TW (1984) Sequence and expression of transcripts of the human T-cell receptor β-chain genes. Nature 312:521–524

Expression of T-Cell Receptor by a Mouse Monoclonal Antigen-Specific Suppressor T-Cell Line

L. ADORINI[1], G. PALMIERI[1], A. SETTE[1], E. APPELLA[2], and G. DORIA[1]

1 Introduction 53
2 Functional Analysis of LH8–105 TsF 54
3 Expression of T-Cell Receptor by LH8–105 T Cells 57
4 Summary 59
References 59

1 Introduction

The antigen receptor expressed by mouse T lymphocytes is composed of a disul-fide-linked dimer of about 85K, resolved under reducing conditions in two sub-units with an apparent M_r of approximately 42K (ALLISON et al. 1982; KAPPLER et al. 1983). The antigen-specific receptor expressed by human T lymphocytes displays a similar structure, but the two subunits, denominated α and β chain, have a M_r of about 51K and 43K, respectively (MEUER et al. 1983; ACUTO et al. 1983).

Genes coding for the α (CHIEN et al. 1984; SIM et al. 1984) and the β (HEDRICK et al. 1984; YANAGI et al. 1984) chains of the T-cell receptor molecule have been identified both in mouse and human T cells. These genes are rearranged and expressed in antigen-specific helper and cytotoxic T-cell hybridomas and T-cell clones. Conversely, no somatic rearrangement of genes coding for the β chain has been observed in most mouse suppressor T-cell hybridomas (HEDRICK et al. 1985). However, human T-cell clones with suppressive activity rearrange and express genes encoding the β chain of the T-cell receptor for antigen (YOSHIKAI et al. 1984; ROYER et al. 1984).

At variance with the antigen receptor described for helper and cytotoxic T cells, the antigen-specific recognition structures expressed by suppressor T-cell clones are still unclear and although a heterogeneous array of antigen-binding soluble factors released by suppressor T cells has been described, their relation-ship to the T-cell surface receptor has not yet been determined.

We have described a cloned T-cell lymphoma line, LH8–105, obtained by radiation leukemia virus-induced transformation of hen egg-white lysozyme (HEL)-specific mouse suppressor T lymphocytes (RICCIARDI-CASTAGNOLI et al.

---

[1] ENEA-Euratom Immunogenetics Group, Laboratory of Pathology, CRE Casaccia, CP 2400, I-00100 Rome A.D.
[2] Laboratory of Cell Biology, NCI, NIH, Bethesda, MD 20205, USA

54   L. Adorini et al.

1981). The LH8–105 suppressor T-cell clone constitutively releases in the culture supernatant products able to specifically suppress the antibody response (ADORINI et al. 1982, 1983) and the delayed-type hypersensitivity (DTH) to HEL (ADORINI et al. 1984).

Since α- and β-chain genes are rearranged and expressed in LH8–105 cells (DE SANTIS et al. 1985) and T-cell receptor structures are present on the surface of LH8–105 cells (BALLINARI et al. 1985), at least some mouse suppressor T cells utilize the same genes as helper and cytotoxic T cells to encode the T-cell receptor α- and β-chains.

Moreover, soluble molecules with HEL-specific suppressive activity constitutively released by LH8–105 cells are bound by rabbit antibodies directed against a $C\beta$ synthetic peptide, indicating a relationship between the T-cell receptor expressed by suppressor T cells and soluble products with suppressive activity.

2   Functional Analysis of LH8–105 TsF

Intraperitoneal HEL-CFA priming in mice of H-2^b haplotype, genetically nonresponder to HEL (HILL and SERCARZ 1975), induces T-suppressor (Ts) cells specific for HEL (ADORINI et al. 1979). From this cell population, enriched in HEL-specific T cells, permanent T-cell lines have been established by radiation leukemia virus-induced transformation (RICCIARDI-CASTAGNOLI et al. 1981). Culture supernatant from LH8–105 T-cell clone is able, when injected into mice, to specifically suppress the antibody response (Table 1) and the DTH reaction induced by HEL (ADORINI et al. 1984). LH8–105 TsF induces suppressive activity only when injected in the afferent phase of the antibody (ADORINI et al. 1982) or DTH (ADORINI et al. 1984) response to HEL and this is therefore a suppressor-inducer factor. Second-order Ts cells are induced by LH8–105 TsF only in HEL-primed mice, indicating the primary role of antigen in the afferent phase of this suppressive circuit.

Suppression of antibody production and DTH induction by LH8–105 TsF injection exhibits fine antigenic specificity restricted to an epitope present in the N-terminal region of the HEL molecule which includes phenylalanine at amino acid residue 3, since injection of LH8–105 culture supernatant induces suppression of anti-lysozyme PFC responses in mice primed with HEL and human lysozyme (HUL), but not in mice primed with ring-necked pheasant egg-white lysozyme (REL) (Table 2).

The recognition by LH8–105 TsF of a determinant present on HEL but absent on REL is confirmed by LH8–105 TsF binding to HEL, but not to REL, immunosorbent (ADORINI et al. 1984). Therefore, the LH8–105 TsF can discriminate between the closely related HEL and REL molecules which differ in 10 out of 129 amino acid residues, whereas it suppresses to the same extent the anti-HUL and the anti-HEL responses.

These two lysozymes differ at 40% amino acid residues, but share an antigenic epitope, including phenylalanine at position 3 critical for inducing suppression. The presence of a suppressive determinant common to HEL and HUL,

Table 1. Suppression of the anti-HEL antibody response by LH8–105 culture supernatant injection

Culture supernatant	Priming	Developed anti-HEL PFC/10^6 PTLN cells	Suppression %	Priming	Developed anti-TNP PFC/10^6 PTLN cells	Suppression %
None	HEL-CFA	21440 (1.09)		TNP-KLH-CFA	2227 (1.44)	
LH8–105	HEL-CFA	9300 (1.35)	57	TNP-KLH-CFA	4256 (1.25)	0

BDF1 mice (5 mice/group) were injected i. p. with 100 μg HEL or TNP-KLH in CFA and developed PFC responses were measured 8 days later in the parathymic lymph node (PTLN) cells. Culture supernatant from LH8–105 cells (1 ml/mouse) was injected i.v. at the same time of antigen priming and for the 2 following days. Values refer to the geometric mean PFC and numbers in parentheses represent a factor by which the mean should be multiplied or divided to give one standard error.

Table 2. Fine antigenic specifity of LH8–105 TsF

LH8–105 TsF injection	Priming	Developed anti-lysozyme PFC/10^6 PTLN cells	Suppression (%)
–	HEL-CFA	17137 (1.30)	
+	HEL-CFA	6095 (1.18)	65
–	REL-CFA	17085 (1.57)	
+	REL-CFA	18591 (1.37)	0
–	HUL-CFA	983 (1.64)	
+	HUL-CFA	265 (1.33)	73

BDF1 mice (5 mice/group) were injected i.p. with 100 μg HEL, REL, or HUL in CFA and PFC responses against the homologous lysozyme were measured 8 days later in the PTLN cells. Culture supernatant from LH8–105 cell clone (1 ml/mouse) was injected for 3 consecutive days and the first injection was given on the same day as antigen priming. PFC values from individual mice are expressed as geometric mean and the numbers in parantheses represent a factor by which the mean should be multiplied or divided to give one standard error.

despite the differences between these two lysozymes, may explain the high HEL HUL cross-reactivity in the immunosuppression exerted by the HEL-specific LH8–105 TsF (ADORINI et al. 1981). The N-terminal regions of HEL and HUL are identical at amino acid residues 1–9, except for glycine at position 4 in HEL which is replaced by glutamic acid in HUL, whereas REL has tyrosine instead of phenylalanine at position 3. Therefore, the LH8–105 TsF displays fine antigenic specificity probably restricted to an epitope including phenylalanine at amino acid residue 3.

To address more directly this issue a synthetic peptide encompassing amino acid residues 1–18 of the HEL molecule and an analogue when phenylalanine has been substituted by tyrosine at position 3 have been prepared by solid-phase synthesis. These two peptides, denominated P_{HEL} and P_{REL}, respectively, have been tested for their ability to induce second-order suppressor T cells in the DTH assay. P_{HEL} as well as HEL and reduced and carboxymethylated HEL (RCM-HEL) are able to induce, in mice injected with LH8–105 TsF, second-order suppressor T cells, as revealed by the transfer of spleen cells into syngeneic HEL-CFA-primed mice. Conversely, P_{REL} priming does not induce detectable suppression in this adoptive transfer system. Moreover, P_{HEL} but nor P_{REL} priming is able to induce suppression of the DTH response in mice injected with LH8–105 TsF (SETTE et al. 1986), thus demonstrating that phenylalanine at amino acid residue 3 is critical for the formation of an epitope able to induce HEL-specific suppressor cells and to mediate information transfer among suppressor T-lymphocyte subsets.

Determinants controlled by genes apparently mapping in the I-J region of the H-2 complex are present on LH8–105 TsF as indicated by binding of molecules with suppressive activity on monoclonal anti-I-J[b] immunosorbent. Determinants recognized by anti-I-J[b] antibodies are also present on LH8–105 cells, as assessed by membrane immunofluorescence (RICCIARDI-CASTAGNOLI et al. 1981) and by radioimmunoassay employing LH8–105 cells as solid phase and monoclonal anti-I-J[b] antibodies revealed by binding of iodinated anti-Ig antibodies (Adorini, unpublished). Moreover, the interaction between LH8–105 TsF and its cellular target is restricted by genes mapping in the I-J region since suppression, both of antibody and DTH responses, is induced in B10. A(3R) (I-J[b]), but not in the I-J congenic B10. A(5R) (I-J[k]) mice. However, molecular biology experiments indicate that I-J exons are not likely to be present between the I-A and I-E subregions of the H-2 complex (KRONENBERG 1983), possibly because the high frequency of multiple cross-overs in H-2 recombinant strains has led to an incorrect map order for the I region or because in the I-J region is contained a regulatory element of a structural gene located elsewhere in the genome (KLYCZEK et al. 1984).

Suppression of the anti-HEL antibody response by LH8–105 TsF is restricted not only by I-J genes but also by Igh-1 genes (ADORINI et al. 1983). Similarly, suppression of the DTH response and induction of second-order Ts cells is also restricted by genes mapping in both the I-J and Igh-1 regions, as determined by cell transfer into I-J and Igh-1 congenic mice.

In conclusion, LH8–105 TsF appears to share most properties with suppressor-inducer molecules. LH8–105 TsF contains I-J-encoded and antigen-binding determinants, suppresses only when injected in the afferent phase of the response, and is able to induce, if injected in antigen-primed mice, second-order Ts cells. Moreover, it displays an exquisitely fine antigenic specificity in immunosuppression which is restricted by I-J and Igh-1 genes. However, in contrast to other suppressor-inducer cell types, LH8–105 cells are Lyt-2[+].

LH8–105 cells, which constitutively produce LH8–105 TsF, do not express the IL-2 receptor and fail to produce IL-2 either constitutively or after stimulation with antigen and antigen-presenting cells, mitogens, or phorbol esters (Adorini, unpublished). In additon, LH8–105 cells do not produce gamma interferon or macrophage-activating factor. Finally, LH8–105 cells are not cytotoxic as revealed by lack of reactivity in short- or long-term assays against different targets even after antigen or lectin approximation.

3 Expression of T-Cell Receptor by LH8–105 T Cells

Relatively few membrane proteins on T cells consist of disulfide-bonded subunits and they can be revealed using a two-dimensional (2-D) polyacrylamide gel electrophoresis (PAGE) in which the proteins migrate according to their molecular mass in the first, nonreduced, dimension and according to the molecular weight of the single subunits in the second, reduced, dimension (PHILLIPS and AGIN 1977). Two-D PAGE analysis of radiolabeled LH8–105 cells reveals five distinct proteins composed of disulfide-linked subunits (BALLINARI et al. 1985); two of them have been analyzed using immunoprecipitation.

The most represented surface molecule with disulfide-bonded structures is the viral product gp70, as determined by immunoprecipitation with anti-gp70 serum.

A disulfide-linked molecule of 84K, resolved in two chains of 42K under reducing conditions, has been positively identified by 2-D PAGE after immunoprecipitation with a rabbit antiserum detecting a family of antigenically and structurally related, T cell-specific, disulfide-linked dimers (McINTYRE and ALLISON 1983). (This antiserum, 8177, was kindly given by Dr. J. P. Allison, University of Texas.) The structure of the molecules immunoprecipitated by the 8177 xenoantiserum from LH8–105 cells closely resembles the 42K dimer isolated from mouse cytotoxic and helper T-cell clones by monoclonal antibodies recognizing clonotypic structures (KAPPLER et al. 1983).

To further assess this issue, rabbit antibodies have been raised against a synthetic peptide desumed from the amino acid sequence predicted by the nucleotidic sequence of a cDNA clone encoding the β chain of a helper T-cell hybridoma. The amino acid sequence predicted for the constant region of a mouse helper T-cell receptor β chain from the 86T1 cDNA clone nucleotide sequence (HEDRICK et al. 1984) has been inspected to identify a sequence with high hydrophilicity and low homology with immunoglobulin constant regions. Local hydrophilicity along the polypeptide chain has been estimated according to KYTE and DOOLITTLE (1982) to identify hydrophilic regions, which are predominantly surface oriented and therefore potentially immunogenic. An hydrophilic sequence exhibiting the lowest degree of homology with the corresponding sequences of other members of the immunoglobulin superfamily has been selected in order to maximize the probability of inducing T-cell receptor-specific antibodies. These two characteristics are present in the peptide corresponding to residues 215–225 of the mouse T-cell receptor β chain. Prediction of the secondary protein structure according to Chou and Fasman indicates that this region in the native molecule most likely corresponds to a β-pleated sheet conformation containing a β turn in position 218. As turns in the protein backbone are likely to correspond to regions of high segmental mobility and this correlates with the location of antigenic determinants, synthetic peptides corresponding to turn-containing regions are suitable candidates for immunogenic epitopes.

The peptide corresponding to amino acid residues 215–225 has been synthesized according to MERRIFIELD (1969), purified using HPLC, and covalently linked to bovine serum albumin (BSA). The rabbit antipeptide antibodies react with

58   L. Adorini et al.

Table 3. Binding of LH8–105 TsF to rabbit anti-Cβ(215–225) immunosorbent

Experiment	Antigen	LH8–105 TsF injection	Developed PFC/10^6 PTLN cells	Suppression (%)
1	HEL-CFA	None	4782 (1.32)	
	HEL-CFA	Unseparated	1305 (1.23)	73
	HEL-CFA	Effluent RαCβ(215–225) Ig	4150 (1.76)	13
	HEL-CFA	Eluate RαCβ(215–225) Ig	1809 (1.73)	62
	HEL-CFA	Effluent NR Ig	2099 (1.30)	56
	HEL-CFA	Eluate NR Ig	4773 (1.09)	0
2	HEL-CFA	None	2447 (1.38)	
	HEL-CFA	Eluate RαCβ(215–225) Ig	372 (1.46)	85
	TNP-KLH-CFA	None	1281 (1.20)	
	TNP-KLH-CFA	Eluate RαCβ(215–225) Ig	1213 (1.32)	5

BDF1 mice (5 mice/group) were injected i.p. with 100 μg HEL or TNP-KLH in CFA and anti-HEL or anti-TNP PFC responses were measured in the PTLN cells. Culture supernatant from LH8–105 cell clone, either unseparated, fractionated on RαCβ(215–225) Ig or normal rabbit (NR) Ig immunosorbents was injected i.v. (0.5 ml/mouse) for 3 consecutive days and the first injection was given on the same day of antigen priming. PFC values from individual mice are expressed as geometric mean and the numbers in parentheses represent a factor by which the mean should be multiplied or divided to give one standard error

surface determinants present on T, but not B cells, as demonstrated by radioimmunoassay on solid-phase linked, glutaraldehyde-fixed cells. LH8–105 suppressor T cells are recognized by this antibody, as well as other RadLV-transformed T-cell clones with suppressive activity. This reactivity is detectable only on fixed cells and unfixed T cells do not bind antibodies directed against this peptide even when incubation is carried out in the presence of 10^{-2} M NaN$_3$ at 4° C, suggesting that glutaraldehyde fixation favors on the plasma membrane the stabilization of a conformation recognized by antipeptide antibodies or, alternatively, renders available for binding a normally nonexposed site.

As previously mentioned, rabbit 8177 antibodies immunoprecipitate from surface-labeled LH8–105 cell proteins resolved using 2-D PAGE under nonreducing/reducing conditions in a molecule of about 84K composed of two disulfide-linked 40K–44K subunits (BALLINARI et al. 1985).

Therefore, the structure of the antigen receptor expressed by LH8–105 suppressor T cells is similar to that described for helper and cytotoxic T cells. Moreover, at least part of the T-cell receptor β-chain constant region appears to be shared between helper and LH8–105 suppressor T cells.

These results are in agreement with the rearrangement in LH8–105 cells of Cα and Cβ genes and the expression of α- and β-chain mRNA species encoding functional transcripts of α and β genes (DE SANTIS et al. 1985).

Expression of T-Cell Receptor 59

The relationship between membrane T-cell receptor and soluble molecules with suppressive activity produced by LH8–105 cells has alos been examined. Culture supernatant from LH8–105 cells eluted from an anti-Cβ(215–225) antibodies immunosorbent specifically suppresses the anti-HEL antibody response (Table 3), indicating recognition by this antibody of both LH8–105 T-cell receptor and T-cell products with suppressive activity. Since suppressive activity is mediated by LH8–105-derived soluble molecules with an apparent M_r of 82K–90K (Ricciardi-Castagnoli et al. 1985) these could represent the released form of the membrane receptor. Studies are currently in progress to verify this hypothesis.

4 Summary

The cloned T-cell lymphoma line LH8–105, obtained by virus-induced transformation of HEL-specific suppressor T lymphocytes, constitutively releases in the culture supernatant products able to specifically suppress the T cell-dependent proliferation, the antibody response, and the delayed-type hypersensitivity to HEL. This suppressive activity is restricted by genes apparently mapping to both the Igh-1 and I-J loci and is specific for a defined epitope in the N-terminal region of the HEL molecule. LH8–105 cells are Thy-1.2^+, Lyt-2^+, I-J$^+$; they produce neither interleukin 2 nor gamma interferon and are not cytotoxic. They express on the cell surface dimers of 84K composed of two 42K subunits immunoprecipitated by rabbit antibodies directed against the T cell receptor constant region s. Antibodies recognizing a synthetic peptide desumed from the amino acid sequence predicted by a cDNA clone sequence encoding the β chain of a helper T-cell hybridoma react with LH8–105 cells. Therefore, the overall structure of the antigen receptor expressed by LH8–105 cells is similar to that described for helper and cytotoxic T cells and at least part of the β-chain constant region is shared between helper and suppressor T cells. LH8–105 cells produce the 1.8 kb α-chain mRNA and the 1.3 kb β-chain mRNA expected for a functional T-cell receptor and they delete both alleles of the $C\beta_1$ gene and rearrange both alleles of the $C\beta_2$ gene, as detected by a $C\beta$ probe from a helper T-cell hybridoma.

Moreover, soluble molecules with HEL-specific suppressive activity released by LH8–105 cells are bound by rabbit antibodies directed against a β-chain synthetic peptide, indicating a relationship between the T-cell receptor and soluble T-cell products with suppressive activity.

Collectively taken these findings indicate that at least some mouse suppressor T cells use the same set of genes as helper and cytotoxic T cells for their antigen receptor and also that soluble products with suppressive activity may represent the released form of the antigen receptor.

References

Acuto O, Hussey RE, Fitzgerald KA, Protentis JP, Meuer SC, Schlossman SF, Reinherz EL (1983) The human T cell receptor: appearance in ontogeny and biochemical relationship of α and β subunits on IL-2 dependent clones and T cell tumors. Cell 34:717–726

60 L. Adorini et al.

Adorini L, Harvey MA, Miller A, Sercarz EE (1979) The specificity of regulatory T cells. II. Suppressor and helper T cells are induced by different regions of hen egg-white lysozyme in a genetically non responder mouse strain. J Exp Med 150:293–306

Adorini L, Harvey MA, Rozycka-Jackson D, Miller A, Sercarz EE (1980) Differential major histocompatibility complex-related activation of idiotypic suppressor T cells. Suppressor T cells cross-reactive to two distantly related lysozymes are not induced by one of them. J Exp Med 152:521–531

Adorini L, Doria G, Ricciardi-Castagnoli P (1982) Fine antigenic specificity and genetic restriction of lysozyme-specific suppressor T cell factor produced by radiation leukemia virus-transformed suppressor T cells. Eur J Immunol 12:719–724

Adorini L, Pini C, De Santis R, Robbiati F, Doria G, Ricciardi-Castagnoli P (1983) Monoclonal suppressor T cell factor displaying V restriction and fine antigenic specificity in immunosuppression. Nature 303:704–706

Adorini L, Colizzi V, Doria G, Ricciardi-Castagnoli P (1984) Immunoregulation of lysozyme-specific suppression. II. Hen egg-white lysozyme-specific monoclonal suppressor T cell factor suppresses the afferent phase of delayed-type hypersensitivity and induces second-order suppressor T cells. Eur J Immunol 14:826–830

Allison JP, McIntyre BW, Bloch D (1982) Tumor-specific antigen of murine T-lymphoma defined with monoclonal antibody. J Immunol 129:2293–2300

Ballinari D, Castelli C, Traversari C, Pierotti MA, Parmiani G, Palmieri G, Ricciardi-Castagnoli P, Adorini L (1985) Disulfide-linked surface molecules of monoclonal antigen-specific suppressor T cells: evidence for T cell receptor structures. Eur J Immunol 15:855–860

Chien Y, Becker DM, Lindsten T, Okamura M, Cohen DI, Davis MM (1984) A third type of murine T cell receptor gene. Nature 312:31–35

De Santis R, Givol D, Hsu P-L, Adorini L, Doria G, Appella E (1985) Rearrangement and expression of the α and β genes of the T cell receptor in functional mouse T suppressor clones. Proc Natl Acad Sci USA 82:8638–8642

Hedrick SM, Cohen DI, Nielsen EA, Davis MM (1984) Isolation of cDNA clones encoding T cell-specific membrane associated proteins. Nature 308:149–153

Hedrick SM, Germain RN, Bevan MJ, Dorf M, Engel I, Fink P, Gascoigne N, Heber-Katz E, Kapp J, Kaufmann Y, Kaye J, Melchers F, Pierce C, Schwartz RH, Sorensen C, Taniguchi M, Davis MM (1985) Rearrangement and transcription of a T cell receptor beta gene in different T cell subsets. Proc Natl Acad Sci USA 82:531–535

Hill SW, Sercarz EE (1975) Fine specificity of the H-2 linked immune response gene for the gallinaceous lysozymes. Eur J Immunol 5:317–324

Kappler J, Kubo R, Haskins K, White J, Marrack P (1983) The mouse T cell receptor: comparison of MHC-restricted receptors on two T cell hybridomas. Cell 34:727–737

Klyczek KK, Cantor H, Hayes CE (1984) T cell surface I-J glycoprotein: concerted action of chromosome 4 and 17 genes forms an epitope dependent on D-mannosyl residues. J Exp Med 159:1604–1617

Kronenberg M, Steinmetz M, Kobori J, Kraig E, Kapp JA, Pierce CW, Sorensen CM, Suzuki G, Tada T, Hood L (1983) RNA transcripts for I-J polypeptides are apparently non encoded between the I-A and I-E subregions of the murine major histocompatibility complex. Proc Natl Acad Sci USA 80:5704–5708

Kyte J, Doolittle RF (1982) A simple method for displaying the hydropathic character of a protein. J Mol Biol 157:105–132

McIntyre BW, Allison JP (1983) The mouse T cell receptor: structural heterogeneity defined by xeno-antisera. Cell 34:739–746

Merrifield RB (1969) Solid-phase peptide synthesis. Adv Enzymol 32:221

Meuer SC, Fitzgerald KA, Hussey RE, Hodgdon JC, Schlossman SF, Reinherz EL (1983) Clonotypic structures involved in antigen-specific human T cell function. Relationship to the T3 molecular complex. J Exp Med 157:705–719

Phillips DR, Agin PP (1977) Platelet plasma membrane glycoproteins. Evidence for the presence of nonequivalent disulfide bonds using nonreduced-reduced two-dimensional gel electrophoresis. J Biol Chem 252:2121–2126

Ricciardi-Castagnoli P, Doria G, Adorini L (1981) Production of antigen-specific suppressive T cell factor by radiation leukemia virus-transformed suppressor T cells. Proc Natl Acad Sci USA 78:3804–3808

Ricciardi-Castagnoli P, Robbiati F, Barbanti E, Colizzi V, Pini C, De Santis R, Doria G, Adorini L (1985) Immunosuppression by cell-free translation products from monoclonal antigen-specific suppressor T cell mRNAs. Eur J Immunol 15:351–355

Royer HD, Bensussan A, Acuto O, Reinherz EL (1984) Functional isotypes are not encoded by the constant region genes of the subunit of the T cell receptor for antigen/major hystocompatibility complex. J Exp Med 160:947–952

Sette A, Colizzi V, Appella E, Doria G, Adorini L (1986) Analysis of lysozyme-specific immune responses by synthetic peptides. I. Characterization of antibody and T cell-mediated responses to the N-terminal peptide of hen egg-white lysozyme. Eur J Immunol 16:1–6

Sim GK, Yagüe J, Nelson J, Marrack P, Palmer E, Augustin A, Kappler J (1984) Primary structure of human T cell receptor α chain. Nature 312:771–775

Yanagi Y, Yoshikai Y, Leggett K, Clark SP, Aleksander I, Mak TW (1984) A human T cell-specific cDNA clone encodes a protein having extensive homology to immunoglobulin chains. Nature 308:145–149

Yoshikai Y, Yanagi Y, Sociu-Foca N, Mak TW (1984) Presence of T cell receptor mRNA in functionally distinct T cells and elevation during intrathymic differentiation. Nature 310:506–508

Somatic Variation of Antigen-Recognition Specificity in H-2^b-TNP-Specific Cytotoxic T-Cell Clones

H. U. WELTZIEN and K. EICHMANN

1 Maintenance of Specificity of CTL Clones Is Due to Selection Rather than to Stability   63
2 Improving Specificity Due to Selection by Antigen   65
3 Discussion   66
References   67

The molecular mechanisms involved in MHC-restricted antigen recognition by T cells are incompletely understood. For example, the strikingly precise ability of certain T-cell clones to distinguish very similar antigens (HURWITZ et al. 1984) is in apparent contrast to the seemingly degenerate specificity of the virgin T-cell repertoire (EICHMANN et al. 1983; FEY et al. 1984). We have therefore considered the possibility that antigen-induced proliferation leads to further somatic diversification of the virgin T-cell pool with subsequent selection of variants with increasingly better antigen recognition properties. We present here results from two experimental systems: (a) We determined the kinetics of the appearance of somatic variants in a long-term CTL clone, cultured with and without its antigen, during short-term exponential growth and (b) we analyzed the changes in the pattern of cross-reactivity in a collection of 42 H-2^b-restricted TNP-specific CTL clones over a period of several months. The data presented here suggest that (a) the antigen recognition structures of in vitro established cloned CTL lines may undergo continuous rapid somatic variation and (b) the selective pressure of antigen stimulation leads to maintenance and/or improvement of the recognition specificity of the CTL clones for the selecting antigen.

1 Maintenance of Specificity of CTL Clones Is Due to Selection Rather than to Stability

For these experiments, we used clone BT7.4.1, derived from a primary in vitro culture of C57B1/6 spleen cells stimulated with trinitrobenzene sulfonic acid (TNBS) modified irradiated syngeneic spleen cells according to the method of Shearer (SHEARER 1974). After repeated restimulation with B6-TNP filler cells in the presence of IL-2 (rat Con A spleen supernatant) clone BT7.4.1 was obtained by three successive statistical clonings, the final one at 0.5 cells/culture.

Max-Planck-Institut für Immunbiologie, Stübeweg 51, D-7800 Freiburg

Current Topics in Microbiology and Immunology, Vol. 126
© Springer-Verlag Berlin · Heidelberg 1986

64   H. U. Weltzien and K. Eichmann

Table 1. Wild-type and variant cells during clonal expansion of clone BT7.4.1

	Fillers +/−TNP	Day 1 2 divisions	Day 2 5 divisions	Day 4 10 divisions
Wild-type cells				
TNP-specific CTL	+	53%	31%	9%
	−		0.8%	0.07%
Variant cells				
Lethal variants	+	33%	58%	81%
	−	57%	96%	99%
Unspecific CTL	+		9%	1.6%
(PHA dependent)	−		4%	0.6%

Clone BT7.4.1 was seeded at a density of 2×10^4 cells/culture in costar wells containing 4×10^6 irradiated C57B1/6 spleen filler cells with or without TNBS modification (3 mM TNBS) in 2 ml RPMI medium, supplemented with fetal calf serum and rat spleen Con A supernatant. Daily, viable cells were counted and limiting dilution cultures initiated on 3×10^5 B6-TNP fillers in round bottom microtiter plates. Limiting dilutions were assayed 6 days later (a) for growth (plating efficiency), (b) for TNP-specific kill, and (c) for lectin-dependent kill. Lethal variants are calculated from the difference of total viable cells in the primary culture minus total growing cells in limiting dilution cultures (from growth frequencies). All numbers are calculated from frequencies in comparison to total cell numbers in the primary cultures

BT7.4.1 is stimulated weekly with syngeneic TNP-spleen cells in the presence of rat Con A supernatant and is strictly TNP-specific, restricted for K^b and without any detectable cross-reactivity on a variety of control targets. This strict specificity has been kept now by BT7.4.1 over a continuous culture period of over 18 months. Antigen-independent sublines could be readily established by withdrawal of antigen. These lines, however, rapidly lost their specificity for $H-2^b$-TNP, maintaining unspecific, i.e., lectin-facilitated cytotoxicity or no activity whatsoever.

In order to study the kinetics of the appearance of these variants, BT7.4.1 cells were cultured on irradiated B6 spleen fillers, modified or not modified with TNBS. Viable cells were counted daily and samples of the parallel cultures were assayed daily by limiting dilution analyses using B6-TNP filler cells. Frequencies were determined for (a) growing cells (plating efficiency), (b) TNP-specific CTL, and (c) lectin-dependent CTL. Results of these assays on days 1, 2, and 4 are given in Table 1.

The conditions were chosen such that growth of BT7.4.1 was exponential between days 1 and 4, with a doubling time of approximately 10 h, i.e., for 10 generations. Viable cell numbers were only slightly lower (30%–50%) on unmodified than on TNP-modified fillers (data not shown). However, upon transfer to limiting dilution cultures, the plating efficiencies of the two populations differed widely (approximately 40-fold lower in absence of antigen) and in both cases steadily declined over the first 4 days of culture. Cells which did not survive the transfer from the original to the limiting dilution culture are termed "lethal variants" in Table 1. Note that the proportions of these lethal variants in the absence of antigen within a period of only 10 cell divisions increased from 57%

to approx. 99% of the cells, whereas the number of TNP-specific CTL dropped to less than 0.1% over the same period. Also in antigen-containing cultures, lethal variants are generated, but at a lower rate (80% after 10 divisions) and a correspondingly lower reduction of TNP-specific CTL is observed. The observation that lethal variants are more frequent in the absence of antigen than in its presence suggests that most cells depend on the recognition of antigen for survival. Both cultures also reveal a significant generation of unspecific, i.e., lectin-dependent CTLs which appear to decrease in number, indicating that they also have a reduced ability to survive. We conclude from these results that somatic variants, both the lethal ones and those which lost their specific antigen recognition, appear at a high rate in clone BT7.4.1 Thus, the results suggest that maintenance of TNP-H-2^b specificity in clone BT7.4.1 is to a large extent due to selection rather than to stability.

2 Improving Specificity Due to Selection by Antigen

A panel of 42 CTL clones with specificity for H-2^b-TNP was isolated by statistical cloning at 0.5 cells/culture from 32 independent cell lines derived from eight individual mice. About 4 weeks after cloning (3 months after explantation), we started to test the specificity of the collection of these clones by monthly ^{51}chromium-release assays on a panel of targets including H-2^b, H-2^d, and H-2^k Con A blasts or tumor lines with and without TNP modification. All of the clones proved to lyse H-2^b-TNP targets, while none of the TNP-free cell types was killed. The clones varied, however, in the type of cross-reactivity with other H-2 haplotypes in the presence of TNP, the most frequent cross-reactivity being for H-2^k-TNP.

We therefore centered our attention on the comparison of H-2^b-TNP vs H-2^k-TNP specific lysis and the changes of this relation over several months of in vitro culture on H-2^b-TNP fillers. The results of this study are summarized in Table 2. It is evident that the number of H-2^k-TNP cross-reactive clones dropped constantly from 37 (1 month after cloning) to 10 (5 months after cloning) and that the number of H-2^b specific noncross-reactive clones increased correspondingly. This improvement of specificity was also reflected in the increase of the mean ratio of H-2^b-TNP over H-2^k-TNP cytotoxicity.

All the clones used in this study were obtained by a single statistical cloning at 0.5 cells/culture. According to Poisson statistics, this infers that 77% or 32 of the 42 clones must have been derived from one single cell while 10 may be derived from two or more cells. This clearly excludes the possibility that the observed changes are a reflection of a nonclonal nature of our in vitro CTL cultures. The pronounced changes in recognition specificity of at least 27 of the 42 clones, therefore, must be due to the acquisition of altered recognition specificities within the clones.

We interpret these results to suggest that selection by antigen not only leads to the maintenance of antigen recognition but, in addition, to its improvement. Although we have no direct evidence that the affinity of the 42 clones for the selecting antigen increased during the period of observation, we think that the loss of cross-reactivity towards other antigens points in this direction.

66 H.U. Weltzien and K. Eichmann

Table 2. Changes in cross-reactivity for $H-2^k$-TNP in $H-2^b$-TNP specific CTL clones from C57B1/6 mice

Timer after cloning[a] (month)	Clones killing $H-2^k$-TNP/Total	%	Ratio (mean $\pm$ SD) $H-2^b$-TNP/$H-2^k$-TNP
1	37/41	90	3.0 ± 2.6
2.5	24/42	57	ND
3	24/42	57	12.4 ± 19.2
4	17/42	40	13.5 ± 15.2
5	10/42	24	21.8 ± 18.2

[a] Cloned at 0.5 cells/well
ND = not determined

A total number of 42 independent, $H-2^b$-TNP-specific CTL clones was assayed in about monthly intervals for specific ^{51}chromium release (split cultures) on RBL5-TNP ($H-2^b$) and RDM4-TNP ($H-2^k$) target cells. Values $> 10\%$ specific lysis were considered positive. The last column represents the average ratio of the percent lysis data on $H-2^b$-TNP over $H-2^k$-TNP targets

3 Discussion

The presented data provide functional evidence that cytotoxic T lymphocytes in long-term in vitro cultures are not necessarily stable, but may be subject to continuous changes in the structures determining their antigen specificity. The molecular basis for these changes is so far unknown. Point mutations in the complementarity determining regions of receptor V_β or V_α genes (as found for V_β by A. Augustin) or sequential rearrangements of different J, D, and V genes (as described by M. Steinmetz, this volume) may be considered. Molecular analyses of the receptor genes isolated from wild type and variant cells may eventually answer these questions. Our findings suggest that such variants exist and can probably be isolated. They also imply, however, that the genetic analysis of such variants may encounter serious problems, since the development of variants appears to be a continuous process and no procedures are presently known to stabilize wild type and variants at any given stage.

The continuous change in the effector specificity of CTL clones in vitro readily explains the finding of many authors (NABHOLZ and MACDONALD 1983) that CTL lines and clones require continuous restimulation with antigen for the maintenance of specificity. We suggest that the presented antigen imposes a strong selective pressure in favor of antigen-recognizing wild-type cells or for variant cells that have an improved antigen recognition. The dependence on antigen recognition for survival may be connected with the dependence on antigen recognition of the expression of receptors for growth factors as described for a number of T-cell clones (ANDREW et al. 1985; LOWENTHAL et al. 1985).

Our observations bear on the results of many studies on the T-cell specificity repertoire by limiting dilution methods. If, as indicated in Table 1, a few cell divisions would indeed provide enough variation to generate new recognition specificities, the results of repertoire analyses would be largely dependent on the selection pressures provided by the culture conditions. Moreover, frequencies may be overestimated due to intraclonal diversification. A method to "freeze" T-cell populations with respect to their antigen-binding structures, as apparently available for B cells in the form of hybridomas, is thus badly needed. Whether or not T-cell hybridomas may serve a similar purpose is not clear, although it seems that in at least some cases stable specificities are observed (KAPPLER et al. 1983).

It remains to be investigated whether somatic variation represents a major mechanism for the generation of the virgin T-cell repertoire in vivo, whether its contribution is restricted to T cells that divide following exposure to antigen, or whether it occurs at all in vivo. In any case, we observe here a further similarity between the receptor systems of T and B cells, and it will be of interest to see whether similar rules apply to T-cell receptor variation as those described for B cells (MCKEAN et al. 1984; SABLITZKY et al. 1985).

References

Andrew ME, Churilla AM, Malek TS, Braciale VL, Braciale TJ (1985) Activation of virus specific CTL clones: antigen-dependent regulation of interleukin 2 receptor expression. J Immunol 134:920–925

Eichmann K, Fey K, Kuppers R, Melchers I, Simon MM, Weltzien HU (1983) Network regulation among T cells; conclusions from limiting dilution experiments. Semin Immunpathol 6:7–32

Fey K, Simon MM, Melchers I, Eichmann K (1984) Quantitative estimates of diversity, degeneracy and connectivity in an idiotypic network among T cells. In: Green MI, Nisonoff A (eds) The biology of idiotypes. Plenum, New York, pp 261–277

Hurwitz JL, Heber-Katz E, Hackett CJ, Gerhard W (1984) Characterization of the murine T_H response to influenza virus hemagglutinin: evidence for 3 major specificities. J Immunol 166:3371–3377

Kappler J, Kubo R, Haskins K, White J, Marrack P (1983) The mouse T cell receptor: comparison of MHC-restricted receptors on two T cell hybridomas. Cell 34:727–737

Lowenthal JW, Tounge C, MacDonald R, Smith KA, Nabholz M (1985) Antigenic stimulation regulates the expression of IL-2 receptors in a cytolytic T lymphocyte clone. J Immunol 134:931–939

McKean D, Huppi K, Bell M, Staudt L, Gerhard W, Weigert M (1984) Generation of antibody diversity in the immune response of BALB/c mice to influenza virus hemagglutinin. Proc Natl Acad Sci USA 81:3180–3184

Nabholz M, MacDonald HR (1983) Cytolytic T lymphocytes. Ann Rev Immunol 1:273–306

Sablitzky F, Wildner G, Rajewsky K (1985) Somatic mutation and clonal expansion of B cells in an antigen-driven immune response. EMBO J 4:345–350

Shearer GM (1974) Cell mediated cytotoxicity to trinitrophenyl-modified syngeneic lymphocytes. Eur J Immunol 4:527–533

The Change of Specificity, Karyotype, and Antigen-Receptor Gene Expression is Correlated in Cytotoxic T-Cell Lines

J.T. EPPLEN, S. ALI, A. RINALDY, and M.M. SIMON

1 Development of Long-Term T-Cell Clones 69
2 Karyotypic Changes in Cultured T-Cell Clones 71
3 Variable Expression of T-Cell Receptor Genes in Cultured T-Cell Clones 72
References 73

It has been postulated, that individual nontransformed vertebrate cells are limited to a finite number of mitotic divisions (HAYFLICK 1965). Beyond that physiological potential the cells either degenerate or transform malignantly. Long-term cultured T-cell clones are intriguing models to test the above postulate. Because of that model character, the karyotypic and molecular genetic analysis of cytotoxic lymphocyte clones (CTLL) and their variants should hint at the genetic and molecular events involved in changes of specificity and function, cellular instability and ultimately malignant transformation.

1 Development of Long-Term T-Cell Clones

The CTLL and their in vitro or in vivo variants described herein were derived from female C57Bl/6 (B6) mice previously primed to male B6 H-Y antigen and correspondingly expressed Thy-1$^+$, Lyt-1$^-$, Lyt-2$^+$, L3T4$^-$, IL-2R$^+$ surface marker phenotypes irrespective of their change in specificity or function (Table 1). H-Y specific CTLL were cloned from in vitro long-term tissue culture lines by standard procedures on irradiated male B6 stimulator cells and supernatant from Con A sensitized rat spleen cells (Con ASN; SIMON et al. 1984a). CTLL maintained under these conditions (CTLL.1) lysed male B6 and other target cells expressing H-Y in the context of H-2D^b determinants and mediated lectin facilitated lympholysis (P815/PHA), but were not cytotoxic when tested on P815 tumor cells or a panel of ten unrelated target cells (tumor lines, Con A blasts) including those from B10.D2 or DBA mice (SIMON et al. 1984a, b and unpublished results). This target cell specificity excluded the presence of H-2D^d cross-reactive anti-H-Y specific clones within the CTLL tested (BOEHMER et al. 1979; KANAGAWA et al. 1982).

Max-Planck-Institut für Immunbiologie, Stübeweg 51, D-7800 Freiburg

Table 1. Development of T-cell lines

		Ag/SN; cloning					
				SN; cloning			
						Medium	
	a H-Y T-cell line	→ CTLL.1	→ CTLL.2	→ CTLL.3	→ CTLL.4	→ ... →	CTLL.5
Surface phenotype		Thy-1$^+$,	Lyt-1$^-$2$^+$,	L3T4$^-$,	JL-2R$^+$		
CML on target	Specific killer		Aged killer			Tumor variant	
B6♂	+	+	±	−	−	−
P815	−	−	±	+	−	−
P815 (PHA)	+	+	+	+	−	−

After prolonged culture periods (4–7 months) all CTLL gradually lost their specific cytotoxic activity and simultaneously gained the ability to lyse P815 tumor cells while retaining cytolytic potential as defined by lectin facilitated lympholysis (Simon et al. 1984a, b; Bevan and Cohn 1976). This change in specificity which seemingly happened to the majority of cells in the cloned population (Simon et al. 1984b) was accompanied by the loss of proliferative capacity of CTLL in response to H-Y antigen and their ability to now grow in Con ASN alone (CTLL.2, CTLL.3, Table 1). CTLL maintained as such rapidly lost all cytotoxic activity for male B6 cells and only killed P815 tumor targets with a frequency close to 1/1 (Simon et al. 1984b). CTLL.3 also did not lyse a panel of other tumor (YAC, RBL5, EL4) and nontumor targets (Con A blasts) (Simon et al. 1984b).

Finally, after continuous culture of CTLL.3 in Con ASN, a variant developed (CTLL.4) which had lost both its cytotoxic activity on P815 tumor targets and its cytotoxic potential as tested by lectin mediated lympholysis (Table 1). This variant cell line could be adjusted to grow in culture medium in the absence of Con ASN. Although in limiting dilution experiments frequencies of 1/3–1/15 were found for T cells growing independently of Con ASN, we have so far been unable to derive T-lymphocyte clones from this line. When transplanted centrally (i.p.) into female B6 mice, CTLL.4 grew progressively in ascites or as a solid tumor in the peritoneum leading to death of the mice. In a certain proportion of recipients, however, this phase was followed by tumor regression resulting in survival of animals. CTLL.4 seemed able to spread to internal lymphoid (spleen, mesenteric, and perithymic lymph nodes) or nonlymphoid organs (uterus, ovary). In contrast to female B6 mice, the outgrowth of CTLL.4 after i.p. inoculation was much less pronounced in male B6 recipients, though in these animals CTLL.4 also showed metastatic capacity by invading internal organs (spleen, lymph node, liver). The derivation of local tumors and individual metastases (CTLL.5) from the in vitro line CTLL.4 was ascertained by phenotype analysis using a Thy-1 congenic mouse strain as recipient as well as by genetic studies (see below).

The data presented so far suggest that it is possible to derive, consistently by in vitro selection pressure, from specific CTLL variants expressing altered specificities and functional activity, and to induce from the same CTLL malignant variants with highly metastatic capacity.

2 Karyotypic Changes in Cultured T-Cell Clones

Since H-Y specific CTLL continuously generate a certain amount of variation affecting general cellular properties, specificity, and functional phenotype, we analyzed the chromosomes of these clones and their variants in different stages as exemplified in Table 2. Thus, the phenotype could be correlated with the karyotype as revealed by conventional and G-banding techniques (RYBAK et al. 1982). CTLL.1 T-cell clones with specificity for H-Y antigen (including one helper T-cell clone) exhibited structurally normal mouse karyotypes with the modal diploid chromosome number of 40 (NESBITT and FRANCKE 1973). As soon as specificity changes were observed (CTLL.2), the chromosome number per metaphase varied dramatically. The distribution of numbers showed two peaks with maxima at 38 and 40. A considerable percentage of hypo- and hypertetraploid metaphases were observed. While in CTLL.2 the morphology of individual chromosomes was intact, further expansion of the clones in the absence of antigen (CTLL.3) was accompanied by multiple rearrangements resulting in altered chromosome structure. Chromosomal abnormalities in long-term cultured T-cell lines have been reported before (e.g., NABHOLZ et al. 1980) and probably are influenced partly by culture components (SANFORD et al. 1979). With time, a growing number of individual chromosomes could not be positively identified in CTLL.3. Several metacentric markers appeared and gaps and breaks were obvious. The longer CTLL.3 cells grew in the presence of Con ASN alone, the more chromosome mutations profoundly restructured the genetic material. This process of continuing genomic reorganization evidently halted in supernatant independent T-cell lines (CTLL.4): The altered banding pattern of individual chromosomes "froze" and comparison of different metaphases showed "stabili-

Table 2. Karyotypes of T-cell lines

Cell type	Number of chromosomes per metaphase	Degree of aneuploidy	Number of metacentric chromosomes	Cromosomal instability
CTLL.1 (2.A4.2.4)	40	$\emptyset$	–	$\emptyset$
CTLL.2 (2.A4.1a)	33–85	++	–	$\emptyset$
CTLL.3 (1.3E6SN)	35–42	++	2–4	++
CTLL.3 (96)	37–43	+++	3–5	+++
CTLL.3 (1.3E6SN)	38–41	+++	5–8	++++
CTLL.4 (1.3E6K1)	39–44	++	3–4	++

72   J.T. Epplen et al.

zation" of the restructured genome. Also the individual metacentric markers were very consistent. Hence the karyotypic evolution can be monitored closely in CTLL and their variants. Compared with other types of permanent cell lines (fibroblasts), the chromosome abnormalities develop very rapidly and might be facilitated by rat Con ASN.

3   Variable Expression of T-Cell Receptor Genes in Cultured T-Cell Clones

Functional T-cell receptor molecules are composed of at least two different subunits (α and β) (HANNUM et al. 1984). The role of a similarly organized and expressed γ chain (SAITO et al. 1984) is not completely clear. Like immunoglobulin genes, expressed T-cell receptor genes are formed by the rearrangement of separately encoded variable and constant region sequences. In the case of the β chain of the T-cell receptor, an optional diversity (D_β) and one of several joining (J_β) elements are used to produce the mRNA which can be translated into polypeptide. The changes in function and specificity of H-Y specific T-cell clones prompted us to investigate the mRNA expression of the T-cell receptor subunits. In Northern-blot hybridization experiments, four lines of evidence could be revealed:

1. In all specific CTLL and their variants, the α, β, and γ chains are expressed in mRNA.

2. With increasing time of CTLL in culture, the expression of α-chain mRNA decreased (CTLL.1 > CTLL.2 > CTLL.3 > CTLL.4 > CTLL.5).

3. In contrast, with increasing time of CTLL in culture, expression of β-chain mRNA increased, reaching significantly higher levels than normal in CTLL.2 (CTLL.1 $\ll$ CTLL.2 < CTLL.3 < CTLL.4, CTLL.5).

4. The γ chain was evenly expressed in all stages except for higher levels in the antigen-independent form CTLL.4.

Hence, specificity and functional alterations in cultured T cells are not only correlated with karyotypic changes, but also with differential alterations in the activity of genes coding for the T-cell receptor.

The loss of a preexisting antigenic specificity and concomitant gain of a new target cell specificity raised the question of whether identical genes coding for the variable region of the T-cell receptor are expressed in the specific CTLL and its variants. From a cDNA clone of CTLL.3, the β-subunit sequence was determined (RINALDY et al. 1985). No somatic mutations were observed comparing cDNA and germline configuration in the V_β region (Epplen et al., in press). In addition several nucleotides at the D_β-J_β junction cannot be accounted for by published germline sequences (SIU et al. 1984). By use of specific oligonucleotide hybridization probes, it was shown that three independently derived CTLL.3 expressed the same variable and D_β-J_β region genes ($V_{\beta AK}$, $D_{\beta AK}$ $J_{\beta AK}$). In contrast the original CTLL.1 was $V_{\beta AK}$ and $D_{\beta AK}$ $J_{\beta AK}$ negative. Southern-blot hybridization data proved the new rearrangement of the $V_{\beta AK}$ germline gene in CTLL.2 and CTLL.3. In preliminary experiments CTLL.4 yielded yet another hybridiza-

Correlation of Changes in Cytotoxic T-Cell Lines 73

tion pattern, which suggests even a third $V_{\beta AK}$ configuration in transformed cells.

Clearly, further experimental evidence is necessary to substantiate the hypothesis that the culture protocol used selects for AK specificity via expression of $V_{\beta AK}$ mRNA. Since the tumorous CTLL.5 is also strongly positive for $V_{\beta AK}$ expression, it will be interesting to reveal any (causal) relationship between the pertubated $V_{\beta AK}$-mRNA expression and transformation events in T cells. In this context it should be noted that in at least one leukemic T-cell line of human origin, a similar and evolutionarily homologous V_β gene is expressed (YANAGI et al. 1984).

In conclusion, changes of function, specificity, karyotype, and molecular genetic aspects are correlated in CTLL and long-term culture derivates which a priori is in accordance with Hayflick's postulate. Although the variation in specificity and function of CTLL as well as their malignant transformation were induced by propagation in vitro, one might speculate that similar phenomena occur in vivo to clones undergoing continuous proliferation, such as those involved in autoimmune or other chronic diseases.

Acknowledgement. We are grateful to F. Bartels, A. Becker, G. Nerz, and M. Prester for excellent technical assistance, and to R. Schneider for typing the manuscript. S.A. is supported by the Alexander-von-Humboldt-Stiftung.

References

Bevan MJ, Cohn M (1975) Cytotoxic effects of antigen- and mitogen-induced T cells on various targets. J Immunol 114:559–565

Epplen JT, Rinaldy A, Becker A, Bartels F, Prester M, Nerz G, Simon MM (1986) Change in antigen specificity of cytotoxic T lymphocytes is associated with the rearrangement and expression of a new T-cell receptor β chain gene. Proc Natl Acad Sci USA (in press)

Hannum CH, Kappler JW, Trowbridge IS, Marrack P, Freed JH (1984) Immunoglobulin-like nature of the α-chain of a human T-cell antigen/MHC receptor. Nature 312:65–67

Hayflick L (1965) The limited in vitro lifetime of human diploid cell strains. Exp Cell Res 37:614–636

Kanagawa O, Louis J, Cerottini J-C (1982) Frequency and cross-reactivity of cytolytic T lymphocyte precursors reacting against male alloantigens. J Immunol 128:2362–2366

Nabholz M, Conzelmann A, Acuto O, North M, Haas W, Pohlit H, Boehmer H von, Hengartner H, Mach J-P, Engers H, Johnson JP (1980) Established murine cytolytic T-cell lines as tools for a somatic cell genetic analysis of T-cell functions. Immunol Rev 51:125–156

Nesbitt MN, Francke U (1973) A system of nomenclature for band patterns of mouse chromosomes. Chromosoma 41:145–158

Rinaldy A, Wallace RB, Simon MM, Becker A, Epplen JT (1985) A highly homologous T-cell receptor β-chain variable region is expressed in mouse and human T cells. Immunogenetics 21:403–406

Rybak J, Tharapel A, Robinett S, Garcia M, Mankinen C, Freeman M (1982) A simple reproducible method for prometaphase chromosome analysis. Hum Genet 60:328–333

Saito H, Kranz DM, Takagaki Y, Hayday AC, Eisen HN, Tonegawa S (1984) Complete primary structure of a heterodimeric T-cell receptor deduced from cDNA sequences. Nature 309:757–762

Sanford KK, Parshad R, Handleman SL, Price FM, Gantt RR, Evans UJ (1979) Serum induced chromosome damage and neoplastic transformation of mouse cells in vitro. In Vitro 15:488–496

Simon MM, Moll H, Prester M, Nerz G, Eichmann K (1984a) Immunoregulation by mouse T-cell clones. I. Suppression and amplification of cytotoxic responses by cloned H-Y-specific cytolytic T lymphocytes. Cell Immunol 86:206–221

Simon MM, Weltzien HU, Bühring HJ, Eichmann K (1984b) Aged murine killer T-cell clones acquire specific cytotoxicity for P815 mastocytoma cells. Nature 308:367–370

Siu G, Kronenberg M, Strauss E, Haars R, Mak TW, Hood L (1984) The structure, rearrangement, and expression of D_β gene segments of the murine T-cell antigen receptor. Nature 311:344–350

von Boehmer H, Hengartner H, Nabholz M, Lenhard M, Schreier MH, Haas W (1979) Fine specificity of continuously growing killer cell clone specific for H-Y antigen. Eur J Immunol 9:592–597

Yanagi Y, Yoshikai Y, Leggett K, Clark SP, Aleksander I, Mak TW (1984) A human T cell-specific cDNA clone encodes a protein having extensive homology to immunoglobulin chains. Nature 308:145–149

Part C: Phenotype and Functional Potential of T-Cell Clones

Introductory Remarks

H. von Boehmer

In this section many facts and possibly artifacts concerning short- and long-term cultured T-cell clones are presented and attempts are made to extrapolate to the in vivo significance. The function of T cells can only be measured after their activation. There is no single-cell assay for most T-cell functions. Consequently the function of the progeny of a single cell is being analyzed. This, however, puts constraints on the validity of the analysis, since cells have to be expanded in vitro under conditions which may or may not deter the functional potential present in the ancestor cells.

The difficulties of such an approach are pointed out by Brooks. What is a sufficient cell number to measure function and after what time in vitro does the functional potential change? Brooks argues that the IL-2 production by $Ly-2^+$ T-cell clones is often not detected simply because in conventional limiting dilution assays the $Ly-2^+$ clones do not reach sufficient clone sizes: $Ly-2^+$ cells produce less IL-2 than $T4^+$ cells and therefore $Ly-2^+$ cells have to be a little more expanded to detect their IL-2 production. This ability of $Ly-2^+$ clones is also reflected in their ability to proliferate after antigenic stimulation. If, however, $Ly-2^+$ cells are kept for prolonged time periods in culture, their ability to synthesize IL-2 and to proliferate is lost. On the basis of these results Brooks argues that in fact every $Ly-2^+$ cell may initially respond with IL-2 production to antigenic stimulation. This could possibly convincingly be shown if one had assays detecting IL-2 mRNA at the single-cell level. In summary, Brooks argues (as do others) that with regard to IL-2 production there is a quantitative rather than a qualitative difference between $Ly-2^+$ or $T8^+$ cells on the one hand and $T4^+$ cells on the other. The ability of $Ly-2^+$ cells to produce IL-2 is in fact reflected in the ability of resting $Ly-2^+$ cells to proliferate autonomously after stimulation by antigen or lectin. This proliferation does not require but can be augmented by $T4^+$ cell-derived IL-2.

With very few exceptions cloned $Ly-2^+$ or $T8^+$ cells are cytolytic (Brooks, Fleischer and Wagner), while the situation with regard to the cytolytic activity of $T4^+$, class II restricted clones is less clear. It is argued by Fleischer and Wagner that the cytolytic activity of the latter clones is always acquired in vitro, since initially all cytolytic T cells isolated from Epstein-Barr virus infected patients are $T8^+$, $T4^-$. Only after propagation of cells for some time in vitro are $T8^-$, $T4^+$ cytolytic clones detected. On the other hand Tite et al. speculate that cytolytic $T4^+$ cells occur in vivo and may cause suppression of antibody formation by lysing an-

---

Basel Institute for Immunology, Grenzacher Strasse 487, CH-4005 Basel

78   H. von Boehmer: Introductory Remarks

tigen presenting B cells. Tite et al. also suggest that the killing by T4[+], class II restricted clones may be distinguished from those of Ly-2[+], class I restricted clones by choice of appropriate targets: certain selected targets are lysed by the latter but not former clones. This analysis should be extended to other T4[+] cytolytic clones, especially those specific for class II antigens as described by Brooks. This may possibly reveal a correlation of surface antigen phenotype and the quality of killing.

Is there any correlation of surface marker and antigen specificity? According to Brooks, such correlation is difficult to demonstrate, i.e., Ly-2[+] and T4[+] clones may recognize class I as well as class II antigens. This does not mean, however, that Ly-2[+] or T8[+] cells are not always able to bind to class I antigens and that T4[+] cells are not always able to bind to class II antigens: their "true" specificity may simply be unknown and by chance they might cross-react on MHC molecules of the inappropriate class. Apart from MHC specific clones it may certainly be said that a correlation between surface markers (Ly-2, T8, or T4) and specificity (class I or class II) exists if MHC-restricted clones are analyzed.

Are there differences in growth requirements of Ly-2[+] or T8[+] clones on the one hand and T4[+] clones on the other? According to Fleischer and Wagner, most T8[+] clones can be grown in media containing IL-2 without antigenic stimulation, while the growth of T4[+] clones requires antigenic stimulation plus IL-2. This is not so with Ly-2[+] clones studied by Brooks: their growth requires periodic stimulation with antigen (required to increase the expression of IL-2 receptors). Even their cytolytic activity increases after antigenic stimulation. This is a common observation mode by many investigators. The constitutive expression of IL-2 receptors by some Ly-2[+] or T8[+] clones is usually associated with chromosomal translocations and may be a step involved with malignant transformation of these cells. Thus, at present there are no well-characterized differences in the growth requirements of Ly-2[+] or T8[+] and T4[+] cells. Both cell types express IL-2 receptors after antigenic stimulation (there may be more stringent conditions for this step with T4[+] cells), both cell types can be expanded in media containing IL-2 and the proliferation is blocked by anti-IL-2 receptor antibodies.

The specificity of Ly-2[+] or T8[+] clones on the one hand and T4[+] clones on the other may degenerate sooner or later during in vitro culture. Shortman shows that under conditions which favor optimal (high frequency) induction and expansion of Ly-2[+] cells, many clones lyse a variety of targets after 7 to 9 days in culture. This problem was not encountered by Larsson (Paris) who, however, reports a lower plating efficiency (personal communication). Whether additional factors were responsible for these apparently opposite results could not be elucidated. The "promiscuous" specificity of short-term (Shortman and Wilson) or long-term (Brooks) Ly-2[+] clones may be divided into two categories, one being "NK-like," the other "aged killer-like." According to Eichmann (personal communication) "aged killers" often lyse P815 mastocytoma non-NK targets. The specificity and even function of T4 clones may also degenerate, resulting in "NK-like" activity and antigen nonspecific suppression (Pawelec et al.). It is unknown whether the changes in specificity are a reflection of changes in antigen-receptor specificity or some other in vitro changes. Without the application of more sophisticated methods one may not see the border between facts and artifacts.

A Study of the Functional Potential
of Mouse T-Cell Clones*

C.G. BROOKS

1   Introduction   79
2   Methods   80
3   Results and Discussion   80
3.1 Characterization of Resting T Cells   81
3.2 Changes in Behavior of T Cells upon Activation   86
4   Conclusions   90
References   91

1 Introduction

The development of techniques for the cloning of single antigen-responsive T cells, and their subsequent expansion to provided large numbers of relatively homogeneous cells, has provided a powerful tool for analysing the biology and biochemistry of T-lymphocyte function. Cloned T-cell lines have played a central role in the acquisition of knowledge of the T-cell antigen receptor and have provided new insights into the recognitive and functional diversity of different T-cell subsets. In the latter area, two general approaches have been utilized. In the first, T cells obtained directly from animals, or following various in vitro manipulations, have been cloned in microplate wells in the presence of appropriate antigen and growth factors, and the activity of the developing clones has been assayed in situ. With the recent development of high efficiency cloning systems (CHEN et al. 1982; MORETTA et al. 1983; PFIZENMAIER et al. 1984), such limiting dilution analysis is potentially an extremely powerful method for dissecting immune responses. However, there are also several problems: the small size of the primary clones severely restricts the number of parameters that can be analyzed; the readout is measured in an all-or-none manner rather than quantitatively, and the frequency of responding cells is often meaningless, as the cloning efficiency, the sensitivity of the detection system, and the antigen specificities of the clones are largely unknown. In the second approach, established T-cell lines are studied in a variety of functional assays, but here there are major problems as to whether a given T-cell clone can be considered "typical" and whether the function of an aged cell line reliably reflects the functional potential of the progenitor cell.

Basic Immunology, Fred Hutchinson Cancer Research Center, 1124 Columbia Street, Seattle, WA 98104, USA

* This work was supported by grant AI-15384 from the National Institutes of Health

80   C.G. Brooks

In an attempt to address some of these problems, we have performed a multiparameter analysis of the functional potential of a large number of mouse T-cell clones freshly isolated by limiting dilution and maintained in a strictly antigen-dependent manner. We found that T-cell function correlated much more closely with cell-surface markers than with the class of MHC product recognized. In addition, we observed that all T-cell clones were capable of expressing both helper and cytotoxic activity, and that the relative proportions of these activities depended upon the activation state of the cells.

2 Methods

Only a brief outline of methods is provided.

T-Cell Cloning. Spleen cells, usually without any prior culture, were cloned at limiting dilution in 96-well plates in Click's medium containing 10% fetal bovine serum (FBS), 10% mouse conditioned supernatant (CS), 50 m M α-methyl mannoside, and irradiated allogeneic stimulator spleen cells. CS was prepared by stimulating spleen cells with 10 μg/ml Concanavalin A (Con A) for 2 days. After 2 weeks, wells with visible clones were transferred to 48-well plates and restimulated with irradiated spleen cells in Click's medium containing 10% FBS and 5% rat CS. After 3–4 days, viable cells were recovered by centrifugation on Ficoll-Hypaque, and cultured a further 3–4 days in the same medium. They were then refed with medium containing 1% rat CS and allowed to rest for at least 1 week prior to restimulation. The clones were maintained in continuous culture by alternate periods of stimulation and rest.

Proliferative Activity. Aliquots of 10^4 cloned T cells were incubated for 2 days in 96-well microplate wells containing Click's/10% FBS and 10^6 irradiated syngeneic or allogeneic stimulator cells with or without a saturating concentration of gene-cloned interleukin 2 (IL-2). Tritiated thymidine was then added to the wells for the last 4 h.

Cytotoxicity Assay. A 4-h chromium release assay, with 5 x 10^3 target cells per V-bottomed microplate well was employed. Effector:target (E:T) cell ratios were either 20:1 or 2:1.

Lymphokine Production. Aliquots of 10^5 cloned T cells were incubated for 24 h in 96-well microplate wells containing Click's/10% FBS with 3 μg/ml Con A. Supernatants were harvested and titrated for IL-2 using the method of GILLIS et al. (1978) or for interferon (IFN) using a VSV/L cell assay. In each assay a reference IL-2 or IFN standard was included.

3 Results and Discussion

Table 1 summarizes the origins of the clones used in this study. All clones were generated against C57BL/6 stimulators, and genetic disparity was varied by using different responder strains. Extensive use was made of B6 mutant mice:

Table 1. Origin of clones

Series	Strain	Culture prior to cloning	Cloned at (cells/well)	Clone frequency	P^a (%)
H	B6-C-H-2^{bm12}/ByJ	1 × MLR	1	1/19	> 95
I	B6-C-H-2^{bm1}/ByJ	None	100	1/900	92
J	CBA/J	None	300	1/1700	90
K	B6-C-H-2^{bm12}/ByJ	None	100	1/1800	92
L	B6-C-H-2^{bm12}/ByJ	2 × MLR	1	1/27	> 95
M	B6-C-H-2^{bm1}/ByJ	None	100	1/1200	> 95

[a] Poisson probability of monoclonality
MLR, mixed lymphocyte reaction with C57BL/6 stimulators

bml mice have an H-2K^b molecule which differs from the wild type in three neighboring amino acids (PEASE et al. 1983); bm12 mice have a mutation affecting three neighboring amino acids in the I-A$_\beta$ chain (MacINTYRE and SEIDMANN 1984). CBA/JKJ mice differ from C57BL/6 mice across the whole H-2 region and also at numerous minor histocompatibility loci. Regardless of strain combinations, clones derived directly from fresh cells arose at a frequency of about 1/1000 nucleated spleen cells (or about 1/300 splenic T cells). If spleen cells were first primed in mixed lymphocyte reaction, the clone frequency rose at least tenfold. In each experiment Poisson analysis indicated that the probability of any given clone being derived from a single progenitor cell was at least 90%.

All clones were maintained on a strict regimen of alternating cycles of antigen and growth factor-induced proliferation followed by resting. The proliferation phase was always restricted to 7 days and the growth factor concentration (5% CS) was the minimum required for active proliferation of growth factor dependent clones. After 7 days the cells were placed in medium containing only 1% CS. Proliferation promptly terminated and the cells became very small and quiescent, as determined by the extremely limited amount of macromolecular synthesis. Cells could be maintained in this state for several weeks or even months before the gradual attrition of cell numbers became severe.

3.1 Characterization of Resting T Cells

Table 2 summarizes the properties of the clones we studied. All experiments were performed with cells which had been in the quiescent state for at least 1 week. The H and I series clones had been maintained in continuous culture for approx. 1 year, and had been recloned at 1 cell/well, prior to this study. The remaining clones were expanded from the limiting dilution plates using the methods described above and, as soon as sufficient numbers of cells became available, they were evaluated for the five sets of parameters described in the table. To avoid operator bias, 6–10 clones were selected at random from the limiting dilution plates in each experiment. About half of these clones failed to maintain proliferative activity and hence were lost. The remaining clones were characte-

82 C.G. Brooks

Table 2. Multiparameter analysis of T-cell clones

Clone	Specificity	Markers		Proliferation[a]				Cytotoxicity[b]			Lymphokines[c]	
		Ly-2	L3T4	Syn	B6	B6+IL-2	%	YAC-1	B6	P-C	IL-2	IFN
H1A	I-A^b	−	+	88	8522	8593	99	0	8	5	<0.005	250
H6B	I-A^b	−	+	88	4277	3589	119	0	6	4	2.4	2×10^3
I1C3A	K^b	+	−	73	5457	4949	110	0	44	3	<0.005	1×10^3
J62	K^b	+	−	279	2348	7768	30	0	34	43	1.2	4×10^3
J69	K^b	+	−	ND	ND	ND	ND	ND	ND	ND	3.3	32×10^3
J96	K^b	+	−	ND	ND	ND	ND	ND	33	ND	0.8	ND
J103	K^b	+	−	56	120	2202	5	ND	7	ND	0.4	4×10^3
J108	K^b	+	−	60	824	4328	19	0	55	58	0.04	32×10^3
J64	I-A^b	+	−	78	656	4236	15	0	16	56	1.6	32×10^3
J119	I-A^b	+	−	88	1337	10871	12	0	17	41	0.6	ND
K1	I-A^b	−	+	148	4590	6674	69	0	20	4	22.0	2×10^3
K2	I-A^b	−	+	137	15019	14246	105	0	2	2	14.5	32×10^3
K3	I-A^b	−	+	69	7630	7715	99	0	0	1	1.6	32×10^3
L1	I-A^b	−	+	127	3351	3476	96	0	0	0	10.0	<32
L2	I-A^b	±	−	74	761	8504	9	0	46	11	0.2	1×10^3
L4	I-A^b	−	+	108	3161	3097	102	0	0	5	2.1	1×10^3
L5	I-A^b	+	−	104	523	14480	3	0	45	10	0.1	ND
L6	I-A^b	±	−	84	557	9788	6	0	28	4	0.2	ND
M7	K^b	+	−	ND	464	13320	3	0	31	71	2.3	4×10^3
M15	K^b	+	−	ND	ND	ND	ND	1	43	35	3.9	2×10^3
M20	K^b	−	+	196	10538	6816	154	0	8	5	19.5	16×10^3
M27	K^b	+	−	196	574	8682	6	0	6	36	4.5	4×10^3

[a] Proliferation was measured after 2 days culture with irradiated syngeneic spleen cells or with irradiated C57BL/6 (B6) spleen cells in the presence or absence of an excess of recombinant human IL-2. Figures show cpm ^{3}H-thymidine uptake and the proliferation to B6 spleen cells alone as a percentage of that to B6 spleen cells plus IL-2.
[b] Figures show percentage cytotoxicity at an E:T ratio of 20:1 on YAC-1, C57BL/6 LPS blasts (B6) und P815 cells coated with Con A (P–C)
[c] Figures show units/ml of lymphokines secreted by 3.3×10^5 cells/ml in the presence of Con A

rized completely or near completely. The set of data displayd in Table 2 should therefore be fully respresentative of clones which can be grown under these culture conditions.

Specificity. The specificity of the clones was determined by (a) blocking proliferation with monoclonal antibodies to class I or class II MHC products, (b) measuring the proliferative response to stimulators bearing recombinant or mutant H-2 haplotypes, or (c) assaying lytic activity on target cells bearing or lacking class II MHC products. All three tests produced concordant results which agreed with the specificities expected from the strain combinations used.

Surface Markers. By indirect microscopy, the expression of Ly-2 and L3T4 markers was found to be mutually exclusive. No double positive or double-negative clones were observed, although clones L2 and L6 gave lower staining for Ly-2 than other Ly-2-positive clones. It has been proposed that surface marker phenotype in some way determines the class of MHC molecule recognized, with

A Study of the Functional Potential of Mouse T-Cell Clones   83

Table 3. Analysis of clone characteristics

A. Surface markers and MHC class recognized

	Ly-2$^+$	L3T4$^+$	
Class I	9	1	$P < 0.03$
Class II	5	7	

B. Helper dependence and MHC class recognized

	Dependent	Independent	
Class I	5	2	$P < 0.18$
Class II	5	7	

C. Helper dependence and markers

	Dependent	Independent	
Ly-2$^+$	10	1	$P < 0.0001$
L3T4$^+$	0	8	

D. Helper dependence and cytotoxicity

	Dependent	Independent	
Cytotoxic	9	2	$P < 0.001$
Noncytotoxic	0	7	

E. Cytotoxicity and MHC class recognized

	Cytotoxic	Noncytotoxic	
Class I	7	1	$P < 0.1$
Class II	6	6	

F. Cytotoxicity and markers

	Cytotoxic	Noncytotoxic	
Ly-2$^+$	12	0	$P < 0.0001$
L3T4$^+$	1	7	

Ly-2$^+$, L3T4$^-$ cells being class I restricted and Ly-2$^-$, L3T4$^+$ cells being class II restricted (Swain 1983). A chi-squared analysis of our result indicated only a weak association between these characteristics (Table 3A). Although most class I reactive clones were Ly-2$^+$, as predicted by the theory, one exception was found (M20); and class II reactive cells were equally likely to be Ly-2$^+$ or L3T4$^+$. It might be argued that the Ly-2 molecule on the Ly-2$^+$, L3T4$^-$ class II specific cells was nonfunctional or that such cells recognized class II determinants in the context of class I MHC products. This latter explanation appears unlikely, however, because the proliferative response of these cells to C57BL/6 stimulators was blocked by class II specific, but not by class I specific, monoclonal antibodies. Thus, although further investigation of these clones is required, results such as those obtained here argue against an obligatory relationship between Ly-2 and class I MHC products and between L3T4 and class II MHC products. In situations where a close correlation has been observed between Ly-2/L3T4 expression and MHC recognition, it may have been that experimental conditions strongly favored responses restricted in this manner. Equally, it is possible that the cloning conditions which we used selected for relatively rare clones. Whichever explanation is correct, it is clear that any theory of T-cell recognition and triggering must be capable of explaining both the apparent association between Ly-2/L3T4 expression and MHC recognition in certain circumstances and the lack of any association in others.

Proliferative Activity. All clones proliferated strongly when exposed to a combination of specific allogeneic stimulator cells and exogenous IL-2. Interestingly, with the exception of J103, the clones also proliferated significantly when presented with allogeneic stimulator cells alone. One explanation of this finding would be that the irradiated stimulator cells secreted IL-2. However, similar levels of proliferation were obtained using stimulator cells treated with anti-Thy-1 and complement to eliminate IL-2-producing cells. The degree of independence from exogenous IL-2 could be quantitated by expressing the proliferative response to antigen alone as a percentage of the response to antigen plus saturating concentrations of exogenous IL-2. From such an analysis it was clear that (a) essentially all T-cell clones displayed some degree of helper independence and (b) there existed a distinct subset of T-cell clones that was completely helper independent.

Taking a response to antigen alone of 50% of the maximal response as the divide between helper-dependent and helper-independent cells, we analyzed the relationship between helper dependence in T-cell clones and other parameters. Table 3B shows that there was no significant relationship with the class of MHC antigen recognized. By contrast, there was an extremely close relationship ($P<0.0001$) with surface phenotype, helper-dependent cells invariably being Ly-2$^+$ and helper-independent cells virtually always being L3T4$^+$ (Table 3C). The only exception to this rule was the aged clone I1C3A. There was also a strong correlation ($P<0.0001$; Table 3D) between helper dependence and the display of cytotoxicity (clones were scored positive for cytotoxicity if they gave greater than 10% lysis on any target; see below). These results argue that the primary relationship in T-cell biology is between surface markers and function, as originally suggested by CANTOR and BOYSE (1977), rather than between surface markers and MHC class (SWAIN 1983), or between MHC class and function (BACH et al. 1976).

Not unexpectedly there was also a high correlation between helper independence and secretion of IL-2 in response to antigen (data not shown). The exceptions to this rule were two aged clones, I1C3A and H1A, which, in the resting state, failed to secrete significant amounts of IL-2 at any time during their response to either alloantigen or Con A. At first sight this might suggest that some clones can proliferate in an IL-2-independent manner. However, as will be discussed below, both I1C3A and H1A could be induced to secrete substantial amounts of IL-2 after exposure to different growth conditions, demonstrating that the IL-2 gene is potentially active in these cells. It is therefore possible that, in response to antigen, IL-2 is produced and is able to trigger cell proliferation by a mechanism which does not require its overt secretion into the medium.

Cytotoxicity. Cytolytic activity was measured at a 20:1 E:T ratio on three key target cells: YAC-1, the mouse prototype NK target; C57BL/6 blast cells obtained by culturing spleen cells with lipopolysaccharide (LPS); and P815 cells coated with Con A. In this manner it was possible to detect intrinsic NK lytic activity, antigen-specific lytic activity, and lectin-dependent lytic activity (LDCC), respectively. In each experiment, syngeneic blast cells and uncoated P815 cells were included, but no significant lysis of these targets by T-cell clones in the quiescent state was ever observed.

None of the clones displayed any NK activity in the resting state. Many clones showed substantial lytic activity against specific blast cell targets, and such clones can be unambiguously classified as cytotoxic. More problematical was the fact that most of the remaining clones displayed low levels of antigen-specific lytic activity, ranging from 2% to 8% specific lysis at a 20:1 E:T ratio. Such lytic activity was at the limits of detection of the assay system and could not be properly quantitated. These clones, which also displayed little or no LDCC, are distinguishable from the overtly cytotoxic clones, and will for the time being be termed noncytotoxic.

When the cytotoxic/noncytotoxic phenotype was compared with other parameters, no significant association was found with the class of MHC recognition (Table 3E): whereas nearly all class I reactive clones were cytotoxic, class II reactive clones could be either cytotoxic or noncytotoxic. By contrast, a very strong correlation ($P<0.0001$) was observed between cytotoxic activity and surface markers, 12/13 cytotoxic clones being Ly-2$^+$ and all 7 noncytotoxic clones being L3T4$^+$ (Table 3F). The only exception was clone K1. These results further support the conclusion that the principal relationship in T cells is between surface markers and function.

A most unexpected finding was that several clones (I1C3A, K1, L4, L6) which had substantial specific lytic activity against LPS blasts displayed little or no LDCC. This result was reproducible and was confirmed in a different assay system in which Con A was present in the assay medium. It has generally been assumed that all cytotoxic T lymphocytes can kill in a lectin-dependent manner. As will be discussed below, this is indeed true, but only when the T cells are in an activated state. In the resting state, many cytotoxic clones can lyse only specific target cells. This finding raises considerable doubt about the validity of using lectin-dependent readout systems to score CTL frequencies in limiting dilution assays.

Conversely, we also observed one example of a clone which had little specific cytolytic activity, but strong LDCC (M27). One explanation would be that LDCC is a more sensitive means of detecting cytolytic activity than antigen-specific cytolysis. However, in light of the findings discussed in the previous paragraph, this is clearly not true for most CTL. Another explanation would be that clones such as these are heteroclitic and recognize the immunizing antigen with insufficient affinity to trigger the cytolytic mechanism. Since these same clones display antigen-specific proliferative responses, it would have to be postulated that higher affinity interaction is required to trigger cytolysis than to trigger proliferation or that the conditions under which proliferation is measured cause the cloned cells to increase their functional affinity. A clone displaying heteroclitic lytic specificity, but the correct proliferative specificity, has recently been described by RUSSELL and DUBOS (1983).

Lymphokine Production. All the young T-cell clones secreted IL-2 when stimulated with Con A. This included cytotoxic T cells and class I reactive T cells which have not generally been regarded as producers of IL-2. There was considerable variation in the amounts of IL-2 secreted, but there appeared to be a distinct subgroup of clones which secreted unusually high amounts (>10 U/ml). All four such clones were L3T4$^+$, helper-independent cells. By contrast only one of three older clones secreted detectable IL-2. This suggests that the ability to secrete IL-2 may decline after long-term culture, and, indeed, preliminary results indicate that the IL-2 production by the younger clones is declining with age.

When low numbers (10^4) of cloned cells were incubated with allogeneic cells, under conditions similar to those used in limiting dilution analysis, most of the low producer clones failed to secrete detectable amounts of IL-2. This observation, coupled with the apparent loss of IL-2 producing capacity after long-term culture and the frequently high IL-2 production by L3T4$^+$, helper-independent clones, probably accounts for the belief that only "helper" T cells can secrete IL-2. The helper-independent cytotoxic T cells (HIT cells) described by WIDMER and BACH (1981) are probably much more common than previously assumed, and, indeed, it may well be that all cytotoxic T cells are capable of secreting IL-2 during certain stages of their life history. Similar conclusions have recently been reached by VON BOEHMER et al. (1984).

All clones tested secreted IFN. The quantities were very variable, but the older clones consistently secreted relatively little, suggesting that lymphokine secretion in general declines after prolonged culture. Interestingly, the secretion of IL-2 and IFN must be independently regulated because (a) there was no correlation between the amounts of IL-2 and IFN secreted, and (b) following activation, the ability to secrete IL-2 in response to Con A could be selectively lost (see below).

3.2 Changes in Behavior of T Cells upon Activation

We have previously shown that when class I reactive mouse T-cell clones are activated by antigen or by culture in medium containing high concentrations of lymphokines, a series of dramatic functional and biochemical changes occurs (BROOKS 1983; BROOKS et al. 1983, 1985).

Within a few hours or days, the clones reversibly acquire a new lytic specificity identical to that of fresh splenic NK cells. This activity eventually broadens into a promiscuous pattern of killing in which many NK-resistant targets are also lysed. In this state, the cells lose all antigen specificity, grow continuously in medium containing lymphokines, and display substantial alterations in membrane glycolipids and glycoproteins. Acquisition of promiscuous lytic activity in limiting dilution cultures has also been described by SHORTMAN et al. (1984).

In order to provide a better understanding of this behavior, we have made a detailed comparison of the functional properties of T-cell clones in the resting state and in the activated state. Cells were activated by culture in medium supplemented with 20% crude BALB/c-derived CS. The first question we addressed was whether such treatment would also alter the lytic activity of class II reactive cells.

Table 4. Activated T cells acquire new lytic specificities

Clone	Day	Y AC-1	P815	P815-Con A	LPS blasts	
					Syn	Allo
K2	0	0	0	0	0	0
	2	0	3	22	0	1
	4	1	0	32	0	0
K3	0	0	0	1	0	0
	2	0	1	12	0	0
	4	0	1	5	0	0
L4	0	0	0	0	0	6
	2	0	1	15	0	1
	4	5	2	15	0	0
L2	0	0	0	5	0	42
	2	8	3	45	18	76
	4	47	50	71	56	70
L5	0	0	0	8	0	44
	2	3	1	34	11	73
	4	23	24	48	35	73
L6	0	0	0	3	0	42
	2	10	3	37	26	75
	4	40	42	58	24	63

Figures show percentage cytotoxicity at an E:T ratio of 2:1

A series of class II reactive clones was cultured in 20% CS for 0, 2, or 4 days, and the lytic activity was measured on (a) YAC-1 and P815 targets to detect NK and promiscuous lytic activity (YAC-1 cells are sensitive to NK and promiscuous killing, P815 cells only to promiscuous killing), (b) P815 cells coated with Con A to detect LDCC, and (c) syngeneic and allogeneic LPS blasts to detect antigen-specific lysis. The results obtained at an E:T ratio of 2:1 are shown in Table 4. In the resting state (day 0), the clones behaved as expected: the L3T4$^+$ clones K2, K3, and L4 had essentially no lytic activity on any target, whereas the Ly-2$^+$ clones L2, L5, and L6 displayed strong lytic activity against specific blast cells, but not against other targets, including the lectin-dependent target P815-Con A. This latter observation emphasizes the point made above, that cytotoxic T-cell clones do not necessarily display LDCC.

After 2 days of activation, significant changes had already occurred. The Ly-2$^+$ clones displayed a marked increase in lysis of specific blasts and a dramatic increase in LDCC. There was also some indication of the acquisition of NK and/or promiscuous lytic activity as revealed by weak lysis of YAC-1 and syngeneic blasts. By day 4, these new activities were strongly expressed.

Over the same time period, the L3T4$^+$ clones did not develop either specific lytic activity or promiscuous lytic activity, demonstrating that the rapid acquisition of promiscuous lytic activity is a function of Ly-2$^+$ cells and not L3T4$^+$ cells. This result was confirmed with the class I reactive M series clones, where the Ly-

2$^+$ lines M7, M15, and M27, but not the L3T4$^+$ line M20, expressed strong promiscuous lytic activity after 7 days culture in 20% CS. It is clear, therefore, that the acquisition of NK and promiscuous lytic activities occurs equally efficiently in both class I and class II reactive T cells provided they are Ly-2$^+$. Once again, there appears to be a much closer relationship between cell function and surface markers than between cell function and the MHC class recognized. The strong association of promiscuous lytic activity with Ly-2$^+$ T cells has also been observed by SHORTMAN et al. (1984) in limiting dilution systems.

A most surprising result was that the L3T4$^+$ clones acquired significant levels of LDCC upon activation, suggesting that perhaps all T cells have some lytic potential. To explore this issue further, we examined the cytotoxicity and lymphokine secretion patterns of a number of T-cell clones subjected to prolonged activation. J62 was used as a typical Ly-2$^+$ clone. As expected, after 13 days of culture in 20% CS, these cells displayed very strong NK lytic activity and LDCC. Interestingly, they also completely lost their ability to secrete IL-2 in response to Con A, but retained normal levels of IFN production. Thus, T cells not only acquire new lytic functions upon activation, but also display selective alterations in the types of lymphokine secreted.

Three L3T4$^+$ T cell lines were also examined: the class II reactive clones K1 and K3, and the class I reactive clone M20. By day 13/14, the only notable change in lytic activity was the acquisition of LDCC. In all three clones, there was a trend towards increased lymphokine secretion, particularly in clone K1 (IL-2 and IFN) and clone M20 (IL-2). By day 26/28, however, a striking alteration in the functional profiles of these clones had occurred. Clone K3 displayed strong NK activity, strong LDCC, and an element of selective lysis against specific blast cell targets. Clones K1 and M20 displayed strong promiscuous lytic activity. In each case, the ability to secrete IL-2 had fallen dramatically and there was also a slight fall in IFN secretion.

Some further examples of the behavior of L3T4 cells in different culture conditions are provided in Tables 5 and 6. The aged helper-independent clone HIA displayed little or no cytolytic activity in the resting state (day 0) and secreted no detectable IL-2. After 18 days of culture in 20% CS, however, the clone had acquired the ability to secrete IL-2. There was also a marked increase in IFN production, but little cytotoxicity. By day 41 there was substantial lectin-dependent lytic activity. The sister clone H6B also had little cytotoxic activity in the resting state, but did secrete IL-2. Thirteen days after placing in 20% CS, LDCC activity had appeared, and by day 18 the cells had strong NK activity, increased IFN production, but reduced IL-2 production. At this point the cells were returned to medium containing 1% CS and within 6 days virtually all NK and LDCC activity had disappeared and the normal capacity to secrete IL-2 had returned. Because both of these lines had been recloned under stringent conditions, the possibility that the observed changes in function were due to a lack of monoclonality is essentially excluded.

Thus, L3T4$^+$ cells, which in their resting state are generally devoid of cytotoxicity, can nonetheless be induced to express high levels of "nonspecific" lytic activity after a prolonged period of activation. At some point in the activation period, there is usually evidence of a low but significant specific lytic activity (for

A Study of the Functional Potential of Mouse T-Cell Clones 89

Table 5. T-cell function after prolonged activation

Clone	Day	Cytotoxicity[a]					Lymphokines[b]	
		YAC-1	P815	P-Con A	Syn[c]	Allo[c]	IL-2	IFN
J62	0	0	2	16	ND	33	2.0	1×10^3
	13	61	8	61	17	30	< 0.01	2×10^3
K1	0	0	1	3	0	20	4.2	1×10^3
	13	5	0	25	2	14	15.3	32×10^3
	26	24	38	54	26	34	0.8	8×10^3
K3	0	0	0	2	0	0	0.6	8×10^3
	13	3	1	13	2	3	0.4	16×10^3
	26	36	13	47	5	19	0.02	8×10^3
M20	0	0	0	4	0	0	1.3	8×10^3
	14	5	0	27	0	6	6.5	16×10^3
	28	59	57	65	46	48	0.01	4×10^2

[a] Measured at an E:T ratio of 2:1
[b] Aliquots of 10^5 cells were stimulated for 1 day with 3 μg/ml Con A. Figures show the units/ml of lymphokine in the supernatants
[c] Syngeneic and allogeneic LPS blasts

Table 6. Sequential alterations in the function of L3T4$^+$ cells caused by changes in culture conditions

Clone	Day	CS (%)	Cytotoxicity[a]					Lymphokines[b]	
			YAC-1	P815	P-Con A	Syn[c]	Allo[c]	IL-2	IFN
H1A	0	1	0	0	1	ND	9	< 0.005	250
	5	20	0	0	8	0	8	< 0.005	1×10^3
	18	20	2	0	8	3	14	1.3	32×10^3
	33	20	5	1	28	0	13	0.6	6×10^3
	41	20	9	6	45	9	23	0.4	4×10^3
H6B	0	1	0	0	2	ND	0	2.4	2×10^3
	13	20	3	1	31	0	0	0.8	32×10^3
	18	20	54	19	39	18	33	0.1	16×10^3
	24	1	3	0	8	4	7	7.8	12×10^3

[a, b, c] See corresponding footnotes in Table 5

example, K1 day 0, K3 day 36, M20 day 14), and, as mentioned earlier, low levels of specific lytic activity are often detectable at high E:T ratios in resting L3T4$^+$ cells. K1 is an extreme example of this phenomenon, which led to its being classified as a cytotoxic cell. Interestingly, recent studies by Janeway and colleagues (see this volume) suggest that specific cytotoxicity by L3T4$^+$ cells is mediated by a different mechanism than is cytotoxicity by Ly-2$^+$ cells. This may provide a qualitative method, rather than the arbitrary quantitative method used here, for classifying cytotoxic function in T-cell subsets. As with Ly-2$^+$ cells, the appearance of NK and promiscuous lytic activity in L3T4$^+$ cells is ac-

90 C.G. Brooks

companied by a drastic reduction in the ability to secrete IL-2 and is preceded by the appearance of LDCC. In both Ly-2$^+$ cells (data not shown) and L3T4$^+$ cells, these changes in function can be reversed.

These observations have profound theoretical and practical implications for our understanding of T-cell organization. The traditional division of T cells into helper, cytotoxic, and suppressor subsets can now be seen to have only restricted validity. Thus, all T cells appear to secrete lymphokines which can help or suppress other lymphocytes. In particular, probably all T cells are capable of secreting IL-2, the quantities secreted by Ly-2$^+$ cells being lower, but overlapping with the spectrum of quantities secreted by L3T4$^+$ cells. It also appears that all T cells have the capacity to display both specific and nonspecific cytotoxic functions. Although in the resting state cytotoxic activity is essentially restricted to Ly-2$^+$ cells and is always antigen-specific, upon activation all T cells show substantial increases in specific lytic activity and develop lectin-dependent, NK, and promiscuous cytotoxic functions. These aspects of T-cell behavior make the clonal analysis of T-cell function by limiting dilution analysis essentially impossible because the relationships between clone size, the level of cell activation, and signal generation are indeterminate. Our studies provide an explanation for many of the cases of "anomalous" behavior in T-cell clones which have been described in the literature, including helper function in Ly-2$^+$ cells, NK-like clones, lymphokine-activated killer cells, and L3T4$^+$ (or T4$^+$ cells in the human) displaying cytolytic activities.

4 Conclusions

A multiparameter analysis of freshly derived mouse T-cell clones has revealed that individual T cells have much greater functional flexibility than previously recognized. In particular all T cells are endowed with the capacity to display both helper and cytotoxic functions. The extent to which these distinctive functions are displayed is determined at two levels – differentiation and environment. The true differentiation status of the cell can be determined with accuracy only in the resting state, and shows an essentially perfect correlation with the surface markers Ly-2 and L3T4 and not with the class of MHC product which the cell recognizes. This differentiation state can be substantially modified by environmental interaction with antigen and/or lymphokines which activate the cells and alter the balance between the helper and cytotoxic (and presumably also suppressor) functions expressed by the cell. The fact that T cells in different activation states have different functions may explain some of the previous difficulties in correlating T-cell function with cell-surface markers and in maintaining T-cell clones in a stable functional state.

Acknowledgements. I would like to thank M. Holscher for outstanding technical assistance in this work, and N. Brooks for carefully typing the manuscript.

References

Bach FH, Bach ML, Sondel PM (1976) Differentiation function of major histocompatibility complex antigens in T lymphocyte activation. Nature 259:273

Brooks CG (1983) Reversible induction of natural killer cell activity in cloned murine cytotoxic T lymphocytes. Nature 305:155

Brooks CG, Urdal D, Henney CS (1983) Lymphokine driven "differentiation" of cytotoxic T cell clones into cells with NK-like specificity: correlations with display of membrane macromolecules. Immunol Rev 72:43

Brooks CG, Holscher M, Urdal D (1985) Natural killer activity in cloned cytotoxic T lymphocytes: regulation by interleukin-2, interferon, and specific antigen. J Immunol 135 (in press)

Cantor H, Boyse EA (1977) Functional subclasses of T lymphocytes bearing different Ly antigens. I. Generation of functionally distinct T cell subclasses in a differentiative process independent of antigen. J Exp Med 141:1376

Chen WF, Wilson A, Scollay R, Shortman K (1982) Limit-dilution assay and clonal expansion of all T cells capable of proliferation. J Immunol Methods 52:307

Gillis S, Ferm MM, Ou W, Smith KA (1978) T cell growth factor: parameters of production and a quantitative microassay for activity. J Immunol 120:2027

McIntyre KR, Seidman JG (1984) Nucleotide sequence of mutant I-Aβ^{bm12} gene is evidence for genetic exchange between mouse immune response genes. Nature 308:551

Moretta A, Pantaleo G, Moretta L, Cerottini JC, Mingari MC (1983) Direct demonstration of the clonogenic potential of every human peripheral blood T cell. J Exp Med 157:743

Pease LR, Schulze DH, Pfaffenbach GM, Nathenson SG (1983) Spontaneous H-2 mutants provide evidence that a copy mechanism analogous to gene conversion generates polymorphism in the MHC. Proc Natl Acad Sci USA 80:242

Pfizenmaier K, Scheurich P, Daubener W, Krönke M, Röllinghoff M, Wagner H (1984) Quantitative representation of all T cells committed to develop into cytotoxic effector cells and/or interleukin 2 activity-producing helper cells within murine T lymphocyte subsets. Eur J Immunol 14:33

Russel JH, Dubos CB (1983) Characterization of a "heteroclitic" cytotoxic lymphocyte clone: heterogeneity of receptors or signals? J Immunol 130:538

Shortman K, Wilson A, Scollay R (1984) Loss of specificity in cytolytic T lymphocyte clones obtained by limit dilution of Ly-2$^+$ T cells. J Immunol 132:584

Swain SL (1983) T cell subsets and the recognition of MHC class. Immunol Rev 74:129

Von Boehmer H, Kieselow P, Leiserson W, Haas W (1984) Lyt-2$^-$ T cell-independent functions of Lyt-2$^+$ cells stimulated with antigen or Concanavalin A. J Immunol 133:59

Widmer MB, Bach FH (1981) Antigen-driven helper-independent cloned cytotoxic T lymphocytes. Nature 294:750

Generation, Propagation, and Variation in Cloned, Antigen-Specific, Ia-Restricted Cytolytic T-Cell Lines*

J.P. TITE, B. JONES, M.E. KATZ, and C.A. JANEWAY, JR.

1 Introduction 93
2 Materials and Methods 94
3 Results 94
4 Summary 99
References 100

1 Introduction

Since the demonstration that B lymphocytes bear surface immunoglobulin (Ig), while helper T lymphocytes are surface Ig negative but bear the T-cell differentiation antigen Thy-1, attempts have been made to correlate the function of a T cell with the expression of differentiation antigens by that cell. In the mouse and in man, it has been found that the majority of helper T cells bear the T4 (or L3T4a) marker, while suppressor and cytolytic T cells bear the T8 or Lyt-2 surface molecule (CANTOR and BOYSE 1976; JANDINSKI et al. 1976; RHEINHERZ et al. 1979). However, many studies, especially those employing cloned T-cell populations, appear to violate these "rules." Thus, cells with helper, suppressor, or cytolytic capabilities have been assigned to either of these populations by several investigators (SWAIN et al. 1981; THOMAS et al. 1981). In this report, we will discuss our current work on cytolytic T cells that are antigen-specific, Ia-restricted, and L3T4a positive (TITE and JANEWAY 1984a, b; TITE et al. 1985). Such cells also manifest at least some of the functions associated with helper T cells. Our studies indicate that the critical determinant of the function of a T cell is the antigen-nonspecific molecules it produces upon activation by antigen:MHC, not its cell surface antigen phenotype or its specificity for a particular self-MHC molecule. We will present evidence that demonstrates that such cells are found amongst normal T cells, and that previous attempts to demonstrate such cells probably failed for technical reasons having to do with assay conditions and target-cell susceptibility.

Howard Hughes Medical Institute, Department of Pathology, Yale University Medical School, 310 Cedar Street, New Haven, CT 06510

* Supported by NIH Grant AI-14579

Current Topics in Microbiology and Immunology, Vol. 126
© Springer-Verlag Berlin · Heidelberg 1986

94   J.P. Tite et al.

2   Materials and Methods

All of the materials and methods employed in these studies have been described in previous publications from this laboratory (TITE and JANEWAY 1984a, b; TITE et al. 1985; JANEWAY et al. 1982; BOTTOMLY et al. 1983).

3   Results

Freshly isolated, antigen-stimulated lymph node T cells can be cytolytic. Mice have been immunized with a variety of antigens injected in complete Freund's adjuvant; 7–10 days later, draining lymph node cells are isolated and stimulated with specific antigen. T-cell blasts isolated from such responses will kill a high percentage of antigen-pulsed B-lymphoma target cells (Table 1), bearing the appropriate Ia antigens (not shown), but do not kill cells bearing the wrong protein antigen or the wrong Ia molecule. Thus, cytolytic function in primed and once-stimulated lymph node T cells is readily demonstrable with several different antigens and MHC genotypes, and is antigen specific and MHC (Ia) restricted.

Cloned, antigen-specific, Ia restricted T-cell lines are cytolytic. When cloned T-cell lines are raised either by cloning in soft agar 3 days after antigen stimulation, or by limiting dilution of T-cell blasts, many of the cloned T-cell lines exhibit cytolytic function. Such cloned T-cell lines allow one to dissect this form of cytotoxicity in detail. As shown in Table 2, such cloned T-cell lines are antigen specific and Ia restricted in helper, proliferation, and cytolytic functions. The data in this table also demonstrate that a single cloned T-cell line can manifest all of these functional capabilities. The behavior of these cloned T-cell lines differs from that of conventional, class I MHC-specific cytolytic T cells; Ia restricted cytolytic T cells can, upon induction with antigen:Ia, kill bystander targets that neither bear antigen nor express Ia molecules (Table 3). Despite this bystander

Table 1.   Freshly isolated, antigen-activated lymph node T-cell blasts kill B lymphoma cells in the presence of specific antigen

Effector:target ratio	Percent specific ^{51}Cr release from targets	
	LK35.2 (H-2^k × H-2^d)	OVA-pulsed LK35.2
10:1	7	70
5:1	5	65
2.5:1	4	41
1.2:1	2	39
0.6:1	1	21

B10.BR (H-2^k) mice were immunized with 50 μg OVA in complete Freund's adjuvant subcutaneously in the base of the tail. After 9–10 days, draining lymph nodes were stimulated for 5 days with 250 μg/ml OVA. T-cell blasts were isolated on one-step LSM density gradients, and used as effector cells in a 6-h ^{51}Cr release assay. Hybrid B-cell lymphoma LK35.2 was made by fusing H-2^k LPS blasts to the H-2^d A20.2J lymphoma. LK35.2 was cultured overnight with 1 mg/1 ml OVA, washed, and labeled with ^{51}Cr

Generation, Propagation, and Variation in Cloned T-Cell Lines   95

Table 2. Cloned, antigen specific, Ia-restricted T-cell lines can help or kill B-cell targets: inhibition by anti-Ia antibodies

Ia-bearing cell	OVA	Effect	Monoclonal antibody	Cloned T-cell line	
				5.5	5.8
Normal B cells	–	Ig secretion	–	790	130
	+		–	15200	10000
Spleen cells	–	T-cell growth	–	2000	400
	+		–	105000	29000
	+		$I\text{-}A^d$	122000	500
	+		$I\text{-}E^d$	9000	23000
B-lymphoma cells	–	Cytolysis	–	0	0
	+		–	40.1	34.2
	+		$I\text{-}A^d$	32.0	3.6
	+		$I\text{-}E^d$	0.9	32.7

BALB/c ($H\text{-}2^d$) OVA-specific cloned T cells were added to normal B cells or mitomycin C-treated spleen cells, or the BALB/c B lymphoma line A20.2J with or without OVA. Monoclonal anti-$I\text{-}A^d$ (MKD6) or anti-$I\text{-}E^d$ (14.4.4) antibodies were used to inhibit assays. Ig secretion were reported as Ig secreting cells per 10^5 B cells; T-cell growth was reported as ^{3}H-thymidine incorporated per 2×10^4 T cells; cytolysis was reported as percent specific ^{51}Cr release at a 5:1 effector:target ratio

Table 3. Cloned, antigen-specific, Ia-restricted cytotoxic T-cell lines kill bystander targets

Bystander target	Percent specific ^{51}Cr release in presence of	
	A20.2J	OVA-pulsed A20.2J
A20.2J ($H\text{-}2^d$, Ia^+)	1.0	31.0
BW5147 ($H\text{-}2^k$, Ia^-)	2.0	15.5

Cloned T-cell line 5.8, specific for OVA:$I\text{-}A^d$, can be stimulated by OVA-pulsed A20.2J ($H\text{-}2^d$) B-lymphoma cells to kill unpulsed BW5147 or A20.2J bystander targets at effector:target ratios of 5:1

cytotoxicity, one can block such cloned cytolytic T cells with unlabeled, antigen-pulsed B cells (Table 4). This suggests that the killing mechanism is saturable, and may apply most strongly to target cells to which the cloned T-cell line can directly bind. The cognate nature of this interaction is also demonstrated by the finding that the target cells preferentially affected by such cytolytic T cells are those bearing the highest density of the relevant Ia glycoprotein on their surface (TITE and JANEWAY 1984b). Thus, although innocent bystander targets can be lysed, there is a pronounced preference for affecting B cells to which the T cell can directly bind by virtue of its antigen:Ia receptor. Finally, as with class I specific cytolytic T cells, mitogenic lectins such as Concanavalin A (Con A) will allow cloned T cells to kill other sensitive targets in addition to the B-cell lymphomas outlined above in the absence of antigen or the appropriate Ia molecules (Table 5). The data in Table 5 show that there are marked differences in the

96   J.P. Tite et al.

Table 4. Blocking of cytolysis with antigen-pulsed, Ia$^+$ cold-target cells

Ratio of cold:hot targets	Percent specific ^{51}Cr release from OVA:A20.2J in the presence of cold target	
	A20.2J	OVA-A20.2J
0	37	37
1.25:1	40	36
2.5 :1	42	31
5 :1	47	15
10 :1	41	6

A20.2J cells were cultured overnight with or without OVA; one aliquot of each was labeled with ^{51}Cr, the other used as a cold target. Cytolysis was mediated by OVA:I-A^d-specific cloned T-cell line 5.8 at an effector target ratio of 5:1 for 6 h

Table 5. Sensitivity of tumor cells to cloned, antigen-specific, Ia-restricted T-cell lines in the presence of mitogenic lectins

Target cell	Percent specific ^{51}Cr release above background in presence of		
	Con A	PHA	Lentil
A20.2J	76	71	83
M12.4.1	20	17	6
WEHI279 1/12	8	13	10
70Z/3.12	77	80	72
BW5147	70	69	72
EL4	36	33	38
P815	96	93	96
P388.D1	81	69	81

Clone 5.9.24, OVA:I-A^d-specific T cells were added to ^{51}Cr-labeled tumor cells at a 5:1 effector:target ratio with 2.5 μg/ml Con A, 3 μg/ml PHA, or 10 μg/ml lentil lectin. Percent specific ^{51}Cr release at 18 h was determined (spontaneous release, 15%–25% for these targets). Background release in the absence of lectins was 4%–18% and has been subtracted

sensitivity of these targets to this lytic effect. These differences are not seen when class I MHC-specific T cells are used with the same target cells.

Cloned, Mls-reactive L3T4a$^+$ T-cell lines can be cytolytic. A number of cloned T-cell lines have been generated that respond by proliferation to Ia bearing stimulator cells of Mls^a or Mls^d genotype (JANEWAY and KATZ 1985; KATZ and JANEWAY 1985). These cloned T-cell lines will help, Mls^{a,d} B cells to proliferate and secrete Ig. As shown in Table 6, these cloned T-cell lines can also kill target cells either in the presence of Con A or as innocent bystanders when the clones are stimulated with Mls^{a,d} spleen cells.

Cloned T-cell lines can be killed by Ia restricted T cells. One puzzling feature of the cytolytic behavior of Ia restricted cloned T-cell lines is their ability to grow despite releasing cytolytic factors as demonstrated above or in assays for lymphotoxin (TITE et al. 1985). Thus, we tested the susceptibility to lysis of various

Generation, Propagation, and Variation in Cloned T-Cell Lines 97

Table 6. Cytolysis mediated by L3T4a$^+$, M1s^{a,d}-reactive cloned T-cell lines

Stimulus	Percent specific ^{51}Cr released by clone IIB
0	4.2
Concanavalin A	85.6
B10.BR spleen cells	9.0
AKR/J spleen cells	77.7

B10.D2 (H-2^d, Mls^b) T cells activated by DBA/2 (H-2^d, Mls^a) spleen cells were cloned by limiting dilution and carried in long-term cultures. Cloned cell lines (5 × 10^4) were tested for cytolysis of ^{51}Cr-labeled A20.2J (H-2^d, Mls^b) targets (1 × 10^4) in the presence or absence of 2.5 μg/ml Con A or 2 × 10^5 B10.BR or AKR/J spleen stimulator cells

Table 7. Susceptibility of cloned T-cell lines to lectin-mediated cytolysis by cloned, Ia-restriced T-cell line 5.9.24

Target cell	Specificity	Cytolytic	Percent specific ^{51}Cr release above background
5.2	OVA:I-E^d	Yes	0
5.5	OVA:I-E^d	Yes	0
5.9.24	OVA:I-A^d	Yes	0
D10.G4.1	Conalbumin:I-A^k	No	67
8D3	OVA:I-A^d	No	58

Cloned T-cell lines were labeled with ^{51}Cr and used as target cells in a 6-h ^{51}Cr release assay. Effector cells were cloned line 5.9.24, specific for OVA:I-A^d. Cytolysis was induced by 2.5 μg/ml Con A. Background cytolysis (0%–5%) in the absence of Con A was subtracted. Spontaneous release was 5%–15%

cloned T-cell lines by other cloned T-cell lines known to be potently cytolytic. As cloned T-cell lines do not express Ia antigens, such experiments were carried out by using ^{51}Cr-labeled cloned T cells either as targets in lectin-dependent cytotoxicity or as bystander targets (not shown). As shown in Table 7, some cloned, antigen-specific T-cell lines are highly susceptible to this form of killing, while many are quite resistant. Of greater interest is the finding that resistant T-cell clones appear to be the most potently cytolytic, while sensitive T-cell clones have no cytolytic function, although they are effective helper T cells in in vitro antibody responses.

Target cell variability in susceptibility to cytolysis by cloned, Ia restricted T-cell lines. We have used a number of normal, cloned, or transformed cell lines as target cells in a variety of ^{51}Cr release assays, and we find they vary widely in their susceptibility to lysis by cloned, Ia restricted T cells. As noted in the previous section, some cloned T-cell lines are highly sensitive to such effects, while others appear to be totally resistant. Where tested, all targets we have examined are equally susceptible to class I MHC-specific cytolytic T cells. In order to analyze resistance in detail, a series of immunoselected variants of the B lymphoma line A20.2J were prepared. We noted that the commonest variant (Type 1) is an Ia

98   J.P. Tite et al.

Table 8. Susceptibility of A20.2J and cytotoxicity-resistant immunoselected variants to growth inhibition by cloned, Ia-restricted T cells and MLR-generated classical CTLs

Target cell		Inhibition index (Ii) in the presence of					^{3}HTdr incorporation in absence of T cells ($\times 10^3$)
		2×10^4 5.9.24 plus				C57BL/6 anti-BALB/c	
Type	Line	Nil	OVA	RaMBr	Con A		
Unselected	A20/2J	1.5	25.8	64.5	64.8	34.8	(387.1)
Type 1	IID-1	1.2	2.7	60.5	72.6	41.2	(363.1)
Type 3	IIA-1.4.1	1.0	113.0	4.5	24.2	59.2	(338.6)
Type 4	IC-1.1	1.0	3.5	5.5	11.8	64.3	(401.9)

A20.2J and sublines selected for resistance to killing by the cloned Ia-restricted T-cell line 5.9.24 activated with antigen (OVA) or rabbit antimouse brain antiserum (RaMBr) were used as target cells for the same cloned, Ia-restricted cytolytic T cells or MLR-generated (C57BL/6J anti-BALB/c) cytolytic T cells. Inhibition of lymphoma proliferation in a 3-day culture was determined and is presented as the inhibition index (Ii). Ii = (mean cpm without T cells) ÷ (mean cpm plus T cells)

antigen low or negative cell which does not effectively present antigen to the cloned T-cell line (Tite and Janeway 1984b). Such variants almost always arise when immunoselection is carried out with cloned Ia restricted T cells and specific antigen.

However, if the same cloned T-cell lines are used to kill FcR-bearing targets, such as A20.2J, by means of the T-cell activating anti-Thy-1 antibodies found in rabbit-antimouse brain antiserum (Jones and Janeway 1981; Jones 1983), two other types of variants arise. The more interesting of these are variants that are now resistant to killing by such cloned T-cell lines even when lectins are used to elicit cytotoxicity (Type 4). Such cloned B-lymphoma variants are resistant to cytolysis as bystander cells, and yet are fully susceptible to conventional class I MHC-specific cytolytic T cells (Table 8). Thus, target cell susceptibility to the lytic mechanism can vary dramatically in this system. These differences in susceptibility to lysis will be very useful in dissecting the mechanism of cell killing in this system.

Expression of cytolytic potential in T-cell lines and cloned T-cell lines is stable. In our experience, the functional phenotype of cloned T cells is stable over long periods of time of continuous culture. Thus, most of the cloned T-cell lines we work with have been in continuous culture for 2–5 years without significant change in functional activity. However, the functional behavior of such lines appears to be quite unstable, especially if one examines cytolytic activity, which appears to decline rapidly with continuous culture of such lines (Table 9). This behavior is probably an expression of the data in Table 7; that is, T cells that make cytolytic molecules and are not resistant to them probably are eliminated, while those that do not make cytolytic molecules survive. Why early cloning might rescue cells which are resistant to the lytic factors they secrete is still not known.

Immunoregulation is performed by cloned, Ia-restricted T-cell lines. We are most interested in the immunoregulatory implications of cloned, cytolytic Ia-restricted T cells. We have previously reported that one such line could function as a suppressor T cell in vitro (Bottomly et al. 1983). This cloned T-cell line, like

Generation, Propagation, and Variation in Cloned T-Cell Lines 99

Table 9. Cytotoxic activity in uncloned antigen-specific T-cell lines

Cytolytic T cell	E:T ratio	Percent specific ^{51}Cr release on day	
		5	28
5.5	5:1	52.1	64.4
Line	5:1	15.9	5.1

BALB/c mice were immunized with OVA as in Table 1. T cells were stimulated weekly with OVA (250 μg/ml) and mitomycin C-treated syngeneic spleen cells. Viable cells were recovered by centrifugation on LSM gradients and tested for cytolytic activity on OVA-pulsed ^{51}Cr labeled A20.2J B-lymphoma cells, 5 and 28 days after culture initiation

the cytolytic T cells, preferentially affected the responses of B cells of the highest Ia antigen density. We do not know, in this case, whether this finding is due to a direct negative effect delivered to the B cell, or whether it reflects an effect on a neighboring helper T cell interacting with the same B cell. Favoring the first interpretation is the finding that LPS-activated normal B cells are susceptible to such cytolytic T cells (TITE and JANEWAY 1984a), while favoring the latter is the finding of ASANO and HODES (1983) that the helper T cell and a suppressor T cell similar to that described by BOTTOMLY et al. (1983) need to interact with the same B cell in order for suppression to occur, and the finding reported here that cloned T cells with helper function are highly susceptible to lysis by such cells.

Recently, one of us (J.T.) has analyzed what may be an in vivo manifestation of these findings. In the immune response of mice to collagen type IV (human), only one MHC genotype gave rise to a strong T-cell proliferative response, while all other strains were negative in this response. However, when antibody responses were examined, the opposite effect was seen. T-cell responsiveness is dominant in this system, but antibody responses are recessive. We are attempting to determine whether T-cell activation in this system favors suppressor/cytolytic, Ia-restricted, antigen-specific T cells over helper T cells.

4 Summary

Cloned, as well as freshly isolated, L3T4a$^+$ T cells can mediate antigen-specific cytolysis that is Ia-restricted. The cytolytic effect, like other functions of such cells, appears to be mediated through the release of soluble, antigen-nonspecific factors. Nevertheless, there is strong preference for such factors to act upon the target cell that is presenting antigen to the cytolytic T cell. Target cells vary markedly in their susceptibility to such cytolytic molecules. The immunoregulatory implications of these findings have been discussed.

Acknowledgements. The authors would like to thank Pat Conrad, Nancy Lindberg, and Barbara Broughton for technical support, our colleagues at Yale for stimulating discussions, and Laurie Hauer for typing the manuscript.

References

Asano Y, Hodes RJ (1983) T cell regulation of B cell activation: cloned Lyt-1$^+$, 2$^-$ T suppressor cells inhibit the major histocompatibility complex-restricted interaction of T helper cells with B cells and/or accessory cells. J Exp Med 158:1178–1190

Bottomly K, Kaye J, Jones B, Jones F III, Janeway CA Jr (1983) A cloned, antigen-specific, Ia-restricted Lyt-1$^+$, 2$^-$ T cell with suppressive activity. J Mol Cell Immunol 1:42–48

Cantor H, Boyse EA (1976) Regulation of cellular and humoral immune responses by T cell subclasses. Cold Spring Harbor Symp Quant Biol 41:23–32

Jandinski J, Cantor H, Tadakuma T, Peavy DL, Pierce CW (1976) Separation of helper T cells from suppressor T cells expressing different Ly components. I. Polyclonal activation: Suppressor and helper activities are inherent properties of distinct T cell subclasses. J Exp Med 143:1382–1390

Janeway CA Jr, Katz ME (1985) The immunobiology of the T cell response to *Mls*-locus disparate stimulator cells. I. Unidirectionality, new strain combinations and the role of Ia antigens. J Immunol 134:2057–2063

Janeway CA Jr, Lerner EA, Conrad PJ, Jones B (1982) The precision of self and non-self major histocompatibility complex encoded antigen recognition by cloned T cells. Behring Inst Mitteilungen 70:200–209

Jones B (1983) Evidence that the Thy-1 molecule is the target for T cell mitogenic antibody against brain-associated antigens. Eur J Immunol 13:678–684

Jones B, Janeway CA Jr (1981) Functional activities of antibodies against brain-associated T cell antigens. I. Induction of T cell proliferation. Eur J Immunol 11:584–592

Katz ME, Janeway CA Jr (1985) The immunobiology of the T cell response to *Mls*-locus disparate stimulator cells. II. Effects of *Mls*-locus disparate stimulator cells on cloned, protein antigen specific, Ia restricted T cell lines. J Immunol 134:2064–2070

Reinherz EL, Kunz PC, Goldstein G, Schlossman SL (1979) Separation of functional subsets of human T cells by a monoclonal antibody. Proc Nate Acad Sci USA 76:4061–4065

Swain SL, Dennert G, Wormsley S, Dutton RW (1981) The Lyt phenotype of a long-term allospecific T cell line. Both helper and killer activates to "IA" are mediated by Ly1 cells. Eur J Immunol 11:175–180

Thomas T, Rogozinski L, Irigoyen OH, Friedman SM, Kung PC, Goldstein G, Chess L (1981) Functional analysis of human T cell subsets defined by monoclonal antibodies. IV. Induction of suppressor cells within the OKT4$^+$ population. J Exp Med 154:459–467

Tite JP, Janeway CA Jr (1984a) Cloned helper cells can kill B lymphoma cells in the presence of specific antigen: Ia restriction and cognate vs non-cognate interactions in cytolysis. Eur J Immunol 14:878–886

Tite JP, Janeway CA Jr (1984b) Antigen-dependent selection of B lymphoma cells varying in Ia density by cloned, antigen-specific L3T4a$^+$ T cells: a possible in vitro model for B cell adaptive differentiation. J Mol Cell Immunol 1:253–264

Tite JP, Powell MB, Ruddle NH (1985) Protein-antigen specific Ia-restricted cytolytic T cells: analysis of frequency, target cell susceptibility and mechanism of cytolysis. J Immunol 135:25–33

Significance of T4 or T8 Phenotype of Human Cytotoxic T-Lymphocyte Clones

B. Fleischer and H. Wagner

1 Introduction   101
2 Functional Analysis of Human T-Lymphocyte Clones   101
3 Cytotoxicity of T4$^+$ T Lymphocytes Can Be Acquired   103
4 Absence of T4$^+$ CTL In Vivo   104
5 T4$^+$ CTL in Short-Term Assays   105
6 Conclusion   107
References   107

1 Introduction

Mature human T lymphocytes can be divided into two mutually exclusive sub-populations by monoclonal antibodies (mAb) to the T4 and T8 markers. On the basis of cell separation experiments, the helper function for B or T lymphocytes, the proliferative capacity to soluble antigens (tuberculin, tetanus toxoid) and to alloantigens has been assigned to the T4/Leu 3 subset, while cytotoxic and sup-pressor functions are associated with the T8/Leu 2 subset (Reinherz and Schlossman 1980; Engleman et al. 1981). Furthermore, T4$^+$ and T8$^+$ T-cell populations exhibit different specificity for either HLA class II or class I anti-gens, both as restriction elements or as target alloantigens. Improved culture conditions and the use of interleukin 2 (IL-2) as T-cell growth factor made it pos-sible to clone human T lymphocytes, enabling cloned T-cell populations to be used to analyze functions and specificities of various T-cell subsets at the single-cell level.

Surprisingly, it was soon realized that the majority of T4$^+$ T-lymphocyte *clones* (TLC) display cytotoxic activity (Moretta et al. 1981), in apparent con-tradiction to the correlation of surface phenotype and function previously ob-served in bulk cultures. In this paper we review our data and those from the literature to discuss the possible significance of the T4$^+$ or T8$^+$ phenotypes in relation to the cytotoxic function of human T lymphocytes.

2 Functional Analysis of Human T-Lymphocyte Clones

After the initial discovery of human CTL with the T4$^+$ phenotype by examina-tion of T cell lines (Krensky et al. 1982; Ball and Stastny 1982) and clones

Department of Medical Microbiology and Immunology, University of Ulm, D-7900 Ulm

Current Topics in Microbiology and Immunology, Vol. 126
© Springer-Verlag Berlin · Heidelberg 1986

102   B. Fleischer and H. Wagner

Table 1. Characteristics of human T4$^+$ and T8$^+$ CTL clones

	T4$^+$ CTL	T8$^+$ CTL
Growth	Antigen dependent	Il-2 dependent, antigen independent
Lytic activity	Mostly low	Always high
Il-2 production	All	Some
Proliferation to antigen	All	Some
Specificity	Mostly class II	Mostly class I

(MORETTA et al. 1981; PAWELEC et al. 1982; SPITS et al. 1982), it was soon realized that T4$^+$ cytotoxic T lymphocyte (CTL) clones were not exceptional but rather common. In some experimental situations even all CTL clones expressed the T4$^+$ phenotype. Exclusively T4$^+$ CTL clones were obtained if T cells were cloned, e.g., after in vitro restimulation with herpes simplex virus (YASUKAWA and ZARLING 1984) or measles virus (JACOBSON et al. 1984). All these clones recognized a class II HLA molecule as restriction element.

Similarly, class II specific T4$^+$ alloreactive T-cell populations could easily be obtained after several in vitro stimulations with stimulator cells sharing only a class II difference, e.g., HLA-DP, with the responder cells (SHAW et al. 1980). The cytotoxicity of these clones and populations could be blocked by mAb against the T4 molecule (BIDDISON et al. 1982). These observations led to the hypothesis (SWAIN 1983) that the T4 or T8 phenotype is associated with the recognition specificity for class II or class I HLA antigens, respectively, rather than with T-cell function. A current model suggests that the T4 or T8 molecules act as additional associate receptors, the ligands of which are the nonpolymorphic parts of the target cell's MHC molecules. This model was supported by the finding that mAb to the T4 or T8 antigen blocked conjugate formation between effector and target cells (BIDDISON et al. 1984).

On the other hand, CTL clones with the T8$^+$ phenotype have been isolated that are specific for the DQ1 determinant on the class I antigen negative Daudi cell line (KRENSKY et al. 1983) in contradiction to the model. Furthermore, class I alloantigen-specific T4$^+$ CTL clones were described (FLOMENBERG et al. 1983), and some of them could be inhibited by anti-T4 mAb (STRASSMAN and BACH 1984). The T4 and T8 phenotype overlap is likewise found with T suppressor-cell clones that can have either phenotype (MINGARI et al. 1982). These findings have led to the conclusion that T4 and T8 molecules are differentiation markers with no relationship to T-cell function and specificity (PAWELEC et al. 1983).

However, a comparison of the properties of T4$^+$ and T8$^+$ CTL clones reveals characteristic differences (Table 1). Though exceptions to all points can be found, the vast majority of clones described in the literature or observed by us clearly exhibit all the properties of one of these categories. Although restimulation is advantageous to maintain long-term growth of T8$^+$ CTL clones, these clones usually grow in medium containing IL-2 alone and do not require antigenic stimulation as opposed by most T4$^+$ CTL clones that do not grow in IL-2 alone for longer than 1 or 2 weeks. Essentially all T4$^+$ CTL clones described so far show proliferative responses in short-term assays to their specific target cells, whereas this is only found with the so-called helper-independent type of T8$^+$ CTL (WEE et al. 1982). Strikingly, the lytic activity of most T4$^+$ CTL is relatively weak, i.e., effector-to-target cell ratios of 10:1 or higher are required for effective lysis. All T8$^+$ CTL we have observed are highly efficient killer cells, bringing about 60%–80% specific lysis at effector-to-target cell ratios of 1 or less. If CTL clones are generated from MLR with class I and class II disparity or after stimulation with the autologous EBV line, T8$^+$ CTL clones are generally class I specific, whereas T4$^+$ CTL clones are specific for class II HLA antigens (MEUER et al. 1982; SPITS et al. 1985). It is interesting that exceptions to this rule are more easily found if the conditions of stimulation are varied. Class II specific T8$^+$ CTL clones are generated if purified T8$^+$ T cells are stimulated with Daudi cells (KRENSKY et al. 1983). Likewise T4$^+$ CTL clones specific for class I alloantigen are generated if T4$^+$ T cells are stimulated with a class I disparity (STRASSMANN and BACH 1984).

3 Cytotoxicity of T4$^+$ T Lymphocytes Can Be Acquired

The controversy described above was held initially under the assumption that phenotype, specificity, and function of clonally expanding T lymphocytes would be stable. However, it has become evident that under the conditions of in vitro cultivation this is not necessarily the case. Whereas, so far, the phenotype of T-cell clones seems to be stable in vitro, human T-cell clones have, e.g., been demonstrated to lose their proliferative capacity and to gain nonspecific suppressive activity (PAWELEC et al. this volume) or they may lose the capacity to produce IL-2 while maintaining other functions (our observation).

For the discussion here, it is relevant that T4$^+$ T-lymphocyte clones with antigen-specific proliferative activity can acquire cytotoxic function (FLEISCHER 1984). This cytotoxicity has the same specificity as the preexisting proliferative response, demonstrating that the new function is also directed and regulated by antigen recognition via the specific receptor. Clearly, acquisition of cytotoxicity is an event taking place within the progeny of a single T cell, as demonstrated by analysis of multiple subclones generated with high cloning efficiency and by the identical pattern of antigen and restriction specificity of preexisting proliferative capacity and acquired cytotoxicity. The proliferative response is not lost upon acquisition of the new function, nor is the phenotype changed. Upon extended cultivation, which in our hands is not limited generally by 30 population doublings (PAWELEC et al. 1983), the cytotoxic activity increases, demonstrated by increased percentage of lysis at constant effector-to-target cell ratios (Fig. 1), though never reaching the efficacy of T8$^+$ CTL clones.

Acquisition of cytotoxic function is not confined to T cells of certain specificity, but can be found with alloreactive PLT clones, with antiviral, class II restricted T8$^+$ clones, and with T4$^+$ lymphocytes specific for soluble antigens such as PPD. It can be found in T lymphocytes activated in vitro by alloantigen or mitogen as well as in T cells activated in vivo, derived and cloned, e.g., directly from

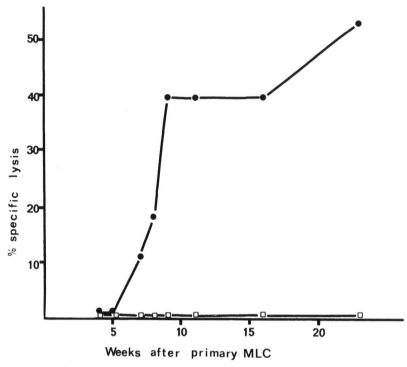

Fig. 1. Development of cytotoxic activity in a T4$^+$8$^-$ alloreactive T-lymphocyte clone. T cells were stimulated in a primary MLC and after 10 days in a secondary MLC. Cloning was performed 4 days after secondary MLC. Clones showing specific proliferative response to stimulator cells were tested for specific cytotoxicity against the stimulator B-LCL cells (●) and the autologous B-LCL cells (□) at various intervals after cloning. Effector to target cell ratio was 5:1 in each assay

the cerebrospinal fluid of patients with infections of the central nervous system (FLEISCHER and BOGDAHN 1983). In our hands, this acquisition is a frequent event, taking place in most experiments in every T4$^+$ T-lymphocyte clone, though at various intervals after cloning. These T4$^+$ clones studied in detail so far all had the capacity to produce IL-2.

Obviously, T4$^+$ T lymphocytes are not terminally differentiated, but have the capacity to express new functional activities. The signals involved in inducing the functional changes remain to be defined. Though our cloning conditions might select for certain subsets of T4$^+$ T lymphocytes, at least in these cells the functional change seems to be invariably programmed.

4 Absence of T4$^+$ CTL In Vivo

The unexpected functional flexibility of T lymphocytes may have important implications for an ongoing immune response. With some of the functional

Table 2. In situ cytotoxic T-cell response to Epstein-Barr virus in infectious mononucleosis

A. Inhibition of cytotoxicity against the autologous B-cell line by monoclonal antibodies

	Inhibition (%)
Anti-class I	73
Anti-class II	0
Anti-T8	98
Anti-T4	2

B. Cytotoxicity in T-cell subsets

$T8^+4^-$ fraction	20% specific lysis (10:1)
$T4^+8^-$ fraction	0% specific lysis (20:1)

A. Without prior in vitro cultivation, T cells from infectious mononucleosis tonsils were purified by E-rosetting and used in a cytotoxicity assay against autologous EBV-transformed B-cell blasts. B. T cells from infectious mononucleosis tonsils were separated in T-cell subsets using fluorescence-activated cell sorting

alterations observed in vitro, however, it is impossible to assess their impact in an immune reaction in vivo, e.g., loss of proliferative activity and gain of natural killer function (PAWELEC et al. 1983). However, since the acquisition of cytotoxic function by a priori noncytotoxic $T4^+$ T lymphocytes is a frequent event in vitro, it should be possible to detect $T4^+$ CTL in vivo.

Only few experiments with primary, in vivo activated human T cells have been reported. In the peripheral blood of patients with acute mumps infection, virus-specific CTL can be found that are restricted by class I HLA antigens and not by HLA-DR antigens (KRETH et al. 1982). Since PHA blasts were used as target cells in these experiments, class II antigen expression on the targets might not be sufficient to detect class II restricted $T4^+$ CTL. Furthermore, in vivo most infected cells may not express class II antigens and therefore precursors of $T4^+$ CTL may not be appropriately expanded. However, the target cells in Epstein-Barr virus infections, the transformed B lymphocytes express abundant class II HLA antigens and therefore should stimulate class II restricted $T4^+$ CTL as well as class I restricted $T8^+$ CTL. Since in infectious mononucleosis the high NK activity in the peripheral blood seems to mask specific CTL activity (SEELEY et al. 1981), we have studied the phenotype and restriction specificity of CTL present in tonsils of acutely infected patients (Table 2). Clearly, at least the majority of CTL present in situ has the $T8^+4^-$ phenotype and is specific for class I HLA antigens as restriction elements. Although both $T4^+$ and $T8^+$ T lymphocytes in situ were activated and expressed IL-2 receptors, cytotoxicity could not be detected in the $T4^+$ fraction.

5 $T4^+$ CTL in Short-Term Assays

The initial assignment of cytotoxic and noncytotoxic capacities to the two phenotypically different major $T4^+$ or $T8^+$ subsets was performed on the basis of separation either before or after in vitro stimulation. If unseparated T lymphocytes from the peripheral blood of normal individuals were separated after a primary MLR, the entire cytotoxic activity resided in the T4⁻ fraction (REINHERZ et al. 1979). Interestingly, if T4⁺ T lymphocytes were stimulated in the absence of T8⁺ T lymphocytes in MLR, significant, although low cytotoxicity could be detected with these responder cells (REINHERZ et al. 1979). In MLR with only class II disparity between responder and stimulator cells, class II specific CTL can be detected only in a minority of cases (BREUNING et al. 1984). The generation of T4⁺ CTL against HLA-DP (former HLA-SB) class II antigens has been extensively investigated. Usually, several restimulations are required to obtain these effector cells (SHAW et al. 1980).

Human secondary antiviral CTL are generally T8⁺ and are restricted by HLA class I antigens (BIDDISON 1980). This has been extensively studied in the influenza virus system (BIDDISON 1980; BIDDISON et al. 1981; MCMICHAEL 1980), but also with mumps and herpes simplex virus (KRESS and KRETH 1982; YASUKAWA et al. 1983). Again, it could be argued that PHA blasts, used as target cells, express little class II antigen and therefore might not be susceptible to lysis by class II restricted T4⁺ CTL. However, the in vitro secondary CTL response against Epstein-Barr virus has been extensively studied, with target cells expressing as much class I as class II HLA antigens. If stimulating conditions are used that only generate the specific CTL response and not the NK-like effector cells, cytotoxicity generated in short-term cultures is only restricted by class I HLA antigens as demonstrated by segregation analysis (MOSS et al. 1981) and blocking with monoclonal antibodies (WALLACE et al. 1981). The effector cells have the T8⁺ phenotype (ZARLING et al. 1981). If, however, Epstein-Barr virus-specific CTL *clones* are generated, cytotoxic clones with either T8⁺ or T4⁺ phenotype will be found, restricted by class I or class II HLA antigens, respectively (MEUER et al. 1983). Surprisingly, 90%–100% of the EBV-specific T4⁺ colonies have cytotoxic activity (MEUER et al. 1983; MISKO et al. 1984).

Cytotoxic T-cell responses can also be generated in vitro against the soluble antigen tuberculin (PPD) in donors showing strong proliferative responses to PPD (HANK and SONDEL 1982). The effector cells are T4⁺ and are restricted by class II antigens (HANSEN et al. 1984).

Taken together, these data show that T4⁺ CTL can be detected in short-term in vitro bulk cultures (Table 3). Apparently, however, this is only possible under conditions in which maximal stimulation and lymphokine production occurs (e.g., the usually vigorous response to PPD or to secondary allostimulation) or under conditions of low IL-2 consumption, if T8⁺ cells are not present or not stimulated. This may indicate that the concentrations of antigen and/or lymphokines in these cultures are critical for the generation of cytotoxic function in the T4⁺ fraction.

These bulk culture experiments allow only a rough estimate of the frequency of CTL in the T4⁺ subpopulation. Recently, by limiting dilution analysis, the frequency of T4⁺ CTL in peripheral blood T lymphocytes after polyclonal activation was determined (MORETTA 1983). Under conditions that allow growth of every human T cell, virtually every T8⁺ T lymphocyte gave rise to a CTL, whereas less than 3% of the T4⁺ cells were CTL precursors. Even when considering

Significance of T4 or T8 Phenotype of Human Cytotoxic T-Lymphocyte Clones   107

Table 3. Detection of T4$^+$ cytotoxic T lymphocytes after activation of human T cells

Mode of activation of resting T lymphocytes	Presence of T4$^+$ CTL
Primary in vivo responses	–
Primary MLC (class I and class II disparity)	–
Primary MLC (class II disparity only)	+/–
Primary MLC (T4$^+$ responder only)	+
Secondary MLC (class II disparity)	++
In vitro secondary antiviral responses	–
In vitro secondary stimulation with PPD	+/++
Limiting dilution	3%
Cloning after in vitro stimulation	50%–100%

this low frequency of CTL in the T4$^+$ fraction, it should be kept in mind that it has been determined under optimal stimulation of the T cells with mitogen and feeder cells and with IL-2 and other lymphokines present in great excess in the cultures.

6   Conclusion

Obviously, analysis of human T lymphocytes directly in vivo or after short-term culture in vitro shows a correlation between phenotype (T8 vs T4), function (cytotoxic vs noncytotoxic) and MH specificity (class I vs class II HLA antigens). If T cells are grown in long-term culture, the correlation of phenotype and the recognition of MHC class (SWAIN 1983) is still the rule. With increasing time of cultivation, however, correlation is no more valid for the T4$^+$ phenotype and absence of cytotoxic function. Though it is striking that the longer T4$^+$ cells are cultivated, the more easily cytotoxicity is generated, it is impossible to assess to what extent cytotoxicity in T4$^+$ T lymphocytes is acquired or due to selective activation and/or preferential expansion from infrequent T4$^+$ CTL precursors. In view of the common characteristics of most T4$^+$ CTL clones described in the literature and those that have acquired their cytotoxic function (Table 1), it is tempting to assume that at least the majority of T4$^+$ CTL are derived from a priori noncytotoxic precursor cells.

It is obvious from the data reviewed here, that this capacity to gain this new functional activity is rarely or not at all realized in vivo. A possible in vivo relevance of similar in vitro alterations of T-lymphocyte behavior might therefore be considered with caution.

References

Ball EJ, Stastny P (1982) Cell-mediated cytotoxicity against HLA-D region products expressed in monocytes and B lymphocytes. IV. Characterization of effector cells using monoclonal antibodies against human T cell subsets. Immunogenetics 16:159–169

108   B. Fleischer and H. Wagner

Biddison WE (1980) The role of the human major histocompatibility complex in cytotoxic T cell responeses to virus infected cells. J Clin Immunol 2:1–9

Biddison WE, Sharrow SO, Shearer GM (1981) T cell subpopulations required for the human cytotoxic T cell response to influenza virus-infected cells: evidence for T cell help. J Immunol 127:487–491

Biddison WE, Rao PE, Talle MA, Goldstein G, Shaw S (1982) Possible involvement of the OKT 4 molecule in T cell recognition of class II HLA antigens: evidence from studies of cytotoxic T lymphocytes specific for SB antigens. J Exp Med 156:1065–1076

Biddison WE, Rao PE, Talle MA, Goldstein G, Shaw S (1984) Possible involvement of the T4 molecule in T cell recognition of class II HLA antigens: evidence from studies of CTL-target binding. J Exp Med 159:783–797

Breuning MH, Beur BS, Engelsma MY, Ivanyi P (1984) Activation of cytotoxic T lymphocytes in HLA-A, -B and -C identical responder-stimulator pairs. I. Variation in generation of anti-class II CTL in primary mixed lymphocyte cultures. Tissue Antigens 24:81–89

Engleman EG, Benike CJ, Grumet FC, Evans RL (1981) Activation of human T lymphocyte subsets: helper and suppressor/cytotoxic T cells recognize and respond to distinct histocompatibility antigens. J Immunol 127:2124–2129

Fleischer B (1984) Acquisition of specific cytotoxic activity by human T4+ lymphocytes in culture. Nature 308:365–367

Fleischer B, Bogdahn U (1983) Growth of antigen-specific HLA-restricted T lymphocyte clones from cerebrospinal fluid. Clin Exp Immunol 52:38–44

Flomenberg N, Naito V, Duffy E, Knowles RW, Evans RL, Dupont B (1983) Allocytotoxic T cell clones: both Leu2+3– and Leu2–3+ T cells recognize class I histocompatibility antigens. Eur J Immunol 11:905–911

Hank JA, Sondel PM (1982) Soluble bacterial antigen induces specific helper and cytotoxic responses by human lymphocytes in vitro. J Immunol 128:2734–2738

Hansen PW, Madsen M, Christiansen SE, Johnsen HE, Kissmeyer-Nielsen F (1984) Cell mediated PPD specific cytotoxicity against human monocyte targets: evidence for restriction by class II HLA antigens. Tissue Antigens 23:171–180

Jacobson S, Richert JR, Biddison WE, Satinsky A, Hartzman RJ, McFarland HF (1984) Measles virus-specific T4+ human cytotoxic T cell clones are restricted by class II HLA antigens. J Immunol 132:754–758

Krensky AM, Reiss CS, Mier JW, Strominger JL, Burakoff SJ (1982) Long-term cytotoxic T cell lines allospecific for HLA-DR6 antigen are OKT4+. Proc Natl Acad Sci USA 79:2365–2369

Krensky AM, Clayberger C, Greenstein JL, Crimmins M, Burakoff SJ (1983) A DC-specific cytotoxic T lymphocyte line is OKT8+. J Immunol 131:2777–2780

Kress HG, Kreth HW (1982) HLA restriction of human secondary mumps virus-specific cytotoxic T lymphocytes. J Immunol 129:844–849

Kreth HW, Kress L, Kress HG, Ott HF, Eckert G (1982) Demonstration of primary cytotoxic T cells in venous blood and cerebrospinal fluid of children with mumps meningitis. J Immunol 128:2411–2414

McMichael AJ (1980) HLA restriction of human cytotoxic T lymphocytes. Sem Immunol Immunopathol 3:3–22

Meuer SC, Schlossman SF, Reinherz EL (1982) Clonal analysis of human cytotoxic T lymphocyte: T4+ and T8+ effector T cells recognize products of different major histocompatibility complex regions. Proc Natl Acad Sci USA 79:4395–4399

Meuer SC, Hogdon JC, Cooper DA, Hussey RE, Fitzgerald KA, Schlossman SF, Reinherz EL (1983) Human cytotoxic T cell clones directed at autologous virus-transformed targets: further evidence for lineage of genetic restriction to T4 and T8 surface glycoproteins. J Immunol 131:186–190

Mingari MC, Melioli G, Moretta A, Pantaleo G, Moretta L (1982) Surface markers of cloned human T cells with helper or suppressor activity on pokeweed mitogen-driven B cell differentiation. Eur J Immunol 12:900–904

Misko IS, Pope JM, Hütter R, Soszynski TD, Kane RG (1984) HLA-DR antigen-associated restriction of EBV-specific cytotoxic T cell colonies. Int J Cancer 33:239–243

Moretta A (1983) Frequency and surface phenotype of human T lymphocytes producing interleukin 2. Analysis by limiting dilution and cell cloning. Eur J Immunol 15:148–155

Significance of T4 or T8 Phenotype of Human Cytotoxic T-Lymphocyte Clones 109

Moretta L, Mingavi MC, Sekaly PR, Moretta A, Chapuis B, Cerottini JC (1981) Surface markers of cloned human T cells with various cytolytic activities. J Exp Med 154:569–574

Moss DJ, Wallace LE, Rickinson AB, Epstein MA (1981) Cytotoxic T cell recognition of Epstein-Barr virus-infected B cells. Specificity and HLA restriction of effector cells reactivated in vitro. Eur J Immunol 11:686–693

Pawelec G, Kahle P, Wernet P (1982) Specificity spectrum and cell surface markers of mono- and multi-functional mixed leukocyte culture-derived T cell clones in man. Eur J Immunol 12:607–615

Pawelec G, Schneider EM, Wernet P (1983) Human T cell clones with multiple and changing functions: indications of unexpected flexibility in immune response networks. Immunol Today 4:275–278

Pawelec G, Busch FW, Schneider EM, Rehbein A, Balko T, Wernet P (1985) Acquisition of suppressive and natural killer-like activities associated with loss of alloreactivity in human "helper" T lymphocyte clones. Curr Top Microbiol Immunol (this volume)

Reinherz EL, Schlossman SF (1980) The differentiation and function of human T lymphocytes. Cell 19:821–824

Reinherz EL, Kung PC, Goldstein G, Schlossman SF (1979) Separation of functional subsets defined of human T cells by a monoclonal antibody. Proc Natl Acad Sci USA 76:4061–4066

Seeley J, Svedmyr E, Weiland O, Klein G, Möller E, Erikson E, Andersson K, van der Waal L (1981) Epstein Barr virus selective T cells in infectious mononucleosis are not restricted to HLA-A and -B antigens. J Immunol 127:293–300

Shaw S, Johnson AH, Shearer GM (1980) Evidence for a new segregant series of B cell antigens that are encoded in the HLA-D region and that stimulate secondary allogeneic proliferative and cytotoxic responses. J Exp Med 152:565–580

Spits H, Yssel H, Terhorst C, de Vries JE (1982) Establishment of human T lymphocyte clones highly cytotoxic for an EBV-transformed B cell line in serum-free medium: isolation of clones that differ in phenotype and specificity. J Immunol 128:95–99

Spits H, Yssel H, Voordouw A, de Vries JE (1985) The role of T8 in the cytotoxic activity of cloned cytotoxic T lymphocyte lines specific for class II and class I major complex antigens. J Immunol 134:2294–2298

Strassman G, Bach FH (1984) OKT4+ cytotoxic T cells can be blocked by monoclonal antibody against T4 molecules. J Immunol 133:1705–1709

Swain SL (1983) T cell subsets and the recognition of MHC class. Immunol Rev 74:129–142

Wallace LE, Moss D, Rickinson AB, McMichael AJ, Epstein MA (1981) Cytotoxic T cell recognition of Epstein-Barr virus-infected B cells. II. Blocking studies with monoclonal antibodies to HLA determinants. Eur J Immunol 11:694–699

Wee SL, Chen LK, Strassman G, Bach FH (1982) Helper cell independent cytotoxic cells in man. J Exp Med 156:1854–1859

Yasukawa M, Zarling JM (1984) Human cytotoxic T lymphocyte clones directed against herpes simplex virus-infected cells. I. Lysis restricted by HLA class II MB or DR antigens. J Immunol 133:422–428

Yasukawa M, Shiroguchi T, Kobayashi Y (1983) HLA-restricted T lymphocyte-mediated cytotoxicity against herpes simplex virus-infected cells in humans. Infect Immun 40:190–197

Zarling JM, Dierckins MS, Sevenich EA, Clouse KA (1981) Stimulation with autologous lymphoblastoid cell lines: lysis of EBV-positive and -negative cell lines by two phenotypically distinguishable effector cell populations. J Immunol 127:2118–2123

Natural and Unnatural Killing by Cytolytic T Lymphocytes

K. SHORTMAN and A. WILSON

1 Introduction 111
2 Kinetics of Development of "Nonspecific" Cytolysis by CTL Clones in Limit-Dilution Culture 112
3 Clone-Splitting Analysis of Specificity 112
4 Nature of Nonspecific Cytolytic Process 113
5 Nature of the Effector Cells 113
6 Origin of the Effector Cells 114
7 Nature of the Target Cell 114
8 Cold-Target Inhibition Analysis of Recognition Patterns 115
9 Mouse Strain Differences in Expression of the Two Recognition Systems 115
10 Conclusions 117
References 118

1 Introduction

Cytolytic T lymphocytes (CTL) are armed with an effective mechanism for killing target cells. Delivery of the lethal hit involves target cell recognition and conjugate formation, and is normally a highly specific process dependent on the clonally distributed, antigen-specific, and MHC-restricted T-cell receptor. The selective aspect of the recognition stage may be bypassed by adding to the cytotoxic assay a lectin (such as phytohemagglutinin [PHA] or concanavalin A [Con A]), in which case CTL will kill most target cells susceptible to the lethal hit mechanism. Until recently this seemed the only way the specificity of the T-cell receptor could be bypassed. However, there are now numerous reports of circumstances where cultured clones of mouse, rat, and human CTL lose specificity, and generally behave as if some lectin had been added to promote killing of a wide range of target cells (SHORTMAN et al. 1983; BROOKS 1983; BROOKS et al. 1983; SIMON et al. 1984; TEH and YU 1983; BINZ et al. 1983; MASUCCI et al. 1980; SANTOLI et al. 1981; TORIBIO et al. 1983; MORETTA et al. 1984; VAN DE GRIEND et al. 1984; BURNS et al. 1984). This report summarizes our analysis of the "unnatural" or "nonspecific" killing by murine CTL, which leads us to the conclusion that two different "broad specificity" receptors may be expressed when CTL develop in culture, additional to the clonally distributed antigen-specific T-cell receptor.

Walter and Eliza Hall Institute of Medical Research, Post Office, Royal Melbourne Hospital, Victoria 3050, Australia

2 Kinetics of Development of "Nonspecific" Cytolysis by CTL Clones in Limit-Dilution Culture

Our results are derived, not from long-term CTL clones, but from limit-dilution culture of normal murine spleen or lymphnode cells, or of sorted Ly-2$^+$ T cells. These are cultured at the level of one T cell per well, in the presence of irradiated spleen filler cells, and are stimulated nonspecifically with Con A. The irradiated filler cells provide most of the growth and differentiation factors needed to maintain clonal expansion for around 9 days; a supplement of a supernatant from Con A stimulated spleen cells is added as well to maintain high cloning efficiency, but is not essential to obtain the findings reported. The cloning efficiency of this system is very high, 70%–95% of all Ly-2$^+$ T cells forming a cytolytic T-cell clone that can be detected in a nonspecific test for cytolytic capacity; this test is usually the PHA-mediated release of ^{111}In from labeled tumor target cells, as detected in a radioautographic assay (WILSON et al. 1982; SHORTMAN and WILSON 1981).

The development of "nonspecific" cytotoxicity can be followed by measuring the incidence of cultures showing direct cytolysis of a tumor target cell, and comparing this to the total incidence of cytolytic cultures measured by lectin-mediated lysis of the same target (SHORTMAN et al. 1984). This is shown in the upper half of Fig. 1, where CBA spleen cells are cultured for various times and assayed on P815 in the presence or in the absence of PHA. At early time points (day 5 or 6) the frequency of clones showing lectin-mediated cytolysis of P815 is 10 to 50 times the frequency of clones showing direct cytolysis of P815. We assume the incidence of k anti-d CTL clones is 0.02 – 0.10 of all CTL clones and that at this point the clones are mainly specific. However, the incidence of clones showing direct cytolysis rises rapidly from day 7, and by day 8–9 most (and sometimes all) CTL clones lyse P815. Since virtually all CTL clones show this phenomenon we have sometimes abandoned clonal analysis at this point, and pooled many hundred cultures to provide enough nonspecific CTL for detailed analysis.

3 Clone-Splitting Analysis of Specificity

These conclusions concerning lytic specificity or nonspecificity, based on the + or – PHA assay, may be checked in a more direct way by splitting cultures into two and assaying on pairs of target cells (SHORTMAN et al. 1984). Examples are given in Table 1. CTL clones in cultures harvested at early time points lyse only one of a given pair of tumor targets, whereas most cultures at day 8 or 9 lyse both members of the pair. It is important to note that the NK target YAC-1 and the non-NK target P815 are *both* lysed by the *same* nonspecific CTL clones derived from 9-day culture of Ly-2$^+$ T cells (Shortman and Wilson, in preparation).

A clone-splitting and reculture approach may also be used to show that the early, specific clones give rise to late, "nonspecific" clones, eliminating the possibility that the two represent independent lineages with separate precursors (SHORTMAN et al. 1984).

Table 1. Split-culture assays for specificity of CTL clones

		Day 6	Day 9
CBA	Total cultures	1056	1056
	Positive on P815	5	72
	Positive on EL4	6	71
	Positive on both P815 and EL4	0	51
	Expected double positives by chance coincidence	0	5
C57BL/6	Total cultures	1056	1152
	Positive on P815	16	90
	Positive on EL4	1	150
	Positive on both P815 and EL4	0	72
	Expected double positives by chance coincidence	0	12

Cultures of CBA or C57BL/6 spleen cells were set up at low responder cell input to reduce coincidence, and split at day 6 or day 9 for separate assay on ^{111}In-labeled P815 or EL4. The results are from SHORTMAN et al. (1984)

4 Nature of the Nonspecific Cytolytic Process

Certain trivial explanations for the direct cytolysis can readily be eliminated (SHORTMAN et al. 1983, 1984). Lysis is not mediated by carry-over of the Con A used to initiate the cultures, as shown by the absence of any blocking by α-methylmannoside. Lysis is not just due to the "cross-reactivity" from an exceptionally high CTL level in the late clones, since the ratio of direct to lectin-mediated lysis is constant with dilution of the effector cell level. Lysis is not mediated by a soluble factor, and is subject to cold-target inhibition. Overall, "nonspecific" killing seems to be a cell-mediated process analogous to normal, specific CTL killing.

5 Nature of the Effector Cells

Morphologically the cells in the nonspecific clones are all large, vacuolated, granular lymphocytes (SHORTMAN et al. 1983; WILSON et al. 1984). Initially this was surprising, since the appearance resembled that of NK cells. However, it is now apparent that cultured CTL often acquire granularity, and this appearance is quite independent of whether the cells are nonspecific or specific (WILSON et al. 1984).

The surface antigenic phenotype of the cells in the CTL clones, and the cells responsible for nonspecific cytolysis, is exactly that expected of normal CTL, namely H-2$^+$ Thy-1$^+$ Ly-2$^+$ L3T4$^-$ (SHORTMAN et al. 1984).

The DNA content and chromosome count of the effector cells is that of normal, dividing murine cells; there is no evidence that nonspecificity is the consequence of polyploidy, or of any of the abnormal cell changes at the DNA level that may be encountered with CTL lines (SHORTMAN et al. 1984; WILSON et al. 1984).

However, nonspecific CTL do appear to be somewhat larger than the average CTL. "Nonspecific" cytolysis of both P815 and YAC-1 is concentrated in the third-largest cells as separated on the basis of low-angle light scatter, whereas lectin-mediated lysis is more evenly distributed over all sizes of cells. Thus, it seems that clones are heterogeneous in capacity for nonspecific cytolysis, only the largest cells showing this effect (Shortman and Wilson, in preparation).

6 Origin of the Effector Cells

Limit-dilution analysis may be used to show that clones of nonspecific CTL are initiated by a single precursor cell, just as are clones of specific CTL. This precursor can be shown, using fluorescence activated cell sorting or cytotoxic procedures, to be a typical, mature, Thy-1$^+$ Ly-2$^+$ L3T4$^-$, T cell (SHORTMAN et al. 1984). The effector cells derive from this single precursor and not from the large excess of irradiated filler cells; this has been shown by growing precursor T cells from one mouse strain on irradiated filler cells derived from another strain differing in Thy-1 allotype, or in H-2 haplotype, then typing the effector cells prior to assay (SHORTMAN et al. 1984). Thus, both precursor and effector cell analysis demonstrates that this anomalous killing is carried out by members of the normal Ly-2$^+$ L3T4$^-$ cytolytic T-cell lineage, and not by some special class of NK cells.

7 Nature of the Target Cell

Are Syngeneic Targets Killed? The nonspecific CTL seem to show no preference for allogeneic as opposed to syngeneic targets. Thus, with cultures from CBA mice the syngeneic tumor R1 is killed, and with cultures of C57BL/6 mice the syngeneic tumor EL4 is killed (SHORTMAN et al. 1983; WILSON and SHORTMAN 1984).

Are Normal Mouse Target Cells Killed? Nonspecific killing is not confined to tumor targets. B-cell blasts (generated by lipopolysaccharide stimulation in culture), T-cell blasts (generated by Con A stimulation in culture), and macrophages (peritoneal exudate cells) are all killed, irrespective of whether they are syngeneic or allogeneic (SHORTMAN et al. 1983; Wilson and Shortman, in preparation).

Are Xenogeneic Target Cells Killed? Of four different human tumor lines which have been tested, none are lysed by nonspecific murine CTL. Two rat tumor cells show only a small degree of lysis in the standard assay. However, several of the xenogeneic lines resistant to lysis nevertheless give cold-target inhibition of the lysis of murine tumor targets, suggesting the xenogeneic targets do present some structure recognized by the nonspecific CTL (Wilson and Shortman, in preparation).

Is Target Cell H-2 Involved? Several lines of evidence suggest that, in contrast to specific killing by CTL, neither surface H-2 nor other MHC antigens are involved in the recognition stage of nonspecific killing by CTL. R1-TL$^-$, a β_2-microglobulin negative and thus H-2 negative variant of the tumor R1 (HYMAN and STALLINGS 1977) is lysed as effectively as the H-2 positive parent line. Although several other H-2 negative murine cell lines are more resistant to lysis, they nevertheless give good cold-target inhibition of lysis of targets such as P815. Thus, even here the lack of surface H-2 had not prevented the initial recognition event, and resistance to lysis presumably represents a limitation at some later stage of the process (SHORTMAN et al. 1983; Wilson and Shortman, in preparation). In line with this observation, nonspecific cytolysis is not blocked by monoclonal anti-Ly-2, in contrast to specific killing by CTL (SHORTMAN et al. 1983).

8 Cold-Target Inhibition Analysis of Recognition Patterns

Most murine target cells cold-target inhibit not only their own lysis, but (to varying degrees) inhibit the lysis of other target cells as well. This suggests that nonspecific CTL have common recognition systems that serve for a range of different target cells. However, the murine tumors YAC-1 (the normal NK target) and P815 (not an NK target) show only limited cross-inhibition, although each of them cold-target inhibit both its own lysis and the lysis of certain other targets, such as EL4 (Wilson and Shortman, in preparation). An example is given in Fig. 2. This difference between recognition of YAC-1 and P815 can also be detected in inhibition studies using the human cell lines K562 and HL60 (Wilson and Shortman, in preparation). Even though these xenogeneic tumors are not lysed by "nonspecific" murine CTL, they nevertheless show selective cold-target inhibition. Thus, the human NK target K562 inhibits lysis by "nonspecific" murine CTL of the murine NK target YAC-1, but not the lysis of P815, whereas HL60 behaves in the converse manner inhibiting lysis of P815, but not the lysis of YAC-1 (Wilson and Shortman, in preparation). The overall conclusion is that "nonspecific" CTL from CBA mice express (in each clone) two distinct broad-specificity recognition systems, one NK-like and one not.

9 Mouse Strain Differences in Expression of the Two Recognition Systems

The loss of CTL-clone specificity, so marked in our CBA and C57BL/6 mice, is not always observed when we culture Ly-2$^+$ cells from other mouse strains. For example, BALB/c spleen cells fail to develop a capacity for direct lysis of P815 (as shown in Fig. 1) or of EL4 (Table 2). However, CTL clones derived from BALB/c mice do develop a capacity to lyse YAC-1 (Table 2), demonstrating that

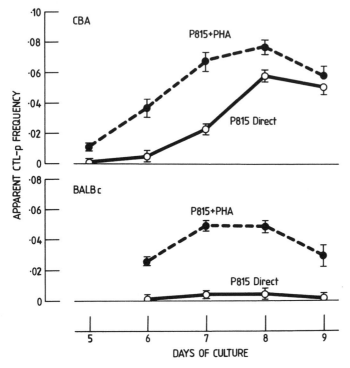

Fig. 1. The kinetics of development of all cytolytic clones and of nonspecific cytolytic clones in Con A stimulated, irradiated filler cell supported, limit-dilution cultures. The data are derived from SHORTMAN et al. (1984); WILSON and SHORTMAN (1984). Limit dilution cultures were set up at levels around 5–10 responder spleen cells per well. Assay for incidence of all cytolytic clones was by ^{111}In release from labeled P815 target cells in the presence of PHA. Assay for the incidence of directly cytolytic clones, mainly nonspecific in the case of CBA cultures, was on the same target cell in the absence of lectin

one of the two broad-specificity recognition systems may be acquired independently of the other (Shortman and Wilson, in preparation).

The ability of cultured CTL clones from different mouse strains to lyse P815, EL4, and YAC-1 is summarized in Table 2, and compared with the NK status of the mouse strain (measured as the ability of uncultured spleen cells to lyse YAC-1 in a 6- to 12-h assay). Some mice produce CTL that become "nonspecific" and lyse all targets (e.g., CBA, C57BL/6), some that remain specific and lyse none (e.g., C57BL/6 bge), while others show loss of specificity towards one, but not the other (e.g., BALB/c). The interesting point from this comparison is that the NK-positive strains develop CTL clones with the ability to lyse the NK target YAC-1, and the NK-negative strains do not. There is no consistent correlation between NK status and the ability of CTL clones to lyse P815. This suggests a strong relationship between NK cells and CTL, both having a YAC-1 recognition receptor under similar genetic control.

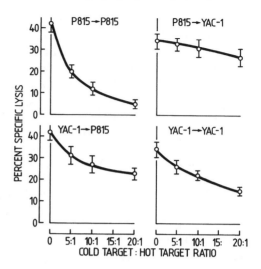

Fig. 2. Limited cross-inhibition between P815 and YAC-1 in cold-target inhibition experiments. Data are from Wilson and Shortman (in preparation). Pooled day 9 CTL clones from limit-dilution culture of Ly-2$^+$ CBA lymphnode T cells were assayed at 5:1 (P815) or 20:1 (YAC-1) effector-to-target ratio, on ^{111}In-labeled tumor targets. In parallel experiments both P815 and YAC-1 caused extensive cold-target inhibition of the lysis of certain third-party target cells, such as EL4

Table 2. Correlation of the NK status of different mouse strains with the propensity to develop "nonspecific" CTL in culture

Strain	H-2	NK STATUS YAC-1 target	Nonspecific cytolysis by CTL clones		
			YAC-1 target	EL-4 target	P815 target
CBA	k	++	++	++	++
AKR	k	+	+	+	+
BALB/c	d	+	+	−	−
DBA	d	−	−	±	±
C57BL/6	b	+	+	++	++
C57BL/6 bge	b	−	−	−	−
A/J	K^{k}D^d	−	−	±	+

The data are summarized from WILSON and SHORTMAN (1984) and Shortman and Wilson (in preparation). NK status was assessed on uncultured spleen cells by a 12-h assay, 50:1 effector:target ratio, on YAC-1. Code: ++, >50%, +, 5%–50%, −, <2%, specific lysis. Nonspecific cytolysis of CTL clones was assessed after a 9-day limit-dilution culture of spleen cells, by comparing the frequency of clones giving direct cytolysis (no PHA present) with the frequency of clones revealed by lectin-enhanced cytolysis of the same target (PHA present).

Code: −, $\frac{+ \text{PHA}}{- \text{PHA}}$ ratio of 10 or more; ±, $\frac{+ \text{PHA}}{- \text{PHA}}$ ratio of 5–10;

+, $\frac{+ \text{PHA}}{- \text{PHA}}$ ratio of 1–5   ++, $\frac{+ \text{PHA}}{- \text{PHA}}$ ratio of 1–3 and extensive cytolysis by most positive clones

10 Conclusions

This line of investigation leads to the conclusion that CTL clones may acquire, as well as the specific T-cell receptor, one or another or both of two different "broad-specificity" recognition systems. One of these recognition systems is NK-like and directed to target structures typical of YAC-1, while the other is distinct from that of NK cells and directed to target structures typical of P815. The almost total "nonspecificity" typical of cultured CBA or C57BL/6 CTL is actually a composite of the effects of these two broad-specificity systems occurring in the one clone. The "NK-like" receptor acquisition by CTL agrees with the studies of Brooks (Brooks 1983; Brooks et al. 1983) on long-term CTL clones, whereas the acquisition of the "P815 receptor" agrees with the "aged-killer cell" CTL-clone killing pattern reported by Simon et al. (1984).

These results present a caveat for the use of limit-dilution cytotoxic cultures to determine the frequency of precursor T cells with a given receptor specificity. It is evident that unless the development of these broad-specificity systems can be eliminated, the results must be considered suspect. Over the years the reported frequency of precursor T cells of certain specificities has been rising, often to embarrassing levels, as culture conditions and growth factor supplements improve. Some part of this rise in apparent precursor frequency has been the increased incidence of induction of "nonspecific" cytolysis by the CTL clones. The judicious choice of mouse strain, together with cold-target inhibition of the nonspecific effect with an appropriate cell, may overcome this problem.

The in vivo significance of this phenomenon of "broad-specificity" killing by CTL is not at all clear. The same might be said of NK cells. Since not all mouse strains readily exhibit the effect, one could argue that it cannot have an essential biological role. Is it entirely a culture artifact? At the target cell level we do have evidence that certain normal mouse cells (albeit activated cells) are potential targets for this sort of killing. As yet we have no evidence that the effector CTL bearing these broad-specificity receptors can be generated in the mouse; if they can we suspect it will only be under conditions where there is an intense and continuous stimulation of Ly-2$^+$ T cells by antigens and growth and differentiation factors. Such "broad-specificity" killing could represent an emergency system functioning only under extreme circumstances. Obviously it could also provide a ready explanation for certain types of immunopathology.

References

Binz H, Fenner M, Frei D, Wigzell H (1983) Two independent receptors allow selective target lysis by T cell clones. J Exp Med 157:1252–1260

Brooks CG (1983) Reversible induction of natural killer cell activity in cloned murine cytotoxic T lymphocytes. Nature 305:155–158

Brooks CG, Urdal DL, Henney CS (1983) Lymphokine-driven "differentiation" of cytotoxic T-cell clones into cells with NK-like specificity: correlations with display of membrane macromolecules. Immunol Rev 72:43–72

Burns GF, Triglia T, Werkmeister JA (1984) In vitro generation of human activated lymphocyte killer cells: separate precursors and modes of generation of NK-like cells and "anomolous" killer cells. J Immunol 133:1616–1663

Hyman R, Stallings V (1977) Analysis of hybrids between an H-2$^+$, TL$^-$ lymphoma and an H-2$^+$, TL$^+$ lymphoma and its H-2$^-$, TL$^-$ variant subline. Immunogenetics 4:171–181

Masucci G, Poros A, Seeley JK, Klein E (1980) In vitro generation of K562 killers in human T-lymphocyte subsets. Cell Immunol 52:247–254

Moretta A, Pantaleo G, Mingari MC, Melioli G, Morella L, Cerottini J-C (1984) Assignment of

Natural and Unnatural Killing by Cytolytic T Lymphocytes 119

human natural killer (NK-like) cells to the T cell lineage. Single allospecific T cell clones lyse specific or NK-sensitive target cells via distinct recognition structures. Eur J Immunol 14:121–131

Santoli D, Francis MK, Trucco M (1981) Phenotypic and functional characterization of allospecific and non-specific (NK- and K-like) cytotoxic T lymphocytes generated in human mixed-lymphocyte cultures from non-cytotoxic precursors. Cell Immunol 65:230–246

Shortman K, Wilson A (1981) A new assay for cytotoxic lymphocytes, based on a radioautographic readout of ^{111}In release, suitable for rapid, semiautomated assessment of limit-dilution cultures. J Immunol Methods 42:135–152

Shortman K, Wilson A, Scollay R, Chen W-F (1983) Development of large granular lymphocytes with anomalous, nonspecific cytotoxicity in clones derived from Ly-2$^+$ T cells. Proc Natl Acad Sci USA 80:2728–2732

Shortman K, Wilson A, Scollay R (1984) Loss of specificity in cytolytic T lymphocyte clones obtained by limit dilution culture of Ly-2$^+$ T cells. J Immunol 132:584–593

Simon MM, Weltzien HU, Buhring HJ, Eichmann K (1984) Aged murine killer T-cell clones acquire specific cytotoxicity for P815 mastocytoma cells. Nature 308:367–370

Teh H-S, Yu M (1983) Activation of nonspecific killer cells by interleukin 2-containing supernatants. J Immunol 131:1827–1833

Toribio ML, de Landazuri MO, Lopez-Botet M (1983) Induction of NK-like cytotoxicity in cultured human thymocytes. Eur J Immunol 13:964–969

van de Griend RJ, Giphart MJ, van Krimpen BA, Bolhuis RLH (1984) Human T cell clones exerting multiple cytolytic activities show heterogeneity in susceptibility to inhibition by monoclonal antibodies. J Immunol 133:1222–1229

Wilson A, Shortman K (1984) Degradation of specificity in cytolytic T lymphocyte clones: mouse strain dependence and interstrain transfer of nonspecific cytolysis. Eur J Immunol 14:951–956

Wilson A, Chen W-F, Scollay R, Shortman K (1982) Semi-automated limit-dilution assay and clonal expansion of all T cell precursors of cytotoxic lymphocytes. J Immunol Methods 52:283–306

Wilson A, Scollay R, Abbot AP, Shortman K (1984) Ly 2 positive cytotoxic T lymphocytes, whether specific or non-specific in lytic activity, may express a large granular, vacuolated lymphocyte morphology. Aust J Exp Biol Med Sci 62:381–401

Acquisition of Suppressive and Natural Killer-Like Activities Associated with Loss of Alloreactivity in Human "Helper" T-Lymphocyte Clones*

G. Pawelec, F.-W. Busch, E.M. Schneider, A. Rehbein, I. Balko, and P. Wernet

1 Characteristics of Alloproliferative Human T Cell Clones 121
2 Modulation of Function in Monoclonal T Cell Populations 121
References 128

1 Characteristics of Alloproliferative Human T Cell Clones

By cloning lymphocyte populations alloactivated in human mixed lymphocyte cultures (MLC), cell lines may be obtained which proliferate in primed lymphocyte typing (PLT) specifically against lymphocyte activating determinants (LADs) associated with different MHC class II gene products. Thus, PLT clones stimulated by HLA-DR, Dw, DQ, DP-like, or DP-associated determinants have been generated (Duquesnoy and Zeevi 1983; Pawelec 1983; Pawelec et al. 1984a). These clones generally carry a $T4^+$ $T8^-$ Leu-8$^-$ phenotype, secrete interleukin 2 (IL-2) on specific stimulation, are not cytotoxic (CTX) against allogeneic or autologous normal, or natural killer (NK)-susceptible, target cells, and the majority do not suppress MLC, PLT, immunoglobulin secretion, or granulocyte-macrophage colony formation (CFU-GM) by normal human bone marrow (BM) cells. In contrast, nonalloproliferative clones from MLC may strongly suppress in these systems, and the majoritiy of such suppressive clones also mediate NK-like CTX on leukemic target cells (Pawelec et al. 1982; Schneider et al. 1985; Falcioni et al. 1985).

2 Modulation of Function in Monoclonal T Cell Populations

It has been noted by several investigators (Malissen et al. 1981; Duquesnoy and Zeevi 1983; Effros and Walford 1984), and studied more fully by ourselves (Pawelec et al. 1984b; Pawelec and Wernet 1985), that the alloproliferative capacity of "helper" clones appears generally unstable, or less stable in culture than CTX or MHC + nominal antigen-specific clones. Indeed, clones with both alloproliferative and CTX activity may lose the former, with retention of the

---

Immunologisches Laboratorium, Medizinische Universitätsklinik, D-7400 Tübingen

* This work was supported in part by SFB 120:A1, A2, C2

latter, after a period in culture (von Boehmer et al. 1984; Wee et al. 1985). On the other hand, MHC class II restricted virus-specific proliferative clones may acquire specific lytic activity on in vitro culture (Fleischer 1984). In part, the apparently greater stability of CTX clones may reflect the selection of a small minority of those long-lived clones which could be used for extended studies. Exact details of longevity, retention of immunological specificity and function, and the proportion of "immortal" clones derived, are rather scarce in the literature (Effros and Walford 1984). Even in the case of CTX cells, there is now accumulating evidence for a high degree of heterogeneity within clonal populations, which may become apparent when culture conditions are modified, or may occur spontaneously. This is particularly the case when periodic restimulation with specific antigen is foregone, and cells are cultured on third-party filler cells, or no filler cells at all. Such clones may develop antiself CTX (Claesson and Miller 1985), CTX against limited ranges of third-party target cells (Simon et al. 1984), or against target cells primarily susceptible to lysis by natural killer (NK) cells (Acha-Orbea et al. 1983; Binz et al. 1983; Brooks et al. 1983). Most probably, even clonal populations are in a permanently "differentiating" state, possibly caused by somatic variation within antigen-receptor genes, constantly generating cells with new antigenic specificities (Augustin and Sim 1984) which are selected for or against according to the culture environment. Even the constant or intermittent presence of specific antigen may not guarantee retention of original clonal specificity and function. Thus, in our hands, alloproliferative PLT clones lost the ability to respond (by proliferation and IL-2 secretion) to stimulatory alloantigen in the absence of IL-2 after about 30 population doublings (PD). This was independent of clonal propagation on specific, autologous, or third-party filler cells, or on use of crude, partially purified, highly purified (Biotest, Lymphocult T-HP) natural IL-2 or recombinant IL-2 (Dr. M. Wrann, Sandoz, Vienna). Despite loss of alloreactivity in the absence of exogenous IL-2, surface phenotypes and karyotypes of the cells remained stable, and growth curves were unaffected. The clones remained completely dependent on filler cells as well as IL-2 for their continued exponential growth. At the time of loss of alloproliferative capacity, those clones which had previously not been suppressive, acquired a nonspecific suppressive effect for lymphoproliferative (LP) responses in MLC and PLT (Pawelec et al. 1984b; Pawelec and Wernet 1985), for Ig secretion (Falcioni et al. 1985), and for CFU-GM (Table 1). The suppressive activity of such ex-PLT clones for CFU-GM was similar in degree and in MHC nonrestriction to that mediated by suppressor-effector clones, and NK-like clones. Thus, clones that had become refractory to antigen-specific stimulation acquired nonspecific suppressive activity in all these different systems.

Stimulation of influenza virus antigen-specific helper clones with high levels of antigen has been found to render them refractory to subsequent stimulation (Lamb et al. 1983). No studies of possible acquired suppressive activities by these "tolerant" clones have thus far been reported (Feldman et al. 1985). In the above system, CD3 molecules were found to be modulated by the tolerogenic process, suggesting the subsequent nonexpression of the T-cell receptor for antigen as an explanation for nonreactivity (Zanders et al. 1983). Our alloreactive clones are maintained in the necessary intermittent presence of antigen, and

Acquisition of Suppressive and Natural Killer-Like Activities 123

Table 1. Suppression of CFU-GM by cloned T cells

Clone added	Number of cloned cells added		
	2×10^5	1×10^5	5×10^4
29-15 (NK-like)	0	25	94
29-23 (NK-like)	0	58	85
29-31 (NK-like)	0	65	99
38-15 (Suppressor)	0	47	81
29-7 (PLT)	100	95	100
29-7 (ex-PLT)	0	26	92
38-32 (PLT)	70	87	100
38-32 (ex-PLT)	0	58	81

Data are given as percent of bone marrow CFU-GM formation measured in the absence of added cloned cells, and represent mean results of three experiments with different donor marrows, all allogeneic to the added clones. The number of colonies per 1×10^5 bone marrow cells varied between 80 and 250

could perhaps be "tolerized" in the same way. However, this may be unlikely in view of their retention of expression of cell-surface CD3 antigens. Indeed, quantitative FACS analysis suggests, if anything, a somewhat increased density of CD3 on ex-PLT cells than on their younger PLT-active counterparts from the same clone. Should CD3 and T-receptor structures have become decoupled on these clones, lack of receptor would still provide an explanation for nonresponsiveness. However, practically all available evidence to date, particularly T-cell antigen-receptor gene transfection experiments, seems to suggest that the expression of CD3 structures and of T-cell receptor structures is mutually dependent. Certainly CD3 and the T receptor appear to be closely associated on the cell surface, and monoclonal antibody (mAb)-, or antigen-dependent modulation of either structure results in concomitant modulation of the other, and reexpression of both structures is concordant (REINHERZ et al. 1983). However, the inability to abrogate CTX function of some CD3$^+$ CTL clones by CD3 modulation has been reported and could be consistent with decoupling of CD3 and the antigen receptor (MORETTA et al. 1984).

When alloproliferative, nonsuppressive PLT clones were purposefully rendered antigen nonreactive by treatment for 18 h with anti-CD3 antibody, followed by 24-h culture in medium with IL-2, they were found to have acquired strong nonspecific suppressive activity for LP responses in MLC (Fig. 1). This treatment and short-term culture protocol resulted in absolutely CD3$^-$ cells, about 80% of which were able to reexpress CD3 after a further 5 days in culture. For those clones where reexpression of CD3 was associated with regained alloreactivity, such cells were no longer suppressive (Fig. 1). A dramatic modulation of PLT clone reactivity by anti-CD3 antibody has been previously reported also by others (SPITS et al. 1985), where non-specific CTX was induced in previously non-CTX cells. It was not investigated whether these clones had also acquired suppressive activity. Murine helper/inducer clones may rapidly down-regulate antigen receptors after stimulation (WILDE and FITCH 1984). Their release of

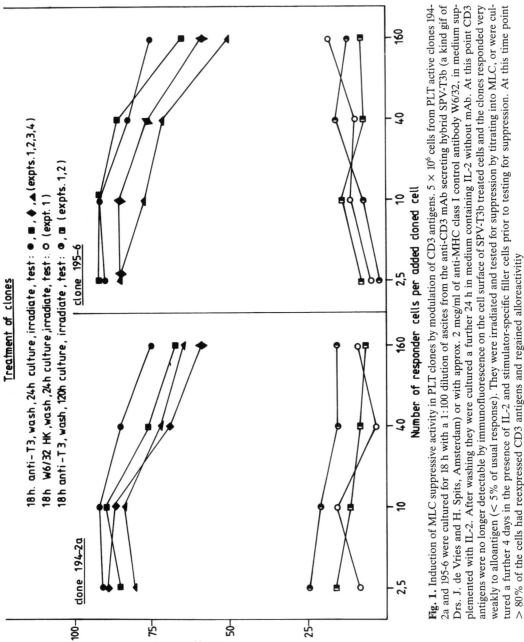

Fig. 1. Induction of MLC suppressive activity in PLT clones by modulation of CD3 antigens. 5×10^6 cells from PLT active clones 194-2a and 195-6 were cultured for 18 h with a 1:100 dilution of ascites from the anti-CD3 mAb secreting hybrid SPV-T3b (a kind gif of Drs. J. de Vries and H. Spits, Amsterdam) or with approx. 2 mcg/ml of anti-MHC class I control antibody W6/32, in medium supplemented with IL-2. After washing they were cultured a further 24 h in medium containing IL-2 without mAb. At this point CD3 antigens were no longer detectable by immunofluorescence on the cell surface of SPV-T3b treated cells and the clones responded very weakly to alloantigen (< 5% of usual response). They were irradiated and tested for suppression by titrating into MLC, or were cultured a further 4 days in the presence of IL-2 and stimulator-specific filler cells prior to testing for suppression. At this time point > 80% of the cells had reexpressed CD3 antigens and regained alloreactivitiy

Acquisition of Suppressive and Natural Killer-Like Activities   125

helper factors for B cells may occur only prior to entering antigen-stimulated cell division, at which time they begin to exert an opposite, inhibiting, effect on B-cell activation (FREEMAN et al. 1983). Human alloproliferative clones similarly modulate their receptors after stimulation with antigen (HAARS et al. 1984). It seems possible that modulation of antigen receptors by antigen or by antibodies may in general result in temporary or permanent refractoriness to further antigen stimulation, associated with acquisition of different, non-"helper"-related functional attributes (for example, suppression or NK-like CTX) by the cells in question.

Because of the association between suppressive and NK-like activity of non-PLT clones, and the reported induction of non-specific CTX by anti-CD3 mAb, the suppressive ex-PLT clones were retested for CTX directly on NK-susceptible target cells, and by cold target cross-competition experiments (PAWELEC and WERNET 1985). Not only was CTX demonstrable for the majority (75%) of ex-PLT clones at between 35 and 40 PD, but blockade of lytic activity by mAb 13.1 (Dr. W. Newman, Ortho Pharmaceutical, New Jersey; NEWMAN 1982; NEWMAN et al. 1984) was identical on ex-PLT effectors, and NK-like clones, as well as freshly prepared, uncultured, peripheral blood NK cells. Thus, effector-cell level inhibition of lysis of erythroleukemic target cells (prototype K562), but not of T leukemic target cells (prototype HSB2) was observed with 10 mcg/ml of 13.1 for all types of effector cells (Fig. 2). This strongly suggested that the same T200-associated NK recognition structures were employed by cultured NK-active cells regardless of their origin, and that these "receptors" were the same as those on uncultured NK cells (PAWLEC and WERNET 1985; PAWELEC et al. 1985a, b).

Clones which had not acquired NK-like CTX by 40 PD failed to acquire it later, whereas NK-like CTX appeared to be a stable trait in clones which had acquired it by 40 PD. NK-like CTX was retained until the eventual demise of the clones, which generally occurred between 60–90 PD. The expression of NK-like CTX was not dependent on the constant presence of high levels of IL-2, in contrast to certain murine CTL clones (BROOKS 1983). Despite this difference, interestingly, the latter displayed altered T-200 phenotypes on acquisition of NK-like CTX (BROOKS et al. 1983). Biochemical analysis of our clones in this context is underway.

The mechanism of the suppressive activity of NK-like and ex-PLT clones was explored. One possible mode of suppression was by the induction of suppressor effectors in normal peripheral blood cells (PBMC). Although all the clones expressed high levels of HLA-DR, DQ, and DP class II antigens, only clones with suppressive activity stimulated early (72-h) LP responses in autologous as well as allogeneic PBMC. Cells stimulated in this way were themselves suppressive when transferred to another MLC (PAWELEC et al. 1984c). Stimulation of early LP responses was associated with the induction of suppression, since irradiation of responding PBMC prevented suppressor induction. MAb inhibition experiments implicated class II, DP-like antigens in the stimulation of proliferation (PAWELEC et al. 1984c). That allogeneic or autologous cells stimulated by suppressive clones were able to inhibit an indicator MLC, again in MHC-unrestricted fashion is shown in Fig. 3. This illustrates the directly measured suppressive effect, suppressor-inducing effect, and LP stimulatory activity of a PLT – ex-PLT

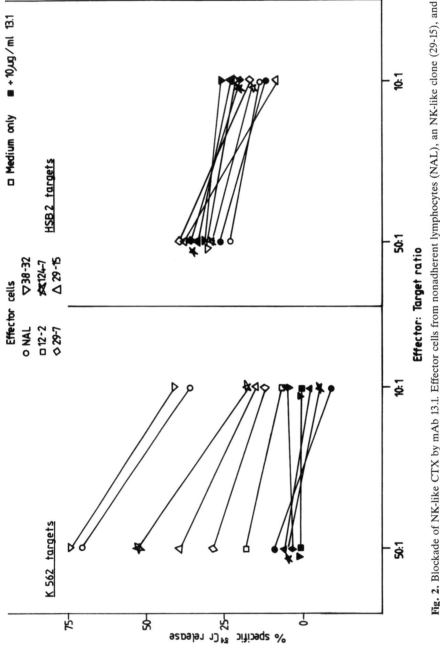

Fig. 2. Blockade of NK-like CTX by mAb 13.1. Effector cells from nonadherent lymphocytes (NAL), an NK-like clone (29-15), and ex-PLT clones (12-2, 29-7, 38-32, and 124-7) were tested in ^{51}Cr-release assays for CTX on K562 or HSB2 target cells in the presence or absence of a saturating quantity (10 mcg/ml) of mAb 13.1 (a kind gift of Dr. W. Newman, Ortho Pharmaceutical, Raritan)

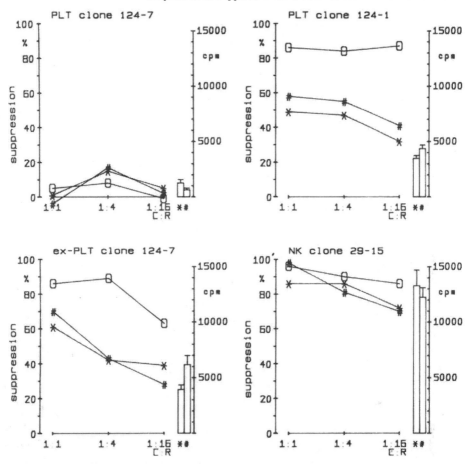

Fig. 3. Mechanism of suppression by cloned T cells. Nonsuppressive PLT clone 124-7, ex-PLT clone 124-7, suppressive PLT clone 124-1 and NK-like clone 29-15 were tested for direct suppressive effects in MLC, for early LP response stimulatory activity, and for suppressor-inducing capacity. The suppressive effects of irradiated cloned cells titrated directly into MLC (O—O) are compared with suppressive effects of normal PBMC previously cocultured for 3 days with irradiated cloned cells prior to transfer to MLC (∗, PBMC autologous to the clone; #, allogeneic PBMC mismatched for MHC class II). The histograms to the *right* of each panel show LP responses elicited by the clones in autologous and allogeneic PBMC after 3 days coculture, as measured by 3H-TdR incorporation

clone pair, a rare PLT-active but concurrently suppressive DR-specific clone 124–1, and a representative NK-like clone. The involvement of class II DP-like molecules also in the induction of suppressor cells by ex-PLT clones has been demonstrated directly by a decrease of suppressor induction in the presence of anti-DR/DP/DP-like mAb TÜ 39 compared with the lack of effect of anti-DR mAb TÜ 34 (PAWELEC and WERNET 1985).

However, it seems certain that at least one other mechanism of suppression exists, since cloned PLT cells stimulated by B-lymphoid cell lines (B-LCL) are also susceptible to suppression by ex-PLT (and NK-like) clones. A CTX activity does not seem to explain these results, since at least in 4-h ^{51}Cr-release assays no kill of activated or quiescent autologous or allogeneic B or T cells could be demonstrated and because mAb 13.1 did not abrogate suppression. IL-2 stimulated growth of factor-dependent T cells was also inhibited by these clones, whereas growth of B-LCL was less sensitive to inhibition by a factor of at least 100.

The presence of mycoplasma contributing to nonspecific suppressive effects must be considered. To claim that cell lines and supernatants are all 100% mycoplasma free is unacceptable due to the difficulties in detecting these organisms. Arguments based on circumstantial evidence must be put forward, the acceptance or rejection of which depend partly on the reader's bias. For example, suppressive activity by the majority of PLT clones is acquired at a defined culture phase, where a delayed effect of, or de novo contamination by, mycoplasma, might be considered unlikely. On the other hand, the "pathological" effect of some species of mycoplasma does seem to appear only after rather a large number of population doublings of the infected cells, although 30 PD still seems to be an excessive number. Possibly one stronger argument parodoxically involves clones which *do* show signs of mycoplasma infection. Even such clones do not lose their PLT activity and acquire suppressive activity until they, too, have reached the critical 30 PD in culture. Conversely, but a less effective argument for reasons of problematic identification, apparently mycoplasma-free clones still lose alloreactivity and begin to suppress at this time. Other arguments against mycoplasma involvement include (a) the inhibition of suppressor induction by some but not all anti-class II mAb, (b) the temporary induction in non-suppressive clones of the same kind of suppressive activity by treatment with anti-CD3 mAb, (c) the mediation of suppressive activity by all NK-like and some non-PLT, non-NK-like clones regardless of age in culture and their derivation from the same experiments as initially nonsuppressive PLT clones, and the fact that only such suppressive clones stimulate early LP responses in PBMC, (d) the lack of detectable mycoplasma contamination in B-LCL exposed to suppressive clones and then allowed to grow further, and (e) the fact that freeze/thaw cell lysates of suppressive clones do not themselves suppress. None of these arguments is definitive, but taken together, we believe them to support the contention that mycoplasma contamination is *not* responsible for the phenomena described here. We would rather suggest that the modifications in functional status of alloreactive clones reflect a longer-term differentiation process where the majority of MLC-derived T cells at 35–40 PD appear fairly homogeneous in their suppressor-effector and class II dependent suppressor-inducing activity, and their T200-dependent NK activity. Whether such a functional phenotype itself represents "end-stage differentiation," somatic mutation of antigen-receptor genes, or perhaps only an arrested phase of the regular antigen/lymphokine-dependent cyclical functional alterations of T cells remains to be seen.

References

Acha-Orbea H, Groscurth P, Lang R, Stitz L, Hengartner H (1983) Characterisation of cloned cytotoxic lymphocytes with NK-like activity. J Immunol 130:2952–2959

Acquisition of Suppressive and Natural Killer-Like Activities 129

Augustin AA, Sim GK (1984) T cell receptors generated via mutations are specific for various histocompatibility antigens. Cell 39:5–12

Binz H, Fenner M, Frei D, Wigzell H (1983) Two independent receptors allow selective target lysis by T cell clones. J Exp Med 157:1252–1260

Brooks CG (1983) Reversible induction of natural killer cell activity in cloned murine cytotoxic lymphocytes. Nature 305:155–158

Brooks CG, Urdal DL, Henney CS (1983) Lymphokine-driven "differentiation" of cytotoxic T cell clones into cells with NK-like specificity: correlations with display of membrane macromolecules. Immunol Rev 72:43–72

Claesson MH, Miller RG (1985) Functional heterogeneity in allospecific cytotoxic T lymphocyte clones. II. Development of syngeneic cytotoxicity in the absence of specific antigenic stimulation. J Immunol 134:684–690

Duquesnoy RJ, Zeevi A (1983) Immunogenetic analysis of the HLA complex with alloreactive T cell clones. Hum Immunol 8:17–23

Effros RB, Walford RL (1984) T cell cultures and the Hayflick limit. Hum Immunol 9:49–65

Falcioni F, Pawelec G, Brattig N, Schneider EM, Berg P, Wernet P (1985) Regulation of lymphoproliferation and Ig secretion by T lymphocyte clones in man. Immunology 54:685–692

Feldmann M, Zanders ED, Lamb JR (1985) Tolerance in T cell clones. Immunol Today 6:58–62

Fleischer B (1984) Acquisition of specific cytotoxic activity by human T4$^+$ lymphocytes in culture. Nature 308:365–367

Freeman GJ, Clayberger C, DeKruyff R, Rosenblum D, Cantor H (1983) Sequential expression of new gene programs in inducer T cell clones. Proc Natl Acad Sci USA 80:4094–4098

Haars R, Rohowsky-Kochan C, Reed E, King DW, Suciu-Foca N (1984) Modulation of T cell antigen receptor on lymphocyte membrane. Immunogenetics 20:397–405

Lamb JR, Skidmore BJ, Green N, Chiller JM, Feldmann M (1983) Induction of tolerance in influenza virus-immune T lymphocyte clones with synthetic peptides of influenza hemagglutinin. J Exp Med 157:1434–1447

Malissen B, Charmot D, Mawas C (1981) Expansion of human lymphocyte populations expressing specific immune reactivities. III. Specific colonies, either cytotoxic or proliferative, obtained from a population of responder cells primed in vitro. Preliminary immunogenetic analysis. Hum Immunol 2:1–13

Moretta A, Pantaleo G, Mingari MC, Moretta L, Cerottini J-C (1984) Clonal heterogeneity in the requirement for T3, T4, and T8 molecules in human cytotoxic T lymphocyte function. J Exp Med 159:921–934

Newman W (1982) Selective blockade of human natural killer cells by a monoclonal antibody. Proc Natl Acad Sci USA 79:3858–3862

Newman W, Targan SR, Fast LD (1984) Immunobiological and immunochemical aspects of the T200 family of glycoproteins. Mol Immunol 21:1113–1121

Pawelec G (1983) Allogeneically primed T lymphocyte clones in the analysis of lymphocyte stimulatory determinants. Hum Immunol 8:239–248

Pawelec G, Wernet P (1985) Loss of alloreactivity associated with acquired suppressive and natural killer-like activities of aged T cell clones. In: Human T cell clones: a modern approach to immunoregulation Feldman M, Lamb J, and Woody JR (eds). Humana, Clifton, NJ pp 327–339

Pawelec G, Kahle P, Wernet P (1982) Specificity spectrum and cell surface markers of mono- and multi-functional mixed leukocyte culture-derived T cell clones in man. Eur J Immunol 12:607–614

Pawelec G, Wernet P, Rosenlund R, Blaurock M, Schneider EM (1984a) Strong lymphoproliferative suppressive function of PLT clones specific for SB-like antigens. Hum Immunol 9:145–153

Pawelec G, Wernet P, Rehbein A, Balko I, Schneider EM (1984b) Alloproliferative human T cell clones primed and cultured in vitro lose proliferative and gain suppressive activity with age. Hum Immunol 10:135–144

Pawelec G, Schneider EM, Wernet P (1984c) Cloned human T lymphocytes with lymphostimulatory capacity preferentially activate suppressor cells. Eur J Immunol 14:335–340

Pawelec G, Newman W, Schwulera U, Wernet P (1985a) Heterogeneity of human natural killer recognition demonstrated by cloned effector cells and differential blocking of cytotoxicity with monoclonal antibodies. Cell Immunol 92:31–40

Pawelec G, Wernet P, Newman W (1985b) Recognitive heterogeneity of NK cells. In: Herberman RB and Callewaert DM (eds) Mechanisms of cytotoxicity by NK cells. Academic, New York pp 655–664

Reinherz EL, Meuer SC, Schlossman SF (1983) The human T cell receptor: analysis with cytotoxic T cell clones. Immunol Rev 74:83–112

Schneider EM, Wernet P, Pawelec G, Busch F-W (1985) Granulocyte-macrophage colony formation by normal bone marrow is suppressed by T cell clones with natural killer-like activity. In: Urbanitz D, Haubeck F (eds) Aktuelle Aspekte der Tumor-Immunologie. Springer, Heidelberg pp 1–11

Simon MM, Weltzien H-U, Bühring H-J, Eichmann K (1984) Aged murine killer T cell clones acquire specific cytotoxicity for P815 mastocytoma cells. Nature 308:367–370

Spits H, Yssel H, Leeuwenberg J, de Vries JE (1985) Antigen-specific cytotoxic T cell and antigen-specific proliferating T cell clones can be induced to cytotoxic activity by monoclonal antibodies against T3. Eur J Immunol 15:88–91

von Boehmer H, Kisielow P, Leisserson W, Haas W (1984) Lyt 2 T cell-independent functions of Lyt 2^+ cells stimulated with antigen of Concanavalin A. J Immunol 133:59–64

Wee S-L, Ochoa AC, Bach FH (1985) Human alloreactive CTL clones: loss and reacquisition of specific cytolytic activity can be regulated by "recombinant" interleukin 2. J Immunol 134:310–313

Wilde DB, Fitch FW (1984) Antigen-reactive cloned helper T cells. I. Unresponsiveness to antigenic restimulation develops after stimulation of cloned helper T cells. J Immunol 132:1632–1638

Zanders ED, Lamb JR, Feldmann M, Green N, Beverley PCL (1983) Tolerance of T cell clones is associated with membrane antigen changes. Nature 303:625–627

Expression and Function of Class II I-A^k Antigens on an Antigen-Specific T-Suppressor Cell Clone*

J. HEUER,[1] E. KÖLSCH,[1] and K. RESKE[2]

1 Introduction 131
2 Biochemical Analysis of I-A^k Molecules Expressed on HF1 Ts Cells 132
3 Functional Analysis of I-A^k Molecules Expressed on HF1 Ts Cells 135
References 137

1 Introduction

The question of whether similar or different modes of Ia-antigen expression exist in different cell classes and mediate different cell type functions is of primary interest to current class II antigen research. Among cells of the lymphoid system in the mouse, class II antigens are primarily expressed on B lymphocytes (SACHS and CONE 1973) and cells of the macrophage lineage (COWING et al. 1978), whereas the majority of T lymphocytes do not seem to express endogenously synthesized class II antigens.

The phenotype analysis of an antigen [bovine serum albumin (BSA)]-specific T suppressor (Ts) cell clone isolated from a CBA/J mouse tolerized to BSA with low doses of antigen has revealed that this Ts cell expresses both I-A^k and I-E^k molecules on its cell surface (HEUER et al. 1982) and that these molecules are synthesized by the cells themselves and in essential features are identical to those from B lymphocytes since they express α, β, and invariant γ (Ii) polypeptides (KOCH et al. 1983).

Expression of the class II molecules on HF1 Ts cells is most likely not an artifact due to an altered gene expression in long-term cultured cells because Ts cells induced in vivo with low doses of BSA can be effectively removed from spleen cells by anti-Ia serum (HEUER et al. 1977) or anti-I-A^k monoclonal antibody (mAb) (BRÜNER et al. 1982) and complement. In this communication we extend the analysis of I-A^k expression on HF1 Ts cells both with respect to biochemical and functional characterization.

---

[1] University of Münster, Department of Immunology, Domagkstraße 3, D-4400 Münster
[2] University of Mainz, Department of Immunology, Hochhaus am Augustusplatz, D-6500 Mainz

* This work was supported by the Deutsche Forschungsgemeinschaft through SFB 104 and SFB 107

2 Biochemical Analysis of I-A^k Molecules Expressed on HF1 Ts Cells

The previous biochemical analysis had shown that principal traits of B-cell Ia are encountered on HF1 Ts cells, yet a few differences were noted (KOCH et al. 1983). In order to reveal their relevance, two types of experiments were performed. In the first one an external ^{125}I-radiolabeling of viable HF1 cells grown in absence of feeder cells was performed as described in HAUSTEIN (1975). I-A^k and I-E^k membrane molecules were immunoprecipitated from radiolabeled cell extract using mAb 10–2.16 (OI et al. 1978) and 14–4–4 (OZATO et al. 1980), respectively, and were subsequently subjected to O'Farrell 2D-gel electrophoresis (O'FARRELL 1975). The essential finding was that surface-labeled I-A^k and I-E^k molecules representing both α and β chains are present on the surface of HF1 Ts cells (Fig. 1). In addition a diffuse and weak appearance of Aα and Aβ in conjunction with the occurrence of distinct forms of Eα and Eβ chains is apparent. This could suggest that altered modes of posttranslational modifications exist for all four subunits and might be expressed on the outer membrane of HF1 Ts cells.

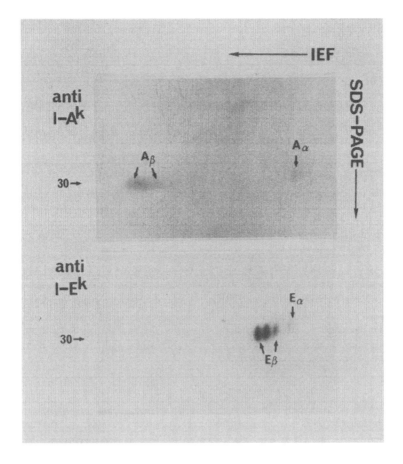

Fig. 1. Ia antigens from ^{125}I surface-labeled HF1 cells

Expression and Function of Class II I-A^k Antigens   133

Earlier pulse-chase studies with biosynthetically labeled spleen cell Ia molecules had indicated that some of the complexity of the 2D-separation patterns resulted from posttranslational processing reactions. Especially the invariant γ-chain and γ-related components were the targets of these modifications (RESKE 1983; ZECHER et al. 1984). Molecules of this category exhibited increasing acidity and a steady increase in molecular weight as compared with the respective primary products. Furthermore, 2D-electrophoretical studies of the kinetics of synthesis of the main component, p35, a processed form of the γ chain, indicated that this modified form appeared approximately 15–30 min after strong γ spots were observed.

Thus, in order to investigate for HF1 cells, the relationship betwen the Ia constituents and posttranslationally generated molecule species, the cells were pulse-labeled with ^{35}S-methionine for 10 min and subsequently chased with an excess of cold methionine (ZECHER et al. 1984). After increasing time intervals I-A^k and I-E^k specific immunoprecipitates were prepared from NP40 extracts of cell aliquots and analyzed using O'Farrell 2D-electrophoresis. The fluorograms obtained are compiled in Fig. 2. The left-hand row of gels represents I-A^k, the right one I-E^k-specific material. Fundamental traits of spleen cell Ia (ZECHER et al. 1984) can be recognized at all time points shown. The similarity is most pronounced immediately after the 10-min pulse (chase time, 0 min) when no processing had as yet occurred. At this time the invariant chain γ and the γ-related components p20, p28 were the key polypeptides seen in I-A^k-specific material. The heavy chain α appeared only weakly labeled and focused as a single spot representing the immature cytoplasmic precursor form of this polypeptide. At longer time intervals this molecule exhibited increasing posttranslational modifications, separating after a chase time of 120 min as a distinct series of five spots, although with immature molecular forms still prevalent. In contrast to the Aα-chain region, the Aβ-chain region is surprisingly complex. However, Aβ itself is barely detectable. This situation applies for the whole chase period and even beyond that. Because of this uncertainty, we avoided an assignment of Aβ spots in Fig. 2. All other spots in the complex Aβ-chain areas except p28 have not been observed before in spleen cell Ia. I-E^k immunoprecipitates had essentially the same characteristics as I-A^k-specific precipitates as shown on the right-hand row of the gels in Fig. 2.

The most remarkable feature of the pulse-chase analysis is apparent when immunoprecipitates at chase time 0 and 30 min are compared. Exceptionally high posttranslational modification can be seen for the invariant γ chain and the components p40 and p20. Thus, for example, the main representative of this series p35, derived from the invariant γ chain, focuses as an array of up to 12 polypeptides spanning a molecular weight range of approximately 5000 daltons and a pH range of about 4 units. Another salient feature of the γ chain and its metamorphic complexity was revealed by the pulse-chase analysis. After 10 min of pulse-labeling, distinct sets of regularly arranged spots (p30, p29, and p18) are resolved in the Aβ- and p20-chain region, respectively. Their regular separation profile, which strongly resembles that of γ, suggests that these components might be variants, possibly glycosylation variants of γ. The fact that they have not been demonstrated previously with spleen cell Ia suggests that they might be

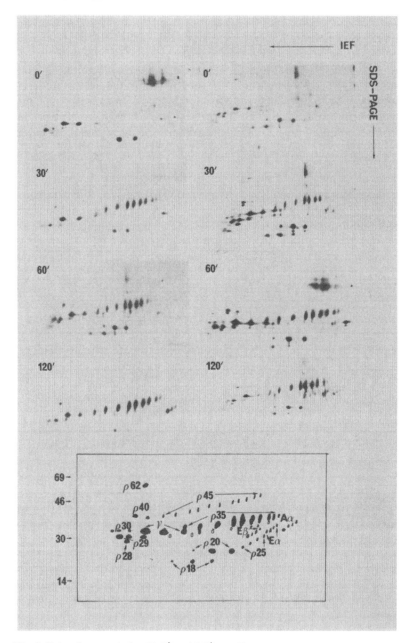

Fig. 2. Pulse-chase analysis of I-A^k and I-E^k specific molecules from HF1 cells

specific for the HF1 cells. Thus this Ts-cell clone might provide a suitable model to study the complex organization of class II molecules in detail, and to test whether preculiarities in the invariant chain structures are related to the function of Ts cells.

3 Functional Analysis of I-A^k Molecules Expressed on HF1 Ts Cells

Expression of I-A^k and I-E^k molecules on the HF1 Ts cells gives the unique opportunity to test their function by probing the effect of anti I-A^k mAb on the proliferation of HF1 Ts cells (HEUER and KÖLSCH 1985).

The experiments to be described required growth of HF1 Ts cells in absence of splenic antigen presenting cells (APC) in order to avoid misinterpretation of data caused by passively absorbed I-A^k molecules. Using the Ts-cell clone HF1 adapted to grow in medium containing syngeneic mouse serum, the fine specificity of antigenic activation of proliferation has been analyzed using various serum albumins as cross-reacting antigens (Table 1). Goat and rabbit serum albumin cross-react strongly with the original antigen BSA, whereas little or no cross-reactivity is found with porcine, dog, and horse serum albumins. Thus, the antigen receptor of HF1 Ts cells discriminates between various mammalian serum albumins.

In subsequent experiments it has been tested whether BSA-specific proliferation is influenced by treating HF1 Ts cells with anti I-A^k mAb (Table 2). Among 11 anti-I-A^k mAb tested, only mAb H118-49 strongly inhibits proliferation of HF1 Ts cells. Since mAb H118–49 in contrast to the other mAb is of the IgM class, it had to be tested whether other IgM anti-I-A^k mAb would also inhibit antigen-specific proliferation of HF1 Ts cells. Table 3 shows that two other IgM anti-I-A^k mAb directed against Ia.m2 do not influence antigen-driven proliferation. The fluorescence profiles on HF1 cells of the inhibitory H118-49 and of three other noninhibitory mAb (B15-124, K25-137, S3-287) are rather similar (HEUER and KÖLSCH 1985). Thus, it is likely that the antigenic specificity of H118-49 mAb is responsible for the blocking capacity. In control experiments it was shown that proliferation mediated by growth factors is not inhibited by this mAb (HEUER and KÖLSCH 1985). The fact that HF1 Ts cells express I-A^k and I-E^k molecules allows in principle that an HF1 Ts cell can present antigen in con-

Table 1. Specificity of antigen-dependent proliferation of HF1 Ts cells

Antigen (serum albumin) in culture	Incorporation of ^{3}H-TdR (cpm ± SEM)
–	309 ± 106
Bovine	18321 ± 1182
Goat	21145 ± 1172
Rabbit	19626 ± 2462
Ovine	7291 ± 541
Dog	1169 ± 73
Porcine	111 ± 74
Horse	1121 ± 325

4×10^3 HF1 Ts cells/well were cultured in 200 μl DME medium supplement with 0.5% syngeneic mouse serum and 5% conditioned medium (CM) in the absence or presence of 200 μg/well of the given serum albumins. Proliferation of responding cells was measured on day 4 by pulsing triplicate cultures with 0.4 μCi ^{3}H-TdR during the last 16 h of the culture periods (for details see reference HEUER and KÖLSCH 1985)

136   J. Heuer et al.

Table 2. Inhibition of BSA-induced proliferation of HF1 Ts cells by mAb H118-49 directed against the private determinant Ia.m1 on I-A^k molecules

mAb[a]		Antigen BSA	Incorporation[b] of ^{3}H-TdR (cpm ± SEM)
Code	Specificity		
H118-49	I-A^k	+	3522 ± 161
H116-32	I-A^k (r)	+	25628 ± 2893
K25-8.7	I-A^{k,b}(j,r,s,q,f)	+	25328 ± 4178
K22-203	I-A^k(f,j,r,s)	+	22454 ± 1258
10.2.16	I-A^k(f,j,r,s)	+	21672 ± 30
H150-13	I-A^k(f,r,s)	+	21037 ± 2196
17/227	I-A^{k,b,d}(v)	+	19600 ± 3190
K25-137	I-A^{k,b}(j,r,s,q,f)	+	19304 ± 152
B15-124	I-A^k	+	14047 ± 856
S3-29	I-A^k(r)	+	21774 ± 2103
S3-287	I-A^k	+	21102 ± 2477
13/18	I-E^{k,d}(p,r,u,v)	+	22038 ± 1692
13/4	I-E^{k,d}(p,r,u,v)	+	17991 ± 1694
H100-30	H-2K^{k,s}(p,r,q)	+	19131 ± 801
B17-263	I-A^{b,d}(q)	+	26937 ± 1147
–	–	+	12427 ± 1264
–	–	–	357 ± 113

[a] For details see reference HEUER and KÖLSCH 1985
[b] 3×10^3 HF1 Ts cells/well were cultured and the proliferation of responding cells was measured on day 3 by pulsing triplicate cultures with 0.4 μCi ^{3}H-TdR during the last 16 h of the culture periods

Table 3. Blockade of BSA-induced proliferation of HF1 Ts cells is not due to the IgM class of the inhibitory mAb H118-49

mAb[a]		Antigen BSA	Incorporation[b] of ^{3}H-TdR (cpm ± SEM)
Code	Specificity and determinant		
H118-49	I-A^k, Ia.m1	+	437 ± 73
26-7-11S	I-A^k, Ia.m2	+	3767 ± 628
26-8-16S	I-A^k, Ia.m2	+	4624 ± 166
–	–	+	4076 ± 947
–	–	–	33 ± 29

[a] For details see reference HEUER and KÖLSCH 1985
[b] 5×10^3 HF1 Ts cells were cultured in flat-bottom microtiter wells and proliferation was measured on day 3. Cultures were pulsed with ^{3}H-TdR during the last 16 h

text with class II structures to other members of the clone. This situation could be named "self-presentation of antigen." The question arises whether self-presentation could be involved in the activation of HF1 cells and whether H118-49 mAb exclusively inhibits such a step. However it has been shown that antigen presentation by APC to class II restricted antigen-primed lymphnode T cells

Expression and Function of Class II I-A^k Antigens 137

(HEUER and KÖLSCH 1985) or antigen-specific T-cell clones (BECK et al. 1982) is inhibited by the majority of anti-I-A^k mAb. Nothing similar to the selective inhibition of proliferation upon interaction between H118-49 mAb and the private Ia.m1 determinant on HF1 cells is found.

Thus, their specific interaction represents a particular phenomenon and shows an involvement of the I-A^k molecules on HF1 Ts cells in the antigen-induced proliferation of this clone. Interaction of mAb with this structure seems to provide an off signal for antigen-induced proliferation. This of course does not imply an inhibitory effect on other cell functions. They could actually be induced by this same signal. It is thus presumed that membrane-bound I-A^k structures, though most likely not the actual antigen receptor (T cell receptor β-chain rearrangement has been found in HF1 Ts cells, Steinmetz, personal communication), are involved with the transmembrane signal transmission upon antigenic stimulation.

From the above data it is intriguing to speculate that T helper (Th) cells might recognize antigen on Ts cells in the same class II restricted fashion as they see it on macrophage APC, yet with two important differences: (a) The T-cell antigen receptor of Ts cells is involved in specific antigen binding; and (b) the cell functions of Ts cells and APC are obviously distinct from each other in many parameters and this should have different consequences on Th-cell differentiation. In principle, however, one would have a competition for class II restricted recognition of antigen by Th cells on macrophage APC and Ts cells. The possible consequences of such an interaction between Ts and Th cells for the modification of the Th repertoire have recently been discussed (KÖLSCH 1984).

References

Beck BN, Frelinger JG, Shigeta M, Infante AJ, Cummings D, Hämmerling G, Fathmann CG (1982) T cell clones specific for hybrid I-A molecules. Discrimination with monoclonal anti I-A^k antibodies. J Exp Med 156:1186–1194

Brüner K, Opitz HG, Kölsch E (1982) The thymus as primary site for antigen-specific T suppressor cells in neonatally induced tolerance to bovine serum albumin. Immunobiology 162:221–228

Cowing C, Schwartz BD, Dickler HB (1978) Macrophage Ia antigens. I. Macrophage populations differ in their expression of Ia antigens. J Immunol 120:378–384

Haustein D (1975) Effective radioiodination by lactoperoxidase and solubilization of cell-surface proteins of cultured murine T lymphoma cells. J Immunol Methods 7:25–31

Heuer J, Kölsch E (1985) Functional studies on the role of I-A molecules expressed by the antigen-specific T suppressor cell clone HF1. J Immunol 134:4031–4034

Heuer J, Stumpf R, Kölsch E, Shen FW, Hämmerling GJ (1977) Suppressor T cells in low zone tolerance. II. Characterization of suppressor T and amplifier cells by physical and serological methods. Eur J Immunol 7:769–775

Heuer J, Brüner K, Opalka B, Kölsch E (1982) A cloned T cell line from a tolerant mouse represents a novel antigen-specific suppressor cell type. Nature 296:456–459

Koch N, Arnold B, Hämmerling GJ, Heuer J, Kölsch E (1983) Structural comparison of I-A antigens produced by a cloned murine T suppressor cell line with B-cell-derived I-A. Immunogenetics 17:497–505

Kölsch E (1984) Interaction of suppressor and helper antigenic determinants in the dominance of either tolerance or immunity. Scand J Immunol 19:387–393

O'Farrel PH (1975) High resolution two dimensional electrophoresis of proteins. J Biol Chem 250:4007–4021

Oi VT, Jones PP, Goding JG, Herzenberg LA, Herzenberg LA (1978) Properties of monoclonal antibodies to mouse Ig allotypes, H-2, and Ia antigens. Curr Top Microbiol Immunol 81:115–129

Ozato K, Mayer N, Sachs DH (1980) Hybridoma cell lines secreting monoclonal antibodies to mouse H-2 and Ia antigens. J Immunol 124:533–540

Reske K (1983) Identification of an invariant chain δ of murine class II antigens and its relationship to the invariant chain γ (Ii). In: Pierce CW, Cullen SE, Kapp JA, Schwartz BD, Shreffler DC (eds) Ir Genes: past, present, and future. Humana, Clifton, NJ p 153–156

Sachs D, Cone JL (1973) A mouse B-cell alloantigen determined by gene(s) linked to the major histocompatibility complex. J Exp Med 138:1289–1304

Zecher R, Ballhausen W, Reske K, Linder D, Schlüter M, Stirm S (1984) The invariant chains of mouse class II antigens: biochemical properties and molecular relationship. Eur J Immunol 14:511–517

Part D: Signal Requirements for T-Cell Activation

Introductory Remarks

H. WAGNER

This section focuses on the signals which induce cytotoxic T-lymphocyte precursors (CTL-P) to clonally develop into CTL. The requirements for cell interactions between antigen-presenting cells (APCs), T-helper cells, and CTL-P was recognized as early as 1973. The use of cell-surface markers to type T-cell subsets, of congeneic mice to define MHC structures involved in T-cell stimulation, of double chamber cultures in which T-helper cells were separated from CTL-P, as well as other approaches have led to the conclusion that in the mouse activated Lyt-2$^-$ L$_3$T$_4^+$ helper cells produce biological activities (lymphokines) that substitute the requirement of L$_3$T$_4^+$ helper T cells in the primary induction of CTL from antigen (mitogen)-reactive CTL-P. Since the description of the T-cell growth factor interleukin 2 (IL-2), results of many investigators support the two-signal concept to explain activation of CTL-P, that is, binding of antigen (mitogen) to reactive CTL-P induces IL-2 receptor (IL-2R) expression, while binding of IL-2 to IL-2R$^+$ CTL-P induces clonal growth and maturation into CTL. Within the framework of this concept the specificity of CTL responses reside in the interaction of antigen with clonally distributed antigen receptors, and clonal growth and maturation into CTL are intimately associated events induced by IL-2. In its original version this concept also implies that activation of IL-2-producing T-helper cells precedes activation of antigen-reactive CTL-P.

The limitation of results obtained in complex bulk culture conditions became clear when it turned out that the function-phenotype correlation of T-cell subsets is less stringent in long-term propagated cloned T cells with defined cell-surface phenotype. Clearly there exist helper-cell independent (bifunctional) CTL clones which upon stimulation produce IL-2 in an autocrine fashion. Furthermore, most cloned T lymphocytes produce more than one lymphokine, for example, IL-2 plus γ-interferon (γ-IFN), and there is clear evidence that IL-2-driven growth of cloned CTL is associated with the secretion of γ-IFN. Thus, even though IL-2 may apparently simultaneously trigger events such as growth and maturation in cloned T cells, the unknown function of autocrine-secreted lymphokines is of major concern. Furthermore, the availability of lymphokines produced by the recombinant DNA technology has eased its in vitro use at high concentrations. However, biological phenomena induced in vitro by high lymphokine concentrations may not necessarily reflect its physiological relevance.

Department of Medical Microbiology and Immunology, University of Ulm, Oberer Eselsberg, D-7900 Ulm

Given these uncertainties, it is not surprising that interpretation of part of the results presented in this section resulted in different conclucions, even though similar experimental approaches were used. In essence, highly purified murine CTL-P were prepared and the frequency of cells was quantitated which, upon exposure to mitogen/antigen (signal 1) and rec. Il-2 (signal 2) expanded clonally and also matured into CTL. The Lausanne group (H.R. MacDonald and Erard) presents clear evidence that upon plating of highly purified, positively selected Lyt-2$^+$ murine T cell into microcultures containing the mitogen Con A plus high concentrations (200 U/ml) of rec. IL-2 (Biogen), up to one of three cells plated expanded clonally, and *all* clonally expanded cells exhibited cytolytic activity. Under these conditions, IL-2 appears to be necessary and sufficient to induce growth *and* maturation of mitogen/antigen activated CTL-P. At variance to this conclusion, the Freiburg group (M. Simon et al.) consistently observed (a) that the frequency of growing/proliferating T cells was 4- to 10-fold higher compared with that of cytolytic T cells, (b) that even though their IL-2 content was equalized, rec. Il-2 was inferior to IL-2 contained in crude supernatant (possibly containing additional lymphokines), and (c) that rec. IL-2 used at lower concentrations appeared preferentially to induce growth while the same IL-2 activity in crude MLC supernatants induced growth as well as maturation into CTL. Results of our own group (Wagner and Hardt) support these observations and point out a heterogeneity within positively selected murine Lyt-2$^+$ T cells in regard to their signal requirements for activation. While our plating efficiency (in the limiting dilution cultures) is 2- to 10-fold lower than that of the Lausanne group, only a minority of positively selected Lyt-2$^+$ can be induced to grow by Con A plus rec. IL-2 (10 U/ml) as compared with those induced by Con A plus IL-2 contained in crude MLC supernatants. We observed that a lymphokine activity termed IL-2 receptor-inducing factor (RIF) and produced by the P388 macrophage cell line substitutes the defective functional activity of rec. IL-2. Thus the majority of resting, Lyt-2$^+$ CTL-P require, besides Con A, the lymphokine RIF in order to become IL-2R positive and thus sensitive to low concentration of IL-2. We feel that these and other open questions will require further experimentations before the precise functional activity of IL-2 during the in vitro induction of CTL from resting CTL-P can definitively be defined.

Heterogeneity of the Signal Requirements During the Primary Activation of Resting Lyt-2$^+$ Cytotoxic T-Lymphocyte (CTL) Precursors into Clonally Developing CTL*

H. WAGNER and C. HARDT

1   Introduction   143
2   Material and Methods   144
3   Results   144
3.1   Distinct Growth Requirements of L3T4 T-Helper Cells as Compared with Lyt-2$^+$ CTL-P   144
3.2   Induction of IL-2 Responsiveness by a Lymphokine Operationally Termed RIF   145
3.3   Frequencies of Lyt-2$^+$ CTL-P Responding to Lectin Plus rec. IL-2 or RIF Plus rec. IL-2, or Rat Con A Sup (RF) Supplemented with rec. IL-2   146
3.4   Conversion of Proliferating, Yet Noncytolytic Lyt-2$^+$ CTL-P into Cytolytic Effector Cells   148
4   Discussion   150
References   152

1 Introduction

The in vitro requirements for cell interactions between antigen-presenting cells, T-helper cells, and cytotoxic T-lymphocyte precursors (CTL-P) for the induction of T-cell mediated cytotoxic responses has been recognized as early as 1973 (BACH et al. 1973; WAGNER 1973; CANTOR and BOYSE 1975). After the discovery of the T-cell growth factor interleukin 2 (IL-2) (MORGAN et al. 1976), it soon became clear that the T-helper cell product IL-2 (WAGNER and RÖLLINGHOFF 1978) was crucial in T-T cell interactions during primary cytotoxic T-cell responses (WAGNER et al. 1980a; SIMON et al. 1981).

Work using in vitro bulk culture systems, purified T-cell subpopulations, and semipurified interleukin batches led to the interleukin model to explain the signal requirements for the primary induction of CTL-P (WAGNER et al. 1980b; SMITH 1980). Accordingly, upon antigen recognition resting CTL-P are induced to express interleukin 2 receptors (IL-2R), while binding of the T-helper cell product IL-2 to IL-2R positive CTL-P controls clonal growth and differentiation into CTL.

Because of the complexity of cell-to-cell interactions occurring in bulk cultures, investigators attempted to define the signal requirements for the activation of CTL-P at the clonal level. This approach became possible with advances in the limiting dilution culture methodology which allows the clonal development

---

Department of Medical Microbiology and Immunology, University of Ulm, Oberer Eselsberg, D-7900 Ulm

* This work was supported by the SFB 112

of few or even individual T cells plated in microcultures, sophisticated cell separation procedures, the availability of pure lymphokine preparations such as IL-2 as provided by modern recombinant DNA technology (rec. IL-2), and monoclonal antibody (MAb) defining the IL-2R. The results obtained in our group indicate that there is a heterogeneity in the activation signal requirements of individual CTL-P and that the concentration of rec. IL-2 used in vitro shapes the function of clonally expanding cells.

2 Material and Methods

The methodology used here has been described in detail elsewhere (HARDT et al. 1985). This includes the preparation of rat concanavalin A supplement (Con A sup), IL-2 receptor-inducing factor (RIF), cytotoxic T-cell differentiation factor (CTDF), cell separation procedures to obtain positively selected murine T cells, Lyt-2$^+$ T cells and L3T4$^+$ T cells, culture conditions, lectin facilitated ^{51}Cr-cytotoxicity assays and pulsing of proliferating cells with ^{3}H-thymidine. The limiting dilution protocol used here follows the description of REIMANN et al. (1985).

3 Results

3.1 Distinct Growth Requirements of L3T4 T-Helper Cells as Compared with Lyt-2$^+$ CTL-P

Peripheral T cells (2×10^3/microculture) separated using flow cytofluorometry in positively selected Lyt-2$^+$ CTL-P and positively selected L3T4$^+$ T-helper cells do not grow in response to the mitogen Con A, presumably because they lack antigen-presenting cells (APCs) (Table 1). However, certain batches of crude Con A sup rich in IL-2 (10 U/ml), but not rec. IL-2 (10 U/ml) induce growth of plated Lyt-2$^+$ CTL-P (Table 1). This contrasts results obtained with L3T4$^+$ T-helper cells. In the latter case only cultures supplemented with accessory cells could be induced to grow. The overall interpretation of this type of results suggests that in mitogen (Con A) driven systems the growth requirements of Lyt-2$^+$ CTL-P can be met by soluble mediators present in Con A sup (rich in IL-2), while L3T4$^+$ T cells require additional signals provided by living accessory cells. In addition, the results indicate that Con A sup rich in IL-2 is superior in providing the growth signals to Lyt-2$^+$ CTL-P triggered by Con A as compared with rec. IL-2. In the latter case the experimental results are variable. In 17 experiments of this type, rec. IL-2 in concentrations equal to that contained in Con A sup (1–10 U/ml) was ineffective. If, however, high concentrations (>50 U/ml) of rec. IL-2 are used, rec. IL-2 appears to become sufficient to induce growth, at least in a subset of the plated Lyt-2$^+$ T cells.

Heterogeneity of the Signal Requirements 145

Table 1. Responsiveness of purified T cells[a] to Con A plus Con A sup or IL-2

Experiment	Mitogen/feeder/ factor added plus Con A	Purified T cells	Proliferative response (cpm ± SD)
1	——	T	340 ± 110
	Con A sup (10%)	T	9400 ± 600
	Syngeneic feeder	T	10450 ± 1300
	——	Lyt-2[+]	370 ± 80
	Con A sup (10%)	Lyt-2[+]	34000 ± 21000
	rec. IL-2 (10 U/ml)	Lyt-2[+]	600 ± 300
	——	L3T4[+]	250 ± 80
	Syngeneic feeder	L3T4[+]	20300 ± 1400
	rec. IL-2 (10 U/ml)	L3T4[+]	540 ± 190
	Con A sup (10%)	L3T4[+]	430 ± 110
2	——	Lyt-2[+]	390 ± 50
	rec. IL-2 (10 U/ml)	Lyt-2[+]	420 ± 70
	rec. IL-2 (100 U/ml)	Lyt-2[+]	560 ± 110
	rec. IL-2 (1000 U/ml)	Lyt-2[+]	3400 ± 1750
	Con A sup (10 U IL-2/ml)	Lyt-2[+]	47000 ± 2400
3	——	Lyt-2[+]	260 ± 180
	Con A sup (10 U IL-2/ml)	Lyt-2[+]	35000 ± 2400
	rec. IL-2 (200 U/ml)	Lyt-2[+]	6400 ± 1800
4	——	Lyt-2[+]	380 ± 140
	Con A sup (10 U IL-2/ml)	Lyt-2[+]	47800 ± 4200
	rec. IL-2 (10 U/ml)	Lyt-2[+]	1900 ± 370
	rec. IL-2 (200 U/ml)	Lyt-2[+]	64000 ± 1200

[a] Responder cells (2×10^3) plus 2.5 μg Con A, ^{3}H-thymidine incorporation (cpm) pulsed with 1 μCi (96–104 h)
T cells: Nylon wool nonadherent CBA or C57Bl/6 LN cells, anti-I-A plus complement treated
L3T4[+] and Lyt-2[+] T cells: positively selected using flow cytofluorometry

3.2 Induction of IL-2 Responsiveness by a Lymphokine Operationally Termed RIF

Because the responsiveness of highly purified Lyt-2[+] CTL-P to Con A plus rec. IL-2 (10 U/ml) can be restored by addition of irradiated APCs, the activity of supernatants of the macrophage cell line P388 was tested. The data detailed in Table 2 detail an extreme case, in which even 10000 U/ml of rec. IL-2 induced only marginal proliferative responses in positively selected Lyt-2[+] CTL-P exposed to Con A. However, addition of 5% (v/v) of crude P388 sup increased the IL-2 (10 U/ml) driven response up to 100-fold. We have described elsewhere that semipurified interleukin-1 (IL-1), γ-interferon (γ-IFN), and colony-stimulating factor (CSF-1) does not substitute for RIF (HARDT et al. 1985), and that RIF increases the IL-2R expression in Lyt-2[+] T cells exposed to Con A (HARDT et al. 1985).

146 H. Wagner and C. Hardt

Table 2. RIF is essential for the induction of proliferative responses by IL-2

rec. IL-2 added	Proliferative responses[a]		Stimulation index
(U/ml)	Without RIF	Plus RIF[b]	(SI)
10000	4.0 ± 2.3	269 ± 19.0	67
1000	2.1 ± 2.0	197 ± 9.6	93
500	0.4 ± 0.1	233 ± 40.0	58
100	4.0 ± 1.5	215 ± 38.0	53.75
50	0.1 ± 0.08	173 ± 19.0	> 300
20	0.3 ± 0.1	86 ± 14.0	286
0	0.5 ± 0.1	0.9 ± 0.3	1.8

[a] Cpm ($\times 10^3$) obtained by culturing 3×10^3 highly purified, high density (HARDT et al. 1985) Lyt-2[+] T cells in the presence of 2.5 μg Con A/ml. Cultured cells were pulsed at day 4
[b] Crude P388 sup, 5% (v/v)

3.3 Frequencies of Lyt-2[+] CTL-P Responding to Lectin plus rec. IL-2, or RIF plus rec. IL-2, or Rat Con A Sup (RF) Supplemented with rec. IL-2

Replicates ($n = 48$) of graded numbers of highly purified Lyt-2[+] T lymphocytes were plated into microwells containing Con A (2.5 μg/ml), plus rec. IL-2 (50 U/ml), or rec. IL-2 (50 U/ml) plus RIF (crude P388 sup, 5% v/v), or rat Con A sup (adjusted with rec. IL-2 to 50 U/ml). After 6 days, 24 microwells per group were pulsed with ^{3}H-thymidine for 20 h. At day 7, the cells of the other 24 microwells were tested for lectin facilitated cytotoxicity. Subsequently the data obtained were subjected to Poisson's distribution. Figure 1 details a representative experiment of the proliferative response obtained, both as dot plot as well as a plot of the number of Lyt-2[+] responder cells and the log of the fractions of negative cultures. Single hit conditions were observed in these limiting dilution experiments indicating that *one* variable, presumably the number of reactive Lyt-2[+] T cells, is rate limiting. As can be seen (Fig. 1), both the magnitude of proliferative responses per microculture as well as the frequency of proliferating cells was low in microcultures containing only Con A plus rec. IL-2, as opposed to microcultures which, in addition, were supplemented with RIF. In fact RIF plus rec. IL-2 (50 U/ml) was functionally as active as rat sup (adjusted with rec. IL-2 to 50 U/ml). In this particular experiment RIF increased the frequency of Con triggered Lyt-2[+] cells responding to rec. IL-2 about 37-fold. It is our experience that the RIF-dependant increase in IL-2 driven proliferative responses appears to be high under conditions where the IL-2 concentration is low. In cultures supplemented with high concentrations of IL-2 (>100 U/ml), RIF appears less rate limiting (Table 3).

Dot plot analysis of the microcultures exhibiting cytolytic activity (Fig. 2) again demonstrate that rat Con A sup (containing 50 U IL-2/ml) is superior in inducing cytolytic activity as compared with rec. IL-2 alone (50 U/ml). Supplementation of rec. IL-2 with RIF increased the frequency of positive microcultures 21-fold – probably due to the overall increase of proliferating microcul-

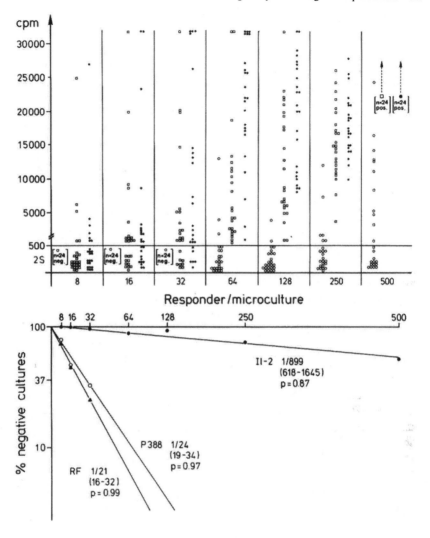

Fig. 1. Dot-plot analysis and frequency estimate of proliferating Lyt-2$^+$ T cells: C57Bl/6 splenic lymphocytes were enriched for T cells by the nylon-wool technique. Out of the nonadherent cells the Lyt-2$^+$ cells were positively selected using flow cytofluorometry (Epics V) using fluoresceinated anti-Lyt-2 antibodies (cl 53-6.7) as described (HARDT et al. 1985). Replicates ($n = 48$) of graded numbers of Lyt-2$^+$ responder cells (500-8 cells/well) were plated into U-shaped microcultures in the presence of Con A (2.5 µg/ml) plus rec. IL-2 (50 U/ml), or rec. IL-2 (50 U/ml) plus RIF (5% v/v), or rat Con A sup adjusted with rec. IL-2 to 50 U IL-2/ml. Proliferative responses of 24 wells were tested after 6 days using the ^{3}H-thymidine uptake technique.
Symbols used in the dot-plot analysis:
–O—O—O–, rec. IL-2 (50 U/ml);
–□—□—□–, rec. IL-2 (50 U/ml) plus RIF (5% v/v);
–●—●—●–, rat Con A sup (50 U IL-2/ml).
  Symbols used in frequency estimation:
–●—●—●–, rec. IL-2 (50 U/ml);
–O—O—O–, rec. IL-2 (50 U/ml) plus RIF (5% v/v);
–▲—▲—▲–, rat Con A sup (50 U IL-2/ml)

148   H. Wagner and C. Hardt

Table 3. Frequencies of precursors of proliferating and cytolytic Lyt-2$^+$ T cells exposed to 2.5 μg Con A

Experiment	Mediator added	IL-2 content	Frequency in Lyt-2$^+$ lymphocytes	
			Proliferating CTL-P	Cytolytic CTL-P
1	rec. IL-2	10 U/ml	1/2500	a
	rec. IL-2	10 U/ml		
	plus RIF		1/ 190	a
	Con A sup	10 U/ml	1/ 89	1/ 110
2	rec. IL-2	50 U/ml	1/ 890	1/2770
	rec. IL-2	50 U/ml		
	plus RIF		1/ 24	1/ 130
	Con A sup adjusted with IL-2R	50 U/ml	1/ 21	1/ 67
3	rec. IL-2	200 U/ml	1/ 12	1/ 15
	rec. IL-2	200 U/ml		
	plus RIF		1/ 7	1/ 12

^{a} All microcultures negative

tures (see Fig. 1). Note that the majority of the proliferating microcultures were not cytolytic (compare Fig. 1 with Fig. 2). The experimental data available so far indicate that the frequency of noncytolytic yet proliferating microcultures becomes high when the microcultures are supplemented with low (10 U/ml) concentrations of rec. IL-2 plus RIF. In contrast, high concentrations (200 U/ml) of IL-2 yield in high frequencies of proliferating *and* cytolytic microcultures (Table 3).

3.4 Conversion of Proliferating, Yet Noncytolytic Lyt-2$^+$ CTL-P into Cytolytic Effector Cells

Positively selected, highly purified Lyt-2$^+$ (1×10^3) were seeded in microcultures supplemented with Con A (2.5 μg/ml), plus RIF, and 10 U/ml rec. IL-2, or with 200 U/ml rec. IL-2 alone. After 5 days proliferative responses were higher in the group of microcultures containing 200 U/ml rec. IL-2. On the other hand, the proliferating cells of the cultures containing only 10 U IL-2/ml exhibited no cytolytic activity. If, however, the latter microcultures were in addition supplemented for the last 2 days with Con A sup depleted of IL-2 by absorption on IL-2 dependent CTLL cells (5% v/v), strong lectin-facilitated cytolytic activity became induced (Table 4). Thus, crude Con A sup appears to contain, besides RIF and IL-2, an additional lymphokine previously designated cytolytic T-cell differentiation factor (CTDF) (WAGNER et al. 1982; HARDT et al. 1985), the functional activity of which is detected provided the cultures are supplemented with low concentrations of rec. IL-2.

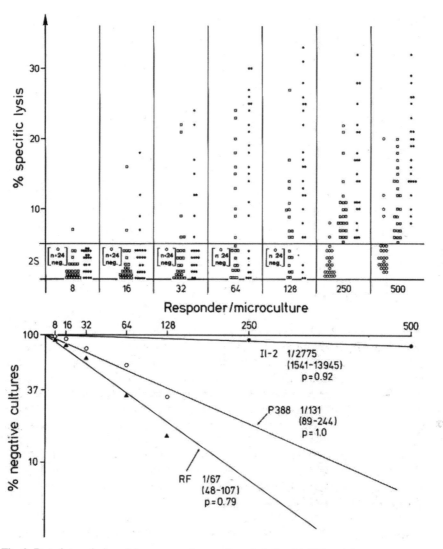

Fig. 2. Dot-plot analysis and frequency estimate of cytolytic Lyt-2$^+$ CTL-p. Microcultures ($n = 24$) of the experiment detailed in Fig. 1 were tested for lectin-facilitated cytolytic activity at day 7 of culture.
Symbols used in the dot-plot analysis:
–O—O—O–, rec. IL-2 (50 U/ml);
–□—□—□–, rec. IL-2 (50 U/ml) plus RIF (5% v/v);
–●—●—●–, rat Con A sup (50 U IL-2/ml).
    Symbols used in frequency estimate:
–●—●—●–, rec. IL-2 (50 U/ml);
–O—O—O–, rec. IL-2 (50 U/ml) plus RIF (5% v/v);
–▲—▲—▲–, rat Con A sup (50 U IL-2/ml)

150 H. Wagner and C. Hardt

Table 4. Conversion of proliferating, noncytolytic Lyt-2$^+$ CTL-P into CTL

Lyt-2$^+$ responder cells suppplemented with Con A, plus	Response induced		
	Proliferative (cpm)	Cytolytic (% lysis)	
		10:1	1:1
rec. IL-2 (200 U/ml)	120000	57	18
rec. IL-2 (10 U/ml)	37000	4	0
rec. IL-2 (10 U/ml) plus CTDF (day 5–7)	42000	46	15
Con A sup (10 U IL-2/ml)	31000	52	19

Replicates of positively selected Lyt-2$^+$ T cells (1×10^3) were incubated with Con A (2 μg/ml), RIF (crude P388 sup, 5% v/v), rec. IL-2 at the concentrations indicated, CTDF (24 h Con A sup depleted of IL-2 by absorption on IL-2 dependent CTLL clones, HARDT et al. 1985). After 5 days, cultures were split and tested either for proliferative or for cytolytic responses

4 Discussion

The experiments described here point out (1) a differential signal requirements for the activation of L3T4$^+$ T-helper cells as opposed to Lyt-2$^+$ CTL-P, (2) a heterogeneity between Lyt-2$^+$ CTL-P in their signal requirements to grow and differentiate into CTL and (3) differential biological effects of rec. IL-2, depending on whether it is used at high or low concentrations. At high concentrations (200 U/ml) IL-2 induces in a subset of Lyt-2$^+$ T cells exposed to Con A both proliferation and maturation into CTL. At concentrations similar to those in crude Con A sup (1–10 U/ml), a factor operationally termed RIF (IL-2 receptor-inducing factor) becomes rate limiting for the growth-inducing effect of IL-2 on resting Lyt-2$^+$ cells exposed to Con A. In addition, the proliferating Lyt-2$^+$ CTL-P exhibit almost no cytolytic potential. However, upon incubation with CTDF (cytotoxic T-cell differentiation factor), cytolytic activity is brought about. Thus, at low IL-2 concentration, the mitogen triggered transition of CTL-P into CTL can be dissociated into steps defining induction, growth, and maturation, each of which is controlled by distinct lymphokines, RIF, IL-2, and CTDF, respectively. If one assumes that in vivo the local concentrations of IL-2 as secreted by L3T4 T-helper cells are limiting, the physiological relevance of RIF and CTDF for the activation of CTL-P, in vivo, becomes apparent.

Previous work (PFIZENMAIER et al. 1984) has shown that in limiting dilution systems T-helper cells can be clonally expanded almost equally as well as Lyt-2$^+$ T cells, provided they are cultured together with syngeneic splenic feeder cells. Without APCs individual L3T4 T-helper cells can not be induced by Con A plus lymphokines such as IL-2 (Table 1). Similar conclusions have been reached by McDONALD and ERARD (1985), and Simon et al. (personal communication). Interestingly, phorbol-ester (PMA) plus Con A render resting L3T4 cells IL-2R positive and sensitive to the growth-promoting effect of rec. IL-2 (MALEK et al. 1985). Since, however, PMA has pleiotropic effects, this observation does not explain the mechanisms of how accessory cells facilitate the activation of resting L3T4 T-helper cells.

There is general agreement that unlike to L3T4 T cells, the activation of Lyt-2^+ T cells can take place, at the clonal level, in the absence of accessory cells (Figs. 1, 2, ERARD et al. 1985a, b; MCDONALD and ERARD 1985; HARDT et al. 1985; SIMON et al. 1985). Thus, mitogen/antigen plus lymphokines present in conditioned medium (Con A sup) appear to be sufficient to induce growth in Lyt-2^+ T cells.

However, whether or not IL-2 alone mediates both growth and maturation in Lyt-2^+ T cells exposed to mitogen/antigen is at present controversial. Because Con A sup contains usually 2–10 U IL-2/ml, and because mediators in Con A sup cause Lyt-2^+ T cells to grow and differentiate into CTL (HARDT et al. 1985), we have tested whether 10 U/ml of rec. IL-2 can substitute the effect of Con A sup containing 10 U/ml. These studies revealed that 10 U/ml of rec. IL-2 are ineffective. Subsequent work led to the conclusion that distinct soluble mediators are contained in crude Con A sup and promote preactivation of CTL-P, clonal growth, and differentiation into CTL, i.e., RIF, IL-2, and CTDF, respectively (HARDT et al. 1985). In contrast, the Lausanne group tested conditions which allowed activation of mitogen/antigen triggered CTL-P *only* by IL-2. Indeed using high concentrations (200 U/ml) of IL-2, both growth and maturation into CTL can be induced in clonally developing CTL-P (ERARD et al. 1985a, b).

Following their protocol, we confirmed this observation (Table 3). Using intermediate concentrations of rec. IL-2 SIMON et al. (1985) noted that Con A sup (10 U IL-2/ml) was superior to rec. IL-2, (70 U/ml) and that rec. IL-2 used at lower concentration failed to induce in proliferating cells maturation into CTL. SIMON et al. (1985) also observed that clonally developing Lyt-2^+ T cells exposed to high concentrations of IL-2 developed cytolytic activity, while those exposed to lower, but still growth-inducing concentrations of IL-2 failed to do so. Thus, a picture is emerging indicating two distinct in vitro activation pathways for resting Lyt-2^+ CTL-P. Once at very high concentrations (200 U/ml), IL-2 can bring about both growth and maturation into CTL in clonally developing CTL-P. It appears as if at very high concentrations IL-2 can upregulate IL-2R expression in target cells which do not respond to lower concentrations of IL-2 (10 U/ml). On the other hand, under conditions defined by low IL-2 concentrations (10 U/ml, yet still at surplus for clonal growth) it is RIF which appears to be mandatory that functional IL-2R expression becomes induced. Since low IL-2 concentrations per se induce no cytolytic activity in clonally proliferating cells, the lymphokine CTDF is required under these conditions to cause the transition of proliferating CTL-P into CTL.

At present, the physiological relevance of either activation pathway appears unclear. Since in vivo high local concentrations of IL-2 may be the exception of the rule, we feel confident that the function of the macrophage product RIF is likely to mirror physiological conditions. Conceptionally, RIF enhances the immunogenicity of antigens presented by APCs. In addition, the dissection of clonal growth and acquisition of cytolytic activity allows, in vivo, the expression of "memory" (clonal expansion) in the absence of cytolytic activity.

152   H. Wagner and C. Hardt

The results obtained using the limiting dilution technique point to a heterogeneity within resting Lyt-2$^+$ T cells in regard to their signal requirements for activation. Intermediate concentrations of IL-2 are sufficient for a low frequent set of Lyt-2$^+$ T cells to be induced to grow and to differentiate into CTL (Figs. 1, 2). While the majority of cells exposed to Con A require RIF to acquire sensitivity to IL-2, only a subset thereof develops cytolytic activity in the absence of CTDF.

Acknowledgement. We thank Dr. Armerding (Sandoz, Vienna) for supplying us with human rec. IL-2. The skilled technical assistance of S. Epple is highly appreciated.

References

Bach FH, Segall M, Zier KS, Sondel PM, Alter BJ, Bach ML (1973) Cell mediated immunity: separation of cells involved in recognitive and destructive phases. Science 180:403

Cantor H, Boyse EA (1975) Functional subclasses of T lymphocytes bearing different Ly antigens. II. Cooperation between subclasses of Ly$^+$ cells in the generation of killer activity. J Exp Med 141:1390

Erard F, Corthesy P, Nabholz M, Löwenthal JW, Zaech P, Plaetink G, MacDonald HR (1985a) Interleukin 2 is both necessary and sufficient for the growth and differentiation of lectin-stimulated T lymphocyte precursors. J Immunol 134:1644

Erard F, Nabholz M, MacDonald HR (1985b) Antigen stimulation of cytolytic T lymphocyte precursors: Minimal requirements for growth and acquisition of cytolytic activity. Eur J Immunol 15:798

Hardt C, Diamantstein T, Wagner H (1985) Signal requirements for the in vitro differentiation of cytotoxic T lymphocytes (CTL): distinct soluble mediators promote preactivation of CTL precursors, clonal growth and differentiation into cytotoxic effector cells. Eur J Immunol 15:472

MacDonald HR, Erard F (1985) Activation requirements for resting T lymphocytes (this volume)

Malek TR, Schmidt JA, Shevach (1985) The murine IL-2 receptor: III. Cellular requirements for the induction of IL-2 receptor expression on T cell subpopulations. J Immunol 134:2405

Morgan DA, Ruscetti FW, Gallo RC (1976) Selective in vitro growth of T lymphocytes from normal human bone marrow. Science 193:1007

Pfizenmaier K, Scheurich P, Däubner W, Krönke M, Röllinghoff M, Wagner H (1984) Quantitative representation of all T cells committed to develop into cytotoxic effector cells and/or interleukin 2 activity producing helper cells within murine T lymphocyte subsets. Eur J Immunol 14:33

Reimann J, Heeg K, Miller RG, Wagner H (1985) Alloreactive cytotoxic T cells. I. Alloreactive and allorestricted T cells. Eur J Immunol 15:387

Simon MM, Edwards AJ, Hämmerling K, McKenzie IFC, Eichmann K, Simpson E (1981) Generation of effector cells from T cell subsets. III. Synergy between Lyt 1 and Lyt 23 lymphocytes in the generation of H-2 restricted and alloreactive cytotoxic T cells. Eur J Immunol 11:246

Simon MM, Landolfo S, Diamantstein T, Hochgeschwender U (1985) Antigen and lectin sensitized cytolytic T lymphocyte precursors require both interleukin 2 and endogenously produced interferon for their growth and differentiation into effector cells. (this volume)

Smith KA (1980) T cell growth factor. Immunol Rev 51:337

Wagner H (1973) Synergy during in vitro cytotoxic allograft responses. Evidence for cell interactions between thymocytes and peripheral T cells. J Exp Med 138:1379

Wagner H, Röllinghoff M (1978) T-T cell interactions during in vitro cytotoxic allograft responses. Soluble products from activated Lyt 1$^+$ T cells trigger autonomously antigen primed Ly 23$^+$ T cells to cell proliferation and cytolytic activity. J Exp Med 148:1523

Wagner H, Röllinghoff M, Pfizenmaier K, Hardt C, Johnscher G (1980a) T-T cell interactions during in vitro cytotoxic T lymphocyte responses. II. Helper factor from activated Lyt 1$^+$ T cells is rate limiting (a) in T cell responses to non immunogenic alloantigen (b) in thymocyte responses to allogeneic stimulator cells and (c) recruits alloreactive or H-2 restricted CTL-precursors from the Lyt 123$^+$ T cell subset. J Immunol 124:1954

Wagner H, Hardt C, Heeg K, Pfizenmaier K, Solbach W, Bartlett R, Stockinger H, Röllinghoff M (1980b) T-T cell interactions during cytotoxic T lymphocyte (CTL) responses: T cell derived helper factor (interleukin 2) as a probe to analyze CTL responsiveness and thymic maturation of CTL progenitors. Immunol Rev 51:215

Wagner H, Hardt C, Rouse BT, Röllinghoff M, Scheurich P, Pfizenmaier K (1982) Dissection of the proliferative and differentiative signals controlling murine cytotoxic T lymphocyte responses. J Exp Med 155:1876

Regulation of Lytic Function
by Recombinant IL2 and Antigen

A.C. OCHOA, G. GROMO, S.-L. WEE., and F.H. BACH

1 Introduction 155
2 Materials and Methods 157
2.1 Recombinant IL2 157
2.2 Lymphoblastoid Cell Lines 157
2.3 Human T Cell Clones 158
2.4 CTL Reversion Protocol 158
2.5 Reactivation Phase 158
2.6 Cell-Mediated Lympholysis Assay 158
3 Results 159
3.1 Primary MLC Sensitization 159
3.2 Clonal Analysis for the Role of IL2 160
4 Discussion 162
References 163

1 Introduction

The study of signals involved in the generation and maintenance of cytotoxic T
lymphocytes (CTLs) has been facilitated by the availability of various techniques
based on the mixed leukocyte culture (MLC) test (BAIN et al. 1964; BACH and
HIRSCHHORN 1964). In addition to the proliferative response in an MLC, CTLs
are generated (HAYRY and DEFENDI 1970; HODES and SVEDMYR 1970; SOLLIDAY
and BACH 1970).

In vitro "secondary" generation of CTLs was accomplished by taking cells
primed in vitro to certain sensitizing antigens, allowing the activated cells to revert to small lymphocytes, and restimulating those cells with the priming antigens (HAYRY 1976). The actual immunogenetic requirements for the regenera-
tion of cytotoxicity came from studies (ALTER et al. 1976; GRILLOT-COURVALIN et
al. 1977) from our own laboratories. We were able to show that following sensitization in the primary MLC to both class I and class II antigens, the primed cells
could be reactivated to generate cytotoxicity against the sensitizing class I antigens either by restimulation of the primed cells with both the class I and the class
II antigens, or by stimulation with the class II priming antigen alone. Our inter-

Immunobiology Research Center, Departments of Laboratory Medicine, Pathology, and Surgery,
University of Minnesota, MN 55455, USA

This is paper # 418 from the Immunobiology Research Center, University of Minnesota, Box 724
Mayo, Minneapolis, MN 55455

Current Topics in Microbiology and Immunology, Vol. 126
© Springer-Verlag Berlin · Heidelberg 1986

Primary Response

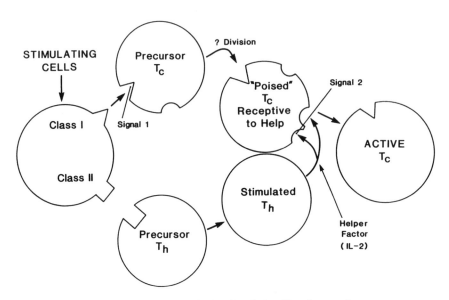

Fig. 1. The stimulating cell carrying both class I and class II antigen evokes separate responses in two T cell populations. The precursor cytotoxic T lymphocyte (T_c) differentiates to a "poised" state in which it is receptive to help, i.e., upregulates expression of receptors for lymphokines(s). In turn the precursor helper cell (T_h) responds to class II antigens and, under the influence of other soluble factors possibly derived from an adherent population, initiates the production of lymphokines(s), including IL-2, which allow for the maturation phase of the poised cell into a cytotoxic cell. (Adapted from BACH et al. 1976)

pretation of those results was based also on kinetic studies in which the class I and class II stimuli were added at different times in "three-cell experiments."

We proposed the following working model (Fig. 1) (BACH et al. 1976): namely, that the precursor CTL recognizes its target, i.e., the class I antigen, which, on the basis of the model for B-cell activation proposed by BRETSCHER and COHN (1970), could be called signal 1 to the precursor CTL. This interaction was not thought to lead to the full generation of a cytotoxic response, but rather to the change from the precursor CTL to a "poised" CTL. We referred to the poised CTL as one that had become "receptive to help." Subsequently, the interaction of the helper T lymphocytes (stimulated by class II antigens) with the poised CTL led to the generation of the full cytotoxic response. The help received by the poised CTL would represent signal 2 to that cell. The concept that signal 1 alone leads to a poised CTL that now has increased expression of receptors for helper factors (1985 terminology has "upregulation of the IL2 receptor") has been generally adopted in the field. We reasoned that the ability to restimulate anti-class I CTLs by reactivation of the primed cells with the sensitizing class II disparity alone was due to stimulation and release by helper T lymphocytes of a factor that would activate the primed CTL; i.e., that only signal 2 was needed for reactivation of primed CTLs. The findings of RYSER et al. (1978) in fact demonstrated that a soluble factor could constitute a substitute for what we had hypothesized as the function of the helper T lymphocyte.

One of the basic observations in bulk culture was that in the primary MLC, cytotoxic cell activity peaked between day 5 and day 8 and subsequently returned to very low levels. Thus, from the data with bulk MLC it was thought that following the cytotoxic phase the CTL "reverted" to a noncytotoxic cell that could be reactivated. Initial results stemming from the analysis of lytic function of both human (ANDREW et al. 1984) and murine (GLASEBROOK et al. 1981; SEKALY et al. 1981) cytotoxic clones were unable to confirm this concept. Cytolytic clones appeared to maintain their function even after removal from IL2-containing medium for various periods of time. Subsequently, it was demonstrated (HOWE and RUSSELL 1983; WIDMER and CLINCHY 1984) that "cyclic changes" in lytic activity of some cloned CTLs did take place if the function of those cells was examined for several days following addition of antigen and IL2-containing medium. Reactivation of activity could be demonstrated by addition of antigen and/or IL2-containing supernatants.

In addition to the role of IL2, several groups (WAGNER et al. 1982; RAULET and BEVAN 1982; KANAGAWA 1983) have suggested that an additional factor is required which, in the terminology of one laboratory, has been referred to as CTL differentiation factor (CDF). The cloning of the IL2 gene (CLARK et al. 1984) led us to investigate which phases of CTL differentiation could be subserved solely by the addition of recombinant IL2. We have studied two systems in which the addition of recombinant IL2 is sufficient for the generation of CTLs and their proliferation; in neither case can we rule out that the cells in culture produce CDF-like factors that are also needed.

2 Materials and Methods

2.1 Recombinant IL2

Recombinant IL2 is a chromatographically purified product of a human IL2 gene obtained by recombinant DNA technology and generously provided by Dr. Robert C. Gallo (Laboratory of Tumor Cell Biology, National Cancer Institute, National Institute of Health, Bethesda, Maryland). Recombinant IL2 was used at a dilution of 1:5000, known to induce maximal growth of the IL2-dependent murine CTLL-20 line as assessed by the standard 24-h thymidine incorporation assay (data not shown).

2.2 Lymphoblastoid Cell Lines

Epstein-Barr virus-transformed lymphoblastoid cell lines (LCL) were produced by the method of SUGDEN and MARK (1977). LCL 526 and the HLA loss mutant 526.41, derived by NICKLAS et al. (1984), were utilized in the experiments of the

158 A.C. Ochoa et al.

present report. The haplotypes of LCL 526 are DPw3, DQw1, DR1, B44, C5, A2/DPw4, DQw4, DR4, B27, Cw2, and A24. LCL 526.41 is a mutant that retained the B27 haplotype, but lost the B44 haplotype. LCL 721.82 is an HLA loss mutant whose HLA specificities are A2, B5, and DPw2 (DeMars et al. 1983).

2.3 Human T Cell Clones

JMAC 28 and KD56 CTLs were derived by using priming and cloning protocols as described by Miyachi et al. (1984) and Ohta et al. (1985). The clones were maintained as follows: cloned CTLs were seeded at 1×10^5 with 1×10^5-irradiated (10000 R) LCL 526 in 2 ml of RPMI-1640 (Gibco Labs, New York), plus 15% human serum which will be referred to as tissue culture medium (TCM), containing recombinant IL2 (1:5000 final dilution) in 16 mm-cluster wells (Costar 3524, Massachusetts). Four days later the contents of each well were split into two wells and replenished with fresh TCM plus recombinant IL2. By day 8 – 9 the cells were harvested and reseeded with antigen (LCL 526) and recombinant IL2. JMAC 28 CTLs usually increased 15- to 30-fold during a weekly cycle, while KD56 CTLs increased by 3- to 5-fold.

2.4 CTL Reversion Protocol

The "reversion" protocol was performed as reported by Wee et al. (1985). Briefly, 4 days after antigenic stimulation in the presence of recombinant IL2, cloned CTLs were washed three times in saline buffered once with phosphate (Gibco-PBS 310-2400 New York), and reseeded at 5×10^5 cells per 6-mm cluster well in 2 ml of either recombinant IL2-supplemented TCM or recombinant IL2-free TCM. Thirty-six hours later, cells were spun in 15-ml conical tubes (Falcon 2095, California) and resuspended in TCM. Viability was determined by trypan blue exclusion. Appropriate numbers of cells were then tested for lytic activity.

2.5 Reactivation Phase

Cells that had lost lytic function (i.e., reverted cells) were reseeded at 5×10^5 in 2 ml of 15% human serum RPMI-1640 containing (a) recombinant IL2 1:5000 dilution, and (b) graded numbers of LCL 526 such that clone : LCL 526 ratios are 1:1, 4:1, 20:1, and 100:1.

2.6 Cell-Mediated Lympholysis Assay

Cytotoxic activity was determined in a 4- to 5-h ^{51}Cr-release assay. The effector to target cell ratios ranged from 30:1 to 1:1, the percentage of specific lysis was calculated as described by Wee et al. (1981). For the lectin-dependent cytotoxic assay (LDCC), phytohemagglutinin-m (PHA-m) was added to the targets at a final concentration of 1%.

3 Results

3.1 Primary MLC Sensitization

Our initial strategy was to generate cytotoxic cells in a primary MLC in which the stimulating cells (a) were irradiated with UV light to abrogate as much as possible the stimulation of proliferation of helper cells and yet to provide the stimulus to precursor CTLs, that is referred to as signal 1 in the introduction, i.e., the antigenic signal, and (b) did not express DR or DQ [HLA loss mutants derived using the approach of KAVATHAS et al. (1980)]. Such a strategy was used to generate poised CTLs, which are receptive to help (see Introduction).

Peripheral blood lymphocytes were isolated from a normal donor and placed in MLC with HLA loss mutant LCL 721.82, which had been treated with UV light, with and without recombinant IL2. Table 1 illustrates the results obtained. Stimulation only with mutant LCL 721.82 treated with UV light did not lead to a detectable proliferative or cytotoxic response. Addition of recombinant IL2 or of supernatant from MLC, however, reconstituted cytotoxic activity. Although the system confirmed to us the importance of IL2 in the generation of cytotoxic activity, the fact that these experiments were done in bulk MLC allowed for the possibility of activation of helper (or other) cells by the recombinant IL2, inducing the production of other lymphokines, such as CDF. It was thus difficult to isolate the role of recombinant IL2 in this system. Similar results have been reported using selected responding cell populations (ERARD et al. 1985).

Table 1. Cytotoxicity of peripheral blood lymphocyte cultures

	E:T ratio			
	30 : 1	10 : 1	3 : 1	1 : 1
1. EB α LCL 721.82 x	40 ± 6	39 ± 10	16 ± 5	9 ± 2
2. EB α LCL 721.82 UV	− 1.5 ± 3	0.2 ± 3	0.6 ± 2	0.1 ± 1
3. EB α LCL 721.82 UV + 20% 1°SN	35 ± 7	28 ± 6	15 ± 9	3 ± 6
4. EB α LCL 721.82 UV + IL2 (1:1000)	25 ± 7	20 ± 7	9 ± 6	4 ± 4
5. EB alone	− 2 ± 6	0.1 ± 4	− 2 ± 2	−2 ± 2
6. EB + 20% 1°SN	1.3 ± 4	2 ± 5	− 0.2 ± 5	2 ± 6
7. EB + IL2 (1:5000)	− 0.4 ± 4	− 2 ± 3	− 1.2 ± 2	−3 ± 6

Peripheral blood lymphocytes from a normal subject (EB) were cultured for 6 days in the presence of LCL 721.82 that had been treated with UV light or x-irradiated. Two IL2 sources were added to some of the LCL 721.82 or stimulated cultures: supernatant from a primary MLC (1°SN) or recombinant IL2 at a final concentration of 1:5000. Cytotoxic activity was tested at the effector:target (E:T) ratios shown above; the results shown represent cytotoxicity (%) ± SD. The target utilized was LCL 721.82. No significant lytic activity was shown to a nonspecific target (data not shown)

3.2 Clonal Analysis for the Role of IL2

Our second strategy was to utilize several of the cytotoxic clones derived in our laboratory which were being maintained in recombinant IL2-containing medium. [Parts of these data have been discussed (WEE et al. 1985; OCHOA et al. 1985).] JMAC 28 is a T3$^+$, T4$^+$, and T8$^-$ CTL clone directed against DR1. At the time it was used it was shown to be able to produce IL2-like activity only when stimulated at responder to stimulator ratios of 5:1 and 10:1 (data not shown). Clone KD56 is a CTL clone with T3$^+$, T4$^+$, and T8$^-$ surface markers which produces detectable IL2-like activity at a responder to stimulator ratio of 1:1. It is directed against class II antigens.

Figure 2 shows the effect of removal of CTL clone JMAC 28 from recombinant IL2-containing medium. There is essentially complete loss of lytic activity in 36 h, paralleled by morphological reversion to small lymphocytes (data not shown). The possibility that the loss of lytic function was not due to changes in the lytic mechanism but rather to changes in the ability to bind to the target was tested by LDCC with the reverted clones. Figure 3 shows that the reverted CTLs are unable to lyse the target even in the presence of PHA-m, while the cells maintained in recombinant IL2 are actively lytic. Similar results were obtained with other clones.

Other CTL clones show only a moderate decline in lytic activity in the first 36 h after removal from recombinant IL2-containing medium (Fig. 4), as compared to the dramatic loss presented by JMAC 28 CTL. Some of these other clones, even after 62 h of recombinant IL2 deprivation, are still significantly lytic. Clone KD56 was tested up to 120 h after removal from recombinant IL2-containing medium and still showed active lytic function (data not shown).

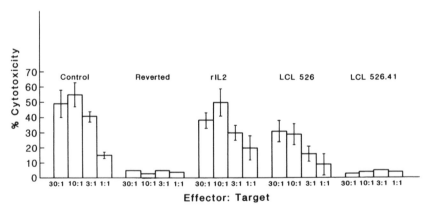

Fig. 2. JMAC 28 CTL reversion and reactivation. JMAC 28 CTL cells were taken on day 4 after stimulation with LCL 526 in TCM plus recombinant IL2 (*rIL2*) at 1:5000, washed three times in phosphate-buffered saline, and recultured at 5 × 10^5 cells/16-mm well (Costar) in TCM plus recombinant IL2 at a dilution of 1:5000 (*control*) or TCM alone. After 36 h cells were tested for cytotoxic activity at the ratios shown in the figure. Reverted cells were then recultured in (a) TCM plus recombinant IL2 (1:5000), (b) TCM plus LCL 526, and (c) TCM plus 526.41, an HLA loss mutant (NICKLAS et al. 1984) not expressing the sensitizing antigen

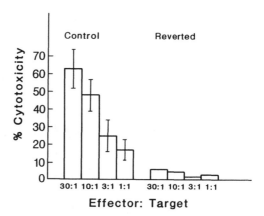

Fig. 3. JMAC 28 CTL maintained continuously in TCM plus recombinant IL2 (*control*) and reverted JMAC 28 CTL were tested for cytotoxic activity in an LDCC. LCL 526.41, which is not lysed by JMAC 28, was used as a target. PHA-m was added at a final concentration of 1%

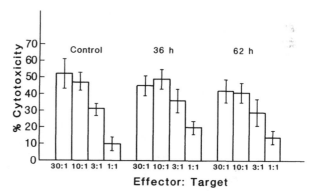

Fig. 4. Cytotoxic activity of clone KD56 after recombinant IL2 deprivation. Cells were taken on day 4 after stimulation with antigen and recombinant IL2, washed three times in phosphate-buffered saline, and plated at 5×10^5 cells/16-mm well in TCM without recombinant IL2. The appropriate number of cells were counted and tested for lytic activity against the specific antigen at the different time intervals shown

Recombinant IL2 was added to the reverted CTL clones to test whether this highly purified lymphokine could reactivate the cells. As shown in Fig. 2, the CTLs showed highly significant lytic activity within 36 h after the readdition of recombinant IL2. The further decrease in the number of cells during the reactivation phase and the fact that the reactivation of lysis was possible after radiation of the reverted cells (MACDONALD et al. 1976; WEE et al. 1985) strengthens the conclusion that this finding cannot be explained simply by the expansion of a subpopulation of CTLs. The number of cells showed an increase only 72 h after reactivation with recombinant IL2.

In addition to the ability of recombinant IL2 to reactivate the cells, specific antigen was tested as a reactivation signal in the absence of overt addition of IL2. Figure 2 shows that a high responder to stimulator ratio (30:1), lytic function is reactivated in an antigen-specific manner, while at low ratios (1:1) there is no reacquisition of cytolytic activity (data no shown). No formal tests have

162   A.C. Ochoa et al.

been conducted to establish whether the fact that the cloned CTLs produced detectable IL2 activity at the high responder to stimulator ratios, but failed to produce detectable IL2 activity at the low ratios, is related to the putative role of IL2 in the reactivation process. During the process of reactivation of the CTLs by the stimulating cells carrying the specific antigen, the cells regained their blast morphology (within 36 h) parallel with the reactivation of their lytic activity. Cells reactivated by antigen did not, however, show an increase in number, which was observed following reactivation with IL2.

4 Discussion

Our goals in the research discussed in this paper were to test to what extent IL2 in the purest form available – that produced by recombinant DNA technology – and antigen would function to allow the development of cytotoxicity of reverted CTLs. In the two systems with which we have worked, recombinant IL2 was sufficed for the development/reinduction of cytotoxicity in cells that showed no detectable cytolytic activity prior to addition of recombinant IL2.

Our results are consistent with the model that we presented several years ago (BACH et al. 1976; Fig. 1 in this study), in which signal 1 to the CTL, i.e., the recognition of specific antigen, leads to a differential change which is not a sufficient stimulus to lead to the full development of cytotoxicity that takes place when both signal 1 (antigen) and signal 2 [lymphokine(s) including IL2] are given. In the primary MLC data, the presentation of signal 1 "alone" was sufficient to render the CTLs responsive to recombinant IL2 presumably by increasing the IL2 receptors, i.e., inducing poised CTLs. Using the cloned CTLs, stimulation with antigen of reverted cells led to the reinduction of cytotoxicity without detectable division of those cells. Addition of recombinant IL2 or recombinant IL2 plus antigen led not only to the reinduction of cytotoxicity, but also to subsequent increases in cell numbers.

The concept that antigen leads to upregulation of the IL2 receptor thus appears to apply also to cloned CTLs. MEUER et al. (1984) have incorporated this concept of an antigen stimulating a CTL to produce more IL2 receptors into their recently published model. They have extended the model to suggest that following prolonged growth in IL2 without antigen, cells become relatively insensitive to IL2 by decreasing the number of IL2 receptors. Our own data (not shown) are in agreement with these findings, i.e., the addition of antigen is necessary to maintain responsiveness to IL2.

Previous reports (GLASEBROOK et al. 1981; SEKALY et al. 1981; ANDREW et al. 1984) that cloned cytotoxic cells maintain their active lytic function when removed from IL2 are consistent with our data on certain CTL clones. Our results demonstrate in addition, however, that there is variation among CTL clones in terms of their reverting to a noncytotoxic status upon withdrawal of IL2. Whether clones fall into two distinct classes in this regard, i.e., those that revert and those that do not, or rather form a continuum in terms of the degree of reversion that takes place, is not known. The findings of ROOPENIAN et al. (1983) from our laboratory that cytotoxic clones fall into a continuum with regard to their ability to proliferate in response to their specific antigen and with regard to their ability to produce IL2-like lymphokines may, we believe, be a good model for the reversion of CTL as well. Insofar as the CTLs do or do not revert according to the amount of IL2 that they produce, there may be a direct parallel between the findings of Roopenian et al. and what may be found when further CTL clones are examined with regard to their reverting to a noncytotoxic status upon withdrawal of IL2.

As already mentioned in the Introduction, our results using activation of cells in primary MLC cannot rule out the fact that other lymphokines such as CDF are needed for the generation of a maximal cytotoxic response. It could be that the recombinant IL2, in combination with antigenic stimulation, led to activation of cells other than the CTLs which produced CDF. We abandoned the bulk culture approach for this reason.

The studies with the cloned cells lead to results that are similar to those obtained with bulk cultures. The fact that a cloned CTL that has reverted following abrupt withdrawal of IL2 from its medium can be reactivated with recombinant IL2 suggests one of the following three possibilities: First, it may be that a cloned CTL is different from a precursor CTL in that the cloned CTL no longer requires CDF for the reacquisition of cytotoxic function. Secondly, it is possible that the cloned CTLs that we have tested all produce CDF, and that in the presence of recombinant IL2 the CTL produces its own CDF. Thirdly, IL2 may be a sufficient signal to stimulate CTLs, in general, to become cytotoxic and proliferate. This issue will probably not be resolved until a reagent is available to detect CDF by a functional assay, availability of a monoclonal antibody, or recombinant DNA techniques. We believe that any of the above possibilities would be an exciting step forward in our understanding of CTL function.

Acknowledgement. This work was supported in part by NIH grants AI 17687, AI 18326, AM 13083, and AI 19007. Siew-Lin Wee is the recipient of the Leukemia Society of America Special Fellow Award.

References

Alter BJ, Grillot-Courvalin C, Bach ML, Zier KS, Sondel PM, Bach FH (1976) Secondary cell-mediated lympholysis: importance of H-2 LD and SD factors. J Exp Med 143:1005

Andrew ME, Braciale V, Braciale T (1984) Regulation of IL-2 receptor expression on murine cytotoxic T lymphocyte clones. J Immunol 132:839–844

Bach FH, Hirschhorn K (1964) Lymphocyte interaction: a potential in vitro histocompatibility test. Science 143:813–814

Bach FH, Bach ML, Sondel PM (1976) Differential function of major histocompatibility complex antigens in T lymphocyte activation. Nature 259:273–281

Bain B, Vas MR, Lowenstein L (1964) The development of large immature mononuclear cells in mixed leukocyte culture. Blood 23:108

Bretscher P, Cohn M (1970) A theory of non-self discrimination. Science 169:1042

Clark CC, Arya SK, Wong-Stael F, Matsumoto-Kobayashi M (1984) Human T-cell growth factor: partial amino sequence, cDNA cloning, and organization and expression in normal leukemic cells. Proc Natl Acad Sci USA 81:2543

DeMars R, Chang C, Rudersdorf RR (1983) Dissection of the D-region of the human major histocompatibility complex by means of induced mutations in a lymphoblastoid cell line. Hum Immunol 8:123

Erard F, Corthesy P, Nabholz M, Lowenthal JW, Zaech P, Plaetinck G, MacDonald MR (1985) Interleukin 2 is both necessary and sufficient for the growth and differentiation of lectin-stimulated cytolytic T lymphocyte precursors. J Immunol 134:1644

164   A.C. Ochoa et al.: Regulation of Lytic Function by Recombinant IL2 and Antigen

Glasebrook AL, Sarmiento M, Loken MR, Dialynas DP, Qunitans J, Eisenberg L, Lutz Ch, Wilde
   D, Fitch FW (1981) Murine T lymphocyte clones with distinct immunological functions. Immunol
   Rev 54:225–241
Grillot-Courvalin C, Alter BJ, Bach FH (1977) Antigenic requirements for the generation of sec-
   ondary cytotoxicity. J Immunol 119:1253–1259
Hayry P (1976) Anamnestic responses in mixed lymphocyte culture-induced (MLC-CML) reaction.
   Immunogenetics 3:417–453
Hayry P, Defendi V (1970) Mixed lymphocyte cultures produce effector cells: Model in vitro for al-
   lograft rejection. Science 168:133
Hodes RJ, Svedmyr EAJ (1970) Specific cytotoxicity of H-2 incompatible mouse lymphocytes
   following mixed culture in vitro. Transplantation 9:470–477
Howe RC, Russell JH (1983) Isolation of alloreactive CTL clones with cyclical changes in lytic ac-
   tivity. J Immunol 131:2141–2146
Kanagawa O (1983) Three different signals are required for the induction of cytolytic T lymphocytes
   from resting precursors. J Immunol 131:606
Kavathas P, Bach FH, DeMars R (1980) Gamma ray-induced loss of expression of HLA and gly-
   oxalase I alleles in lymphoblastoid cells. Proc Natl Acad Sci USA 77:4251
MacDonald HR, Sordat B, Cerottini JC, Brunner KT (1976) Generation of cytotoxic T lymphocytes
   in vitro. IV. Functional activation of memory cells in the absence of DNA synthesis. J Exp Med
   142:622
Meuer SC, Hussey R, Cantrell D, Hodgdon JC, Schlossman SF, Smith K, Reinherz E (1984) Triggering of the T3-Ti antigen-receptor complex results in clonal T-cell proliferation through an in-
   terleukin-2 dependent autocrine pathway. Proc Natl Acad Sci USA 81:1509
Miyachi Y, Wee S-L, Chen L-K, Grumet FC, Bowman RH, Taurog JD (1984) A cytolytic human T
   lymphocyte clone differentially recognizing HLA-B27 subtypes. Hum Immunol 10:237
Nicklas JA, Miyachi Y, Taurog JD, Wee S-L, Chen L-K, Grumet FC, Bach FH (1984) HLA loss
   variants of a B27+ lymphoblastoid cell line: genetic and cellular characterization. Hum Immunol 11:19–30
Ochoa AC, Wee SL, Bach FH (1985) Loss and re-acquisition of lytic function by cloned cytotoxic T
   lymphocytes: role of specific antigen and interleukin 2 (IL2). (submitted for publication)
Ohta N, Anichini A, Reinsmoen NL, Strassman G, Wernet P, Bach FH (1985) Analysis of human
   class II antigens by cloned cytolytic T cell reagents: antibodies detecting the HLA-DP prod-
   uct(s). Hum Immunol (in press)
Raulet DH, Bevan MJ (1982) A differentiation factor required for the expression of cytotoxic T-cell
   function. Nature 296:754
Roopenian DC, Widmer MB, Orosz CG, Bach FH (1983) Helper cell-independent cytolytic T lym-
   phocytes specific for a minor histocompatibility antigen. J Immunol 130:542
Ryser J-E, Cerottini J-C, Brunner KT (1978) Generation of cytolytic T lymphocytes in vitro. IX. In-
   duction of secondary CTL responses in primary long-term MLC by supernatants from secondary
   MLC. J Immunol 120:370
Sekaly R, MacDonald H, Zaech P, Glasebrook A, Cerottini J-C (1981) Cytolytic T lymphocyte func-
   tion is independent of growth phase and position in the mitotic cycle. J Exp Med 154:575
Solliday S, Bach FH (1970) Cytotoxicity: specificity after in vitro sensitization. Science 170:1406–
   1409
Sugden W, Mark W (1977) Clonal transformation of adult human leucocytes with Epstein-Barr virus.
   J Virol 23:503
Wagner H, Hardt C, Rouse BT, Rollinghof M, Schevrich P, Pfizenmaier K (1982) Dissection of the
   proliferative and differentiation signals controlling murine cytotoxic T lymphocyte responses. J
   Exp Med 155:1876
Wee SL, Wu S, Alter BJ, Bach FH (1981) Early detection and specificity analysis of human cytolytic
   T lymphocyte (CTL) colonies generated in soft agarose culture: a potential assay for definition
   of CTL defined (CD) determinants. Hum Immunol 3:45–56
Wee SL, Ochoa AC, Bach FH (1985) Human alloreactive CTL clones: loss and re-acquisition of spe-
   cific cytolytic activity is dependent on interleukin 2. J Immunol 134:310
Widmer MB, Clinchy B (1984) Independent regulation of cytolysis and proliferation in antigen-
   driven CTL clones. J Cell Biochem 8A:111

The Target Structure for T11: A Cell Interaction Molecule Involved in T-Cell Activation?

T. Hünig

1 Introduction 165
2 Isolation of a mAb to the Target Structure Recognized by T11 (T11TS) 165
3 Cellular Distribution of T11TS 166
4 Identification of T11TS by Radioimmunoprecipitation 168
5 Partially Purified T11TS Blocks the E Receptor 168
6 Blocking of Mixed Lymphocyte Reaction by mAb to T11TS 168
7 Conclusions 170
References 172

1 Introduction

Human T lymphocytes bind sheep red blood cells (SRBC) via the "E receptor," a single-chain polypeptide with a molecular weight of about 50000 serologically defined by T11 and related markers (Howard et al. 1981; Kamoun et al. 1981; Bernard et al. 1982; Verbi et al. 1982). Recently, it has been shown that some monoclonal antibodies (mAbs) to the E-receptor block T-cell activation and T-cell-mediated cytolysis (Palacios and Martinez-Maza 1982; Martin et al. 1983; Krensky et al. 1983), and other anti-T11 mAbs as well as the E-rosetting procedure itself activate T cells polyclonally (Meuer et al. 1984; Larsson et al. 1978). These findings are compatible with the hypothesis that the E receptor is a cell interaction molecule involved in T-cell activation and function. Its interaction with SRBC could then be due either to fortuitous cross-reactivity, or to the fact that SRBC express the sheep form of the "physiological" ligand, which would cross-react with the human homologue. If the molecule recognized by the E receptor on red blood cells should indeed be the hypothetical cell interaction molecule recognized by T11, it should also be found on nucleated cells, where it could participate in the cellular interactions involved in T-cell responses.

2 Isolation of a mAb to the Target Structure Recognized by T11 (T11TS)

Eighty-six anti-SRBC mAbs, kindly provided by M. Lohoff of the Institute for Virology and Immunobiology in Würzburg, were screened for inhibition of E ro-

Institute for Virology and Immunobiology, Versbacher Strasse 7, D-8700 Würzburg

Present address: Laboratorium für molekulare Biologie, Genzentrum an der Universität München, Am Klopferspitz, D-8033 Martinsried

166   T. Hünig

Table 1. Inhibition of autologous and xenogeneic E rosettes by mAb and by partially purified T11TS

	Inhibition (%) of E rosettes formed between		
Addition to tests	Human PBL/SRBC	Human PBL/RBC	STBL/SRBC
Normal mouse IgG (2 μg)	0	0	0
anti-T11: 1:25	100	100	0
1:125	100	100	0
1:625	59	58	nd
1:3125	3	6	nd
Fab L180/1			
2000 ng	100	0	100
400 ng	100	0	100
80 ng	100	nd	100
16 ng	100	nd	100
3 ng	45	nd	49
Partially purified T11TS			
2000 ng	100	nd	nd
500 ng	100	nd	nd
125 ng	87	nd	nd
31 ng	49	nd	nd

nd, not done; PBL, peripheral blood lymphocytes; STBL, sheep T cell blasts; NM, normal mouse

settes. Table 1 shows that amounts in nanograms of antigen-binding is fragments (Fab) of mAb L180/1, the only positive mAb identified, completely abrogate rosette formation between human peripheral blood lymphocytes (PBL) and SRBC, and between sheep T-cell blasts (STBL) and SRBC. This indicates that the same cell surface component on the SRBC membrane is recognized by sheep T cells in autologous, and by human T cells in xenogeneic, E-rosetting. Similarly, anti-T11 mAb blocks the attachment of both autologous (human) and xenogeneic (sheep) RBC to human PBL, indicating that the same E receptor is functioning in the binding of human RBC and SRBC. On the other hand, the anti-T11 mAb used does not bind to sheep T cells, and mAb L180/1 does not react with human RBC (not shown). As expected, no rosette inhibition was observed in these combinations. It appears, therefore, that the anti-T11 mAb employed and mAb L180/1 recognize species-specific determinants on the E receptor and on its target, respectively.

3   Cellular Distribution of T11TS

The failure of mAb L180/1 to react with human red blood cells has limited our investigation of the cellular distribution and functional involvement of T11TS to the sheep system. Figure 1 shows that mAb L180/1 stains SRBC, sheep white

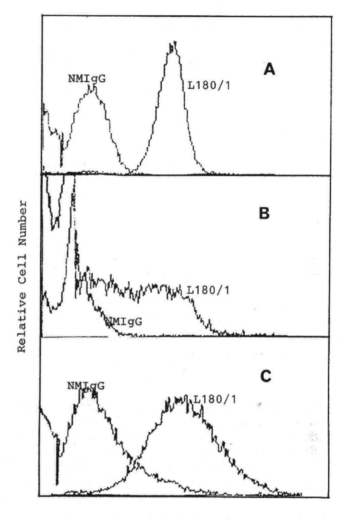

Fig. 1A-C. Expression of the antigen recognized by mAb L180/1 on sheep red and white blood cells. **A** SRBC; **B** SWBC; and **C** STBL. First antibody was L180/1 or normal mouse IgG (*NM IgG*; 4 μg/ml); second antibody was fluorescein isothiocyanate-(FITC)-conjugated goat antimouse Ig. Analysis of 2×10^4 cells was performed on an EPICS V flow cytometer, using a forward angle light scatter gate. **A** and **C** are from the same experiment, **B** from a separate one

bloods cells (SWBC), and concanavalin A-induced STBL propagated in IL2. This could mean either that T11TS as detected by mAb L180/1 is expressed on both red and white blood cells or that the mAb binds to a sheep-specific carbohydrate antigen expressed on various glycoproteins (GP) and/or glycolipids.

168 T. Hünig

4 Identification of T11TS by Radioimmunoprecipitation

In order to identify the molecule bearing the L180/1 determinant on sheep red and white blood cells, radioimmunoprecipitation and sodium dodecyl sulfate-polyacrylamide gel electrophoresis (SDS-PAGE) was performed. Figure 2 shows that a protein with an apparent molecular weight of about 42000 is specifically immunoprecipitated from detergent lysates of surface-iodinated SRBC. A band of the same apparent molecular weight is visible after immunoprecipitation of detergent lysates of ^{3}-H-leucine-labeled STBL with mAb L180/1. In addition, immunoprecipitates from both SRBC and STBL lysates undergo the same shift in molecular weight after neuraminidase treatment (not shown). Carbohydrate labeling, endoglycosidase digestion, and trypsin digestion have proved the GP nature of T11TS (not shown).

5 Partially Purified T11TS Blocks the E Receptor

We have also used insolubilized mAb L180/1 to enrich for T11TS by affinity chromatography, using the lysate of 100 ml of packed SRBC as starting material. While such preparations still contain some contaminating proteins as detected by coomassie blue stains of SDS-PAGE (not shown), they seemed sufficiently enriched to permit investigation of whether this material interacted with the E receptor of human T cells. E rosette inhibition by partially purified T11TS (Table 1) suggests that the column eluate does indeed contain the SRBC membrane molecule that reacts with the E receptor. This is more directly demonstrated by the experiment shown in Fig. 3. Here, partially purified T11TS was used to block the binding of anti-T11 mAb to the E receptor as assessed by indirect immunofluorescence. Binding of anti-T3 mAb was not affected.

6 Blocking of Mixed Lymphocyte Reaction by mAb to T11TS

The above findings suggest that mAb L180/1 does indeed detect the sheep form of the molecule recognized by the E receptor. The expression of this GP on white blood cells is in line with the above hypothesis that the E receptor and its ligand are complementary cell interaction molecules. Since blocking of the E receptor with some mAbs to T11 had been shown by others to inhibit T-cell activation, tests were conducted to; is determine whether the same would be true for mAb to T11TS as well. Table 2 sums up a characteristic experiment. Mixed lymphocyte reaction (MLR) was initiated between white blood cells from two outbred sheep, and purified mAb L180/1 or normal mouse (NM) Ig were added at various concentrations. Inhibition, though not complete, was indeed observed with as little as 0.4 μg mAb L180/1 per milliliter. In contrast, the response of SWBC to human recombinant IL2 without intentional antigenic stimulation

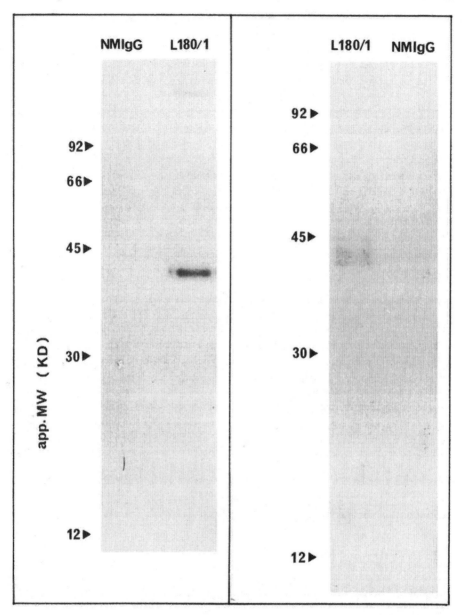

Fig. 2. SDS-PAGE of radioimmunoprecipitates stained with mAb L180/1. *Left panel*: SRBC lysate, surface-iodinated. *Right panel*: concanavalin A-binding fraction of the lysate from ^{3}H-leucine-labeled STBL. Slab gels of 12% acrylamide were run under reducing conditions. Apparent molecular weights are given in kilodaltons

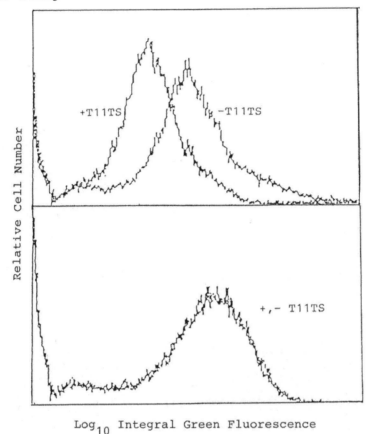

Fig. 3. Partially purified T11TS inhibits the binding of anti-T11 mAb to human PBL: 2.5×10^5 PBL were pretreated for 30 min with 1 μg protein eluted from the L180/1 affinity column. They were then washed and stained with anti-T11 (*upper panel*) or anti-T3 (*lower panel*) mAb, followed by goat anti mouse FITC

was not affected by the presence of the antibody, indicating that after the acquisition of IL2 reactivity and in the presence of sufficient IL2, T-cell proliferation is resistant to blocking with mAb to T11TS.

7 Conclusions

The results summarized in this chapter show that the expression of the cell surface molecule recognized by the E receptor of T lymphocytes in E-rosetting is not restricted to RBC. Furthermore, preliminary evidence is presented for the functioning of this molecule, which we have termed T11 target structure

The Target Structure for T11: A Cell Interaction Molecule Involved in T-Cell Activation? 171

Table 2. Inhibition of alloantigen-induced but not of IL2-driven sheep T-cell proliferation by mAb L180/1

Responders	Stimulators	Human re-combinant IL2	Purified IgG	^{3}H-thymidine incorporation (cpm $\times 10^{-3}$) (pulsed day 4 – 5)
5×10^5	–	–	–	6.67
5×10^5	5×10^5	–	–	58.76
5×10^5	5×10^5	–	10 μg NM IgG/ml	60.33
5×10^5	5×10^5	–	2 μg NM IgG/ml	51.48
5×10^5	5×10^5	–	0.4 μg NM IgG/ml	68.87
5×10^5	5×10^5	–	10 μg L180/1/ml	18.90
5×10^5	5×10^5	–	2 μg L180/1/ml	17.18
5×10^5	5×10^5	–	0.4 μg L180/1/ml	23.09
5×10^5	–	5 units/ml	–	47.50
5×10^5	–	5 units/ml	10 μg NM IgG/ml	54.95
5×10^5	–	5 units/ml	2 μg NM IgG/ml	45.21
5×10^5	–	5 units/ml	0.4 μg NM IgG/ml	46.82
5×10^5	–	5 units/ml	10 μg L180/1/ml	42.12
5×10^5	–	5 units/ml	2 μg L180/1/ml	41.30
5×10^5	–	5 units/ml	0.4 μg L180/1/ml	45.17

(T11TS), as a cell interaction molecule in T-cell activation. While the latter point will require confirmation in better defined systems than the sheep MLR, the present findings may provide a common basis for our understanding of the classical E-rosetting phenomenon and the recent demonstrations of the functional involvement of the T11 molecule in T-cell responses. Thus, T11TS may serve its true function on WBC (and possibly on other nucleated cells) as an acceptor for the T11 molecule. Its presence on RBC may have little or no functional relevance, a situation possibly similar to the expression of major histocompatibility complex (MHC) class I molecules on mouse RBC.

It is of particular interest that activation of T lymphocytes through the E receptor has recently been demonstrated in immature thymocytes that do not express the T3/T-cell receptor complex (Fox et al. 1985). This finding could provide a basis for understanding the regulation of T-cell proliferation in early T-cell development. In this context, the present demonstration that T11TS is expressed on activated T lymphocytes could perhaps indicate that cells of the T lineage provide the signal that stimulates early thymocyte proliferation through the E receptor. We hope to be able to test this hypothesis by developing anti-T11TS mAb in experimental systems more amenable to cellular analysis.

Acknowledgements. I thank Rita Mitnacht for excellent technical assistance, M. Lohoff for his collection of SRBC-specific hybridomas, Dr. Fiers and Dr. Devos for a gift of recombinant human IL2, Dr. A. Schimpl and Dr. E. Wecker for helpful discussions, and Christel Stoppe for typing this manuscript. This work was supported by the Deutsche Forschungsgemeinschaft through SFB 105, Würzburg.

172   T. Hünig

References

Bernard A, Gelin C, Raynal B, Pham D, Grosse C, Boumsell IS (1982) Phenomenon of human T-cells rosetting with sheep erythrocytes analysed with monoclonal antibodies. J Exp Med 155:1317–1333

Fox DA, Hussey RE, Fitzgerald KA, Bensussan A, Daley JF, Schlossman SF, Reinherz EL (1985) Activation of human thymocytes via the 50-KD T11 sheep erythrocyte binding protein induces the expression of interleukin 2 receptors on both T3$^+$ and T3$^-$ populations. J Immunol 134:330–335

Howard FD, Ledbetter JA, Wong J, Bieber CP, Stinson EB, Herzenberg LA (1981) A human T-lymphocyte differentiation marker defined by monoclonal antibodies that block E-rosette formation. J Immunol 126:2117–2122

Kamoun M, Martin PJ, Hansen JA, Brown MA, Siadeck AW, Nowinski RC (1981) Identification of a human T-lymphocyte surface protein associated with the E-rosette receptor. J Exp Med 153:207–212

Krensky AM, Sanchez-Madrid F, Robbins E, Nagy JA, Springer TA, Burakoff SJ (1983) The functional significance, distribution, and structure of LFA-1, LFA-2, and LFA-3: cell surface antigens associated with CTL-target interactions. J Immunol 131:611–616

Larsson EL, Andersson J, Coutinho A (1978) Functional consequences of sheep red blood cell rosetting for human T-cells: gain of reactivity to mitogenic factors. Eur J Immunol 8:693–696

Martin PJ, Longton G, Ledbetter JA, Neumann W, Braun MP, Beatty PG, Hansen JA (1983) Identification and functional characterization of two distinct epitopes on the human T-cell surface protein tp 50. J Immunol 131:180–185

Meuer SC, Hussey RE, Fabbi M, Fox D, Acuto O, Fitzgerald KA, Hodgdon JC, Protentis JP, Schlossman SF, Reinherz EL (1984) An alternative pathway of T-cell activation: a functional role for the 50-KD T11 sheep erythrocyte receptor protein. Cell 36:897–906

Palacios R, Martinez-Maza O (1982) Is the E-receptor on human T-lymphocytes a "negative signal receptor"? J Immunol 129:2479–2485

Verbi W, Greaves M, Schneider C, Konbek K, Janossy G, Stein H, Kung P, Goldstein G (1982) Monoclonal antibodies OKT11 and OKT11A have pan-T reactivity and block sheep erythrocyte "receptors". Eur J Immunol 12:81–86

Antigen- and Lectin-Sensitized Murine Cytolytic T Lymphocyte-Precursors Require Both Interleukin 2 and Endogenously Produced Immune (γ) Interferon for Their Growth and Differentiation into Effector Cells

M.M. SIMON[1], S. LANDOLFO[2], T. DIAMANTSTEIN[3], and U. HOCHGESCHWENDER[1]

1   Introduction   173
2   Results   174
2.1   Recombinant Human IL2 and Lectin Induce Growth and Effector Function in Lyt-2+ but not Lyt-2− Lymphocytes   174
2.2   Precursor Frequency Analysis of Lyt-2+ Lymphocytes Induced by Lectin or Antigen and Recombinant Human IL2   175
2.3   Monoclonal Antibodies Specific for the IL2 Receptor Interfere With Induction of CTL-P by Varying Conventional Lymphokine Sources   180
2.4   Endogenous IFN-γ Participates in the Maturation of CTL-P   180
3   Conclusions   183
References   184

1 Introduction

The transition of precursor cells of cytolytic T lymphocytes (CTL) into effector cells is induced by antigen/lectin and through cooperation between T-cell subsets (CANTOR and BOYSE 1975; SIMON et al. 1981). The discovery that the synergistic effect of lymphocytes during CTL development can be replaced by soluble mediators (lymphokines) secreted by T cells (ALTMAN and COHEN 1975; PLATE 1976; WAGNER and RÖLLINGHOFF 1978) and the availability of clonally derived lymphokine sources (GLASEBROOK et al. 1982) prompted a series of studies on the role of these factors in CTL induction. From these investigations, two types of lymphokine emerged which seemed to be essential for the generation of CTL from their precursor cells (CTL-P): interleukin 2 (IL2), which provides signals for the proliferation of activated CTL-P (SMITH 1980; GULLBERG et al. 1983), and one or more CTL differentiation factors (CDF), which are considered to induce maturation in developing CTL-P (RAULET and BEVAN 1982; WAGNER et al. 1982; FOLK et al. 1983; KANAGAWA 1983). However, the exact roles of soluble mediators in CTL induction could not be ascertained because of the difficulties to purify lymphokine preparations to homogeneity and the finding that even lymphokine sources from cloned T-cell lines contained multiple biological activities.

    With the advent of recombinant DNA technology, pure lymphokine preparations have been obtained in sufficient quantities to enable closer examination of

---

[1] Max-Planck-Institut für Immunbiologie, Stübeweg 51, D-7800 Freiburg
[2] Institute of Microbiology, University of Torino, I-Torino
[3] Immunologische Forschungseinheit, Klinikum Steglitz, Freie Universität, D-1000 Berlin

Current Topics in Microbiology and Immunology, Vol. 126
© Springer-Verlag Berlin · Heidelberg 1986

174   M.M. Simon et al.

their involvement in T-cell activation. In the present study we have used highly purified murine T-cell subsets, recombinant sources of lymphokines (IL2, IFN-γ), and monoclonal antibodies (moAb) specific for either lymphokine (IFN-γ) or lymphokine receptors (IL2R) to ask the following questions:

1. Is IL2 sufficient to drive lectin- or antigen-sensitized Lyt-2$^+$/Lyt-2$^-$ lymphocytes into effector cells?

2. How many cells can be induced under these conditions in both T lymphocyte subpopulations?

3. Are other factors distinct from IL2 involved in the generation of CTL, and what is their function?

4. Do precursor cells themselves contribute lymphokines to the development of CTL into effector cells?

A preliminary account of these studies has been presented recently (HOCH-GESCHWENDER and SIMON 1985).

2   Results

2.1   Recombinant Human IL2 and Lectin Induce Growth and Effector Function in Lyt-2$^+$ but not Lyt-2$^-$ Lymphocytes

The analysis by flow cytofluorometry (FCF) of C57BL/6 lymph node T cells previously treated with moAb anti-Lyt-2.2 (moAb 19/178, kindly provided by Dr. U. Hämmerling, Sloan-Kettering-Cancer Center, N.Y., N.Y.) followed by fluoresceinated goat antimouse immunoglobulin revealed a positive and a negative subpopulation which could easily be separated (Fig. 1). In more than ten experiments, a mean of 41% of T cells expressed the Lyt-2.2 marker. After FCF sorting, both populations – Lyt-2$^+$ and Lyt-2$^-$ – were at least 94% pure by the criterion of staining reciprocally with moAb specific for either L3T4 or Lyt-2 determinants (CEREDIG et al. 1983), and did not contain detectable amounts of adherent cells (as defined by histochemical staining with nonspecific esterases; BURSTONE 1957, data not shown).

Both selected and unselected T-cell populations were incubated without accessory cells (non-T, radioresistant spleen cells) and sensitized with concanavalin A (Con A) in the presence of exogenous IL2 sources (recombinant human IL2, rec. hIL2; supernatant of Con A-activated rat spleen cells, Con A-SN), or with either lectin or lymphokine sources alone, and tested for proliferation and for cytotoxic activity in a lectin-dependent lympholysis assay on P815 tumor target cells and phytohemagglutinin (PHA). As seen in Fig. 2, Lyt-2$^+$ lymphocytes were induced to proliferate and to develop into CTL in the presence of Con A and rec. hIL2 or Con A-SN, but not when incubated with either Con A or lymphokine sources (rec. hIL2, Con A-SN) alone. Proliferative and cytotoxic responses of Con A-activated Lyt-2$^+$ cells were similar in cultures with rec. hIL2 or Con A-SN previously adjusted to contain the same amount of IL2 activity, and were comparable to those of unselected T cells. As expected from previous studies, no cytotoxic activity was generated from Lyt-2$^-$ lymphocytes, but neit-

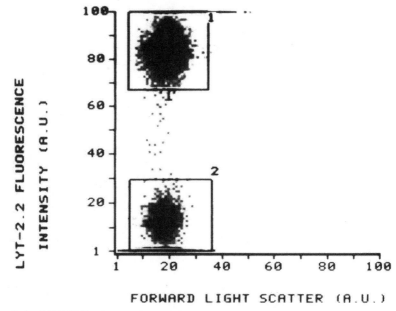

Fig. 1. FCF analysis of C57BL/6 nylon wool-purified lymph node T cells stained with monoclonal antibody anti-Lyt-2.2 and fluorescein-conjugated antigen-binding fragment F(ab')$_2$ goat antimouse immunoglobulin on an Orthocytofluorograph 50 H (Ortho Diagnostic Systems, Westwood, Calif.). Correlation of forward light scatter and the fluorescence intensity (given in arbitrary units, A.U.) of 20000 individual cells are shown. Numbers 1 and 2 define areas selected for sorting of Lyt-2$^+$ and Lyt-2$^-$ lymphocytes

her were they induced to proliferate under these conditions. In addition, only marginal IL2 activity was detected in FCF-selected Lyt-2$^-$ populations stimulated with Con A alone (data not shown). These results indicated that IL2 directly induces growth and maturation in Con A-activated Lyt-2$^+$ lymphocytes without the assistance of other accessory cells or factors, and suggested that Lyt-2$^-$ cells require either different or additional signals for their induction. The possibility that Lyt-2$^+$ lymphocytes were only reactive to lectin and IL2 because of their previous binding of moAb anti-Lyt-2.2 was excluded in experiments leading to similar results (data not shown) in which responder cells were sorted by FCF according to the L3T4 marker which is reciprocally expressed with Lyt-2 on mouse T cells (CEREDIG et al. 1983).

2.2 Precursor Frequency Analysis of Lyt-2$^+$ Lymphocytes Induced by Lectin or Antigen and Recombinant Human IL2

The frequencies of FCF sorted Lyt-2$^+$ and Lyt-2$^-$ precursor cells that respond to lectin and rec. hIL2 in the absence of accessory cells by growing (GTL-P, as determined by visual examination) and development of CTL (CTL-P) were determined in a limiting dilution (LD) system (SIMON et al. 1984). In Table 1 only the

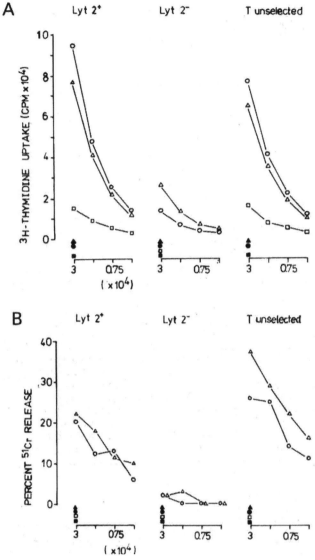

Fig. 2. A Proliferative and **B** cytotoxic activities of FCF-sorted C57BL/6 Lyt-2[+] and Lyt-2[−] lymphocytes and unselected T cells generated in response to Con A and IL2-containing lymphokine sources. Microcultures (3 × 10[4] cells/well; six wells/group) were set up in RPMI-1640 medium supplemented with L-glutamine (2 mM), kanamycin (100 μg/ml), tyrosine (10 μg/ml), hydroxyethylpiperazine ethanesulfonic acid (HEPES) buffer (25 mM), 2-mercaptoethanol (2 × 10^{-5} M), and 10% selected fetal calf serum; nylon wool-purified and FCF-sorted Lyt-2[+] and Lyt-2[−] lymphocytes or unselected T cells were cultured in the presence or absence of Con A (3 μg/ml) and/or lymphokine sources (100 units IL2/ml; see legend to Table 1), and incubated at 37 °C in a humidified atmosphere of 5% CO$_2$. Addition to culture: none ■; Con A □; rec. hIL2 ●; Con A-SN ▲; Con A + rec. hIL2 ○; Con A + Con A-SN △). Proliferation (**A**) was measured on day 3 after a ^{3}H-thymidine pulse for the last 12 h. Cytotoxic activity (**B**) was determined on day 3 by titrating effector cells on 2 × 10^3 ^{51}Cr-labeled P815 tumor target cells in the presence of 4% PHA in a 4-h asssay. Each *point* represents the mean of triplicate wells. Numbers on the *abscissa* indicate the number of responder cells (x 10^4) cultured on day 0, the descendants of which were tested on day 3. The percentage-specific ^{51}Cr release was calculated by the equation: ^{51}Cr release (%) = $(x-y/z-y) \times 100$, in which x is the counts per minute in the supernatant (SN) of target cells mixed with effector cells; y is the cpm in the SN of target cells incubated alone; and z is the cpm after lysis of target cells in 1N-HCl

Antigen- and Lectin-Sensitized Murine Cytolytic T Lymphocyte 177

Table 1. Frequencies of precursor cells in FCF-sorted Lyt-2$^+$ lymphocytes that grow and develop into CTL in response to lectin and rec. hIL2

Experi-ment	Culture condition		Frequency in Lyt-2$^+$ lymphocytes of	
			GTL-P	CTL-P
1	Con A + rec. hIL2	(70 units)	1/17 (1/12–1/29)	1/79 (1/57–1/129)
	Con A		^{a})	^{a})
2	Con A + rec. hIL2	(70 units)	1/11 (1/8–1/17)	1/86 (1/24–1/133)
	Con A + Con A-SN	(70 units)	1/4 (1/3–1/6)	1/28 (1/18–1/56)
3	Con A + rec. hIL2	(60 units)	1/8 (1/6–1/13)	1/29 (1/21–1/49)
	Rec. hIL2	(60 units)	^{a})	^{a})
4	Con A + rec. hIL2	(70 units)	1/10 (1/7–1/16)	1/44 (1/33–1/68)
	LA + rec. hIL2	(70 units)	1/19 (1/13–1/35)	1/72 (1/32–1/116)
5	Con A + rec. hIL2	(70 units)	1/9 (1/7–1/13)	1/33 (1/22–1/63)
	Con A + rec. hIL2	(8 units)	1/39 (1/23–1/125)	^{a})
	Con A + MLC SN	(8 units)	1/8 (1/4–1/16)	1/35 (1/23–1/69)

^{a}) All cultures negative; LA, leukoagglutinin

Graded numbers of FCF-sorted C57BL/6 Lyt-2$^+$ responder cells (1000 cells – 2.5 cells/well) were set up in culture medium in groups of 24 microcultures (0.2 ml) and were sensitized to lectin (Con A, 3 μg/ml; LA, 1 μg/ml) and the indicated lymphokine sources (numbers of units/ml in parentheses refer to the activity of IL2 as reveled by probit analysis (GILLIS et al. 1978) in comparison to a standard titration curve obtained with rec. hIL2 on a lymphokine-dependent line, CTLL-2. For rec. hIL2, 1 unit of biological activity, which produces 50% of the maximal response, corresponds to 0.2 μg protein. After 8–10 days, growth in each well was identified by microscopic inspection. Cytotoxic activity was tested on days 8–10 for each well by incubating effector cells with 2×10^{3} ^{51}Cr-labeled P815 tumor target cells in the presence of PHA (4%) in a 4-h assay. Minimal estimates of frequencies were calculated by the minimum χ^2 method from the Poisson distribution relationship between the number of responder cells and the logarithm of the fraction of negative cultures (TASWELL 1981), accepting experiments with P > 0.05 (95% confidence limits are given in parentheses)

data for Lyt-2$^+$ lymphocytes (results from five representative experiments) are given. In general, Lyt-2$^-$ lymphocytes were not activated under these conditions and the low number of GTL-P occasionally detected in this population – about 30- to 100-fold fewer than those in the Lyt-2$^+$ subset – suggests the activation of contaminating Lyt-2$^+$ cells rather than the induction of Lyt-2$^-$ lymphocytes. It is obvious from the data in Table 1 that high proportions of GTL-P and CTL-P were activated in Lyt-2$^+$ lymphocytes responding to Con A and rec. hIL2, ranging between 1/8 and 1/12 for GTL-P and between 1/29 and 1/86 for CTL-P (as detected by lectin mediated lysis of P815 tumor target cells). Frequencies of GTL-P and CTL-P similar to those with Con A were also found in Lyt-2$^+$ lymphocytes responding to rec. hIL2 and another lectin, leukoagglutinin (LA; experiment 4 in Table 1). The admixture of both lectins to cultures did not further increase the frequency of responding cells (data not shown), suggesting that Con A and LA act on the same rather than on distinct Lyt-2$^+$ target cells (KANAGAWA 1983).

No induction of any precursor cell was observed in cultures containing Lyt-2$^+$ cells and either Con A (experiment 1) or rec. hIL2 (experiment 3) alone, thus excluding contaminating preactivated Lyt-2$^+$ lymphocytes (DEVOS et al. 1984)

178 M.M. Simon et al.

Table 2. Correlation between the amount of IL2 activity and the generation of CTL from FCF-sorted and Con A-activated Lyt-2$^+$ lymphocytes

Titration of rec. hIL2 (units/0.2 ml)	Cytolytic activity (lytic units/10^4 cells) of Lyt-2$^+$ lymphocytes cultured in	
	Rec. hIL2	Rec. hIL2 + MLC-SN
200	214.2	214.2
100	214.2	315
50	54	153
25	15	60
12.5	0.6	35.4
6.25	0.3	15
0	0	15

Microcultures (1×10^3 cells/well, 0.2 ml) were set up in culture medium in triplicate with FCF-sorted C57BL/6 Lyt-2$^+$ lymphocytes, Con A (3 μg/ml), various concentrations of rec. hIL2 (units/0.2 ml) in the absence or presence of a fixed concentration of MLC-SN (25%), or with MLC-SN (25%) alone. On day 7 cytotoxic activity was determined by titrating effector cells on ^{51}Cr-labeled P815 tumor cells in the presence of PHA (4%) in a 4-h assay. For each lymphocyte population tested, a dose-response curve was established and the number of lytic units per 10^4 cells was calculated. In this experiment, 1 lytic unit was arbitrarily defined as the number of lymphocytes plated at day 0, the descendants of which are required to achieve 50% lysis of 2×10^3 ^{51}Cr-labeled target cells within 4 h

and again emphasizing the necessity for both signals (Con A and IL2) in the induction of resting CTL-P. Visual examination of individual cultures seeded with low numbers of cells showed quite heterogeneous growth characteristics for activated Lyt-2$^+$ lymphocytes, resulting in colonies which differed significantly in clone size. Though initially the growth rate was fairly consistent between various clones, some of them ceased to grow after several days in culture or even died after 2–6 divisions. These findings, which are reminiscent of previous studies on the growth characteristics of preactivated T-cell subsets (KUPPERS et al. 1984), may reflect an inherent heterogeneity of CTL-P in the Lyt-2$^+$ population and warrant further examination.

The finding that the frequencies of mitogen-reactive GTL-P were always higher than those of CTL-P is probably due to the lower sensitivity of the cytotoxic assay rather than reflecting qualitative differences of precursor cells. This assumption is also supported by the observation that pooled effector populations derived from LD micro cultures seeded with either high or low responder cell numbers showed similar cytolytic activities (data not shown), and indicates that CTL-P do not require extensive expansion in order to express their cytolytic activity.

Although adjusted to the same IL2 activity, consistently higher frequencies for GTL-P, and particularly for CTL-P, were found in lectin-driven Lyt-2$^+$ populations cultured with Con A-SN or supernatant from secondary mixed lymphocyte cultures (MLC-SN) than with rec. hIL2 (Table 1, experiments 2, 5). However, when rec. hIL2 was used at IL2 concentrations higher than those in conventional sources, similar numbers of GTL-P and CTL-P were induced (Table 1, experiment 5). The same effect was seen when rec. hIL2 was titrated to cultures

Antigen- and Lectin-Sensitized Murine Cytolytic T Lymphocyte   179

Table 3. Frequencies of precursor cells in FCF-sorted Lyt-2$^+$ lymphocytes that grow and develop into CTL in response to P815 tumor cells and rec. hIL2

Ex-peri-ment	Culture condition	Frequency in Lyt-2$^+$ lymphocytes of		
		GTL-P	PTL-P	CTL-P
1	P815 + rec. hIL2 (70 units)	1/70 (1/56–1/93)	1/142 (1/109–1/203)	1/275 (1/219–1/372)
2	P815 + rec. hIL2 (70 units)	1/59 (1/44–1/82)	nd	1/131 (1/100–1/193)
	P815 + Con A-SN (70 units)	1/44 (1/32–1/71)	nd	1/83 (1/65–1/116)
	P815 + MLC-SN (10 units)	1/25 (1/17–1/50)	nd	1/90 (1/71–1/124)
3	P815 + rec. hIL2 (10 units)	1/99 (1/78–1/134)	1/879 (1/591–1/1711)	1/3094 (1/2060–1/6213)
	P815 + rec. hIL2 (100 units)	1/72 (1/59–1/94)	1/121 (1/91–1/180)	1/278 (1/232–1/347)
	P815 + MLC-SN (10 units)	1/62 (1/48–1/88)	1/71 (1/55–1/100)	1/153 (1/120–1/212)

nd, not done

Graded numbers of FCF-sorted C57BL/6 Lyt-2$^+$ responder cells (5000–38 cells/well) were set up in culture medium in groups of 24 microcultures (0.2 ml) and were incubated with 5×10^3 irradiated (8000 rad) P815 tumor cells and various lymphokine sources (numbers of units/ml in parentheses refer to the activity of IL2 present in each lymphokine source, and were determined as described in the legend to Table 1). Growth, proliferation, and cytotoxic activity were tested from the same cultures. Growth in each well was identified by microscopic inspection on day 8. Proliferation was measured following the ^{51}Cr release assay on day 9 after a previous 20-h ^{3}H-thymidine pulse of microcultures. Cytotoxic activity was tested on day 9 for each well by incubating effector cells on 2×10^3 ^{51}Cr-labeled P815 tumor target cells in a 4-h assay. Minimal estimates of frequencies were calculated as described in the legend to Table 1 (95% confidence limits are given in parentheses)

containing Lyt-2$^+$ lymphocytes and Con A in the presence or absence of a fixed concentration of MLC-SN (Table 2). In the absence of or at low concentrations of rec. hIL2 (6.25–12.5 units), significant CTL activity was only observed in cultures which in addition received MLC-SN (25% ≙ 8 units IL2/ml). At intermediate doses of rec. hIL2 (25–50 units), higher lytic units were always found in cultures which also contained MLC-SN, and only at very high concentrations of rec. hIL2 (100–200 units) were similar CTL activities observed irrespective of the presence of MLC-SN. At present it is not clear whether the biological activity detected in MLC-SN (or Con A-SN) is due to another factor distinct from IL2, or whether the different activation potential of IL2 in the three lymphokine sources [human IL2 (rec. hIL2) vs rat IL2 (Con A-SN) vs mouse IL2 (MLC-SN)] is due to their differential affinity to the mouse IL2 receptor. However, the possibility that conventional IL2 sources were superior to rec. IL2 because of a differential degradation of natural vs recombinant IL2 in culture was excluded (data not shown).

Experiments 1–3 in Table 3 demonstrate that in the presence of allogeneic stimulator cells (H-2^d), C57BL/6 Lyt-2$^+$ cells were induced by rec. hIL2 for growth (GTL-P, 1/59–1/99; determined by visual examination) and proliferation (PTL-P, 1/121–1/879; as determined by ^{3}H-thymidine incorporation), and for generation of specific CTL (CTL-P, 1/131–1/3094). In these studies P815 tumor cells were used as stimulator cells to avoid a possible contribution of accessory cells during activation. Thus, as for lectin, specific induction of Lyt-2$^+$ effector cells by alloantigens is independent of accessory cells and only requires additional signals provided by IL2. As shown before, frequencies for antigen-specific GTL-P (PTL-P), and CTL-P induced in Lyt-2$^+$ populations were higher in Con A-SN or MLC-SN than in rec. hIL2, provided all three lymphokine sources contained comparable IL2 activities (Table 3, experiments 2, 3), but were similar when rec. hIL2 was used at a higher concentration (Table 3, experiment 3). Lyt-2$^-$ cells could not be stimulated by P815 tumor cells for growth, which is not surprising in view of their deficiency in class II H-2 antigens (KIESSLING et al. 1975), but also did not respond to another tumor line of B10A origin expressing I-A allo antigens (CH-1.1; KOCH et al. 1984) under the same conditions (HOCHGE-SCHWENDER and SIMON 1985, and data not shown). In our hands, the activation of Lyt-2$^-$ lymphocytes by either lectin or antigen and rec. hIL2 always required in addition accessory cells.

2.3 Monoclonal Antibodies Specific for the IL2 Receptor Interfere With Induction of CTL-P by Varying Conventional Lymphokine Sources

In order to test whether IL2 is the only lymphokine able to induce growth and effector function in lectin-sensitized CTL-P, Lyt-2$^+$ cells were incubated with Con A and cultured in various lymphokine sources (Con A-SN, MLC-SN, rec. hIL2) in the presence or absence of monoclonal antibodies to the IL2 receptor (IL2R) known to specifically inhibit the binding of IL2 to its membrane receptor (AMT-13, OSAWA and DIAMANTSTEIN 1984). It is obvious from the data in Table 4 that in the presence of antibody AMT-13 for the entire period of culture, CTL responses were totally inhibited irrespective of the lymphokine source used. Together with the finding that AMT-13 also interfered with the development of CTL when the antibody was only present for the first 24 –48 h of culture (not shown), the data do not provide evidence for the existence of other factor(s) with IL2-like activity and support the conclusion that IL2 delivers signals for both proliferation of activated CTL-P and, most importantly, also those essential for the induction of resting CTL-P.

2.4 Endogenous IFN-γ Participates in the Maturation of CTL-P

Because of the notion that IFN-γ is involved in the development of CTL (SIMON et al. 1979; LANDOLFO et al. 1985), we tested the effect of recombinant mouse IFN-γ (rec. mIFN-γ) on the polyclonal induction of cytotoxic responses from Lyt-2$^+$ cells. It is shown in Fig. 3b that IFN-γ alone at concentrations from 7–900 units did not induce any CTL activity from Con A-sensitized Lyt-2$^+$ cells, and

Table 4. Effect of monoclonal antibody (mAb) AMT-13 on the induction of CTL from FCF-sorted Lyt-2$^+$ lymphocytes sensitized with Con A and different lymphokine sources

Addition to culture		Percentage ^{51}Cr Release Effector to target cell ratio			
Lymphokine source	mAb AMT-13	10	5	2.5	1.25
–	–	0	0	0	0
Con A-SN	–	32.4	22.0	14.3	9.7
Con A-SN	+	0	0	0	0
MLC-SN	–	23.5	14.3	6.1	3.8
MLC-SN	+	0	0	0	0
Rec. hIL2	–	14.5	2.1	5.0	2.5
Rec. hIL2	+	0	0	0	0

Microcultures (1 × 10^3 cells/well) were set up in culture medium with FCF-sorted C57BL/6 Lyt-2$^+$ lymphocytes, Con A (3 µg/ml), and the indicated lymphokine sources [Con A-SN (10%, or 30 units IL2/ml); MLC-SN (25%, or 10 units IL2/ml); and rec. hIL2 (30 units IL2/ml)] in the absence or presence of monoclonal antibody AMT-13 (1:100, final dilution). Cytotoxic activity was tested for each group on day 8 by titrating effector cells on 2 × 10^3 ^{51}Cr-labeled P815 tumor cells in the presence of PHA (4%) in a 4-h assay. Numbers given for effector to target ratio indicate the number of responder cells plated on day 0, the descendants of which were tested on day 8

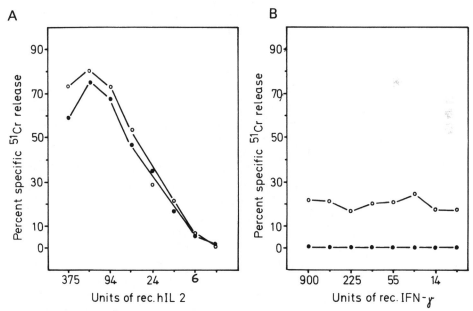

Fig. 3A, B. Contribution of rec. hIL2 and rec. mIFN-γ to the generation of CTL from FCF-sorted Lyt-2$^+$ cells responding to Con A. Microcultures (1 × 10^3 cells/well) were set up in culture medium in triplicate with FCF-sorted C57BL/6 Lyt-2$^+$ responder cells, Con A (3 µg/ml), and either **A** increasing concentrations of rec. hIL2 in the absence (●) or presence (○) of a fixed amount of rec. mIFN-γ (100 units/well) or **B** increasing concentrations of rec. mIFN-γ in the absence (●) or presence (○) of a fixed amount of rec. hIL2 (20 units/well). Cytotoxic activity was determined on day 7 by incubating effector cells with 2 × 10^3 ^{51}Cr-labeled P815 tumor target cells in the presence of 4% PHA in a 4-h assay. Each *point* represents the mean of triplicate cultures. For calculation of percentage-specific ^{51}Cr release see legend to Fig. 2

182   M.M. Simon et al.

Table 5. Inhibition of generation of CTL from FCF-sorted Lyt-2^+ lymphocytes responding to Con A and rec. hIL2 in the presence of monoclonal antibody AN-18

Addition of monoclonal antibody	Effector to target cell ratio			
	10	5	2.5	1.25
	Percentage ^{51}Cr release			
–	33.8	22.8	13.8	7.5
AN-18 (1:5)	0.3	0	0.1	0.5
AN-18 (1:10)	3.4	1.2	0.2	0.4
AN-18 (1:50)	21.2	15.6	8.7	4.3

Microcultures (1×10^3 cells/well) were set up in culture medium with FCF-sorted C57BL/6 Lyt-2^+ lymphocytes, Con A (3 μg/ml), and rec. hIL2 (60 units/ml final concentration) in the absence or presence of monoclonal antibody AN-18 (at the indicated dilutions 1:5, 1:10, 1:50). Cytotoxic activity was tested for each group on day 8 by titrating effector cells on 2×10^3 ^{51}Cr-labeled P815 tumor cells in the presence of PHA (4%) in a 4-h assay. Numbers given for effector to target cell ratio indicate the number of responder cells plated on day 0, the descendants of which were tested on day 8

did not significantly alter the inducing effect of a fixed concentration of rec. hIL2 (20 units, Fig. 3b) or of increasing amounts of IL2 (titrated in the range from 3 to over 300 units; Fig. 3a). At first glance these data suggested that IFN-γ has no direct effect on Lyt-2^+ lymphocytes, but that it elicits biological activity via other T-cell subsets (Lyt-2^-) or nonlymphoid cells (macrophages). On the other hand, we have found that a considerable proportion of lectin- or antigen-activated Lyt-2^+ lymphocytes that developed into CTL also secreted IFN-γ. In a representative experiment the frequencies of Lyt-2^+ precursor cells that responded to lectin or antigen and rec. hIL2 with development of CTL or with secretion of IFN-γ (IFN-γ-P) were 1/52 (CTL-P) and 1/144 (IFN-γ-P) for Con A-reactive cells, and 1/577 (CTL-P) and 1/1427 (IFN-γ-P) for P815-reactive cells. Thus, it is still possible that IFN-γ is involved in the maturation of CTL-P and is secreted in sufficient amounts by the precursor cells themselves. This possibility was tested by incubating Lyt-2^+ cells with Con A and rec. hIL2 and adding to cultures moAb with specificity for IFN-γ (AN-18, PRAT et al. 1984). As seen in one (out of four) representative experiments, depicted in Table 5, moAb AN-18 strongly inhibited the generation of CTL at concentrations between 1:5 and 1:10, and still reduced cytolytic activity considerably at a dilution of 1:50. In further experiments it was found that the same moAb only inhibited CTL responses when present for up to 48 h, but not when added later, thus excluding mere toxic effects of the reagent (data not shown). The specificity of the moAb AN-18 used was simultaneously ascertained by its capability to inhibit in vitro the reduction of viral infectivity and of NK boosting activity mediated by IFN-γ (PRAT et al. 1984). The data are therefore in accordance with the assumption that IFN-γ is endogenously produced during activation of Lyt-2^+ cells and is necessary for the development of CTL from their precursor cells. It remains to be determined whether the same lymphocyte produces and consumes IFN-γ at the same time.

3 Conclusions

The data reviewed in this paper reveal that IL2 acts directly on lectin- and antigen-sensitized Lyt-2$^+$ CTL-P, and is sufficient for the induction of growth and generation of CTL. In contrast, Lyt-2$^-$ lymphocytes are not activated under these conditions to divide and to develop effector functions. The use of IL2 produced by recombinant DNA technology excludes other lymphokines as effector molecules. This is further supported by the finding that moAb to the IL2R inhibit the development of CTL from CTL-P responding to lectin in the presence of conventional (Con A-SN, MLC-SN) or recombinant (IL2) lymphokine sources. It also indicates that the Con A-SN or MLC-SN tested did not contain other soluble mediators with biological activities similar to those of IL2. Therefore, the signals provided by IL2 are responsible for both activation and expansion of CTL-P, but it is not clear whether there is a qualitative difference in the induction of the two events.

The present study strongly indicates that the transition of antigen- or lectin-stimulated CTL-P into effector cells in the presence of IL2 does not require the assistance of other cell types. Together with their restriction specificity (class I major histocompatibility gene complex antigen), this property allows CTL-P to be activated by foreign antigens appearing on the membrane of virtually all cells in the body, including neoantigens on any transformed cell, and to develop into CTL with exogenous help. Our results are not compatible with a previous study from HÜNIG et al. (1983) indicating that induction of IL2 responsiveness by Con A is accessory cell-dependent, though it was not determined whether this is true for all T-cell subsets. However, they confirm recent findings by ERARD et al. (1985) obtained in a similar system and suggesting that the two signals provided by lectin and IL2 are sufficient for induction and maturation of CTL-P.

At present we find it difficult to explain why only a fraction of Lyt-2$^+$ lymphocytes can be activated by lectin and rec. hIL2 in LD. It is possible that this population contains more than one T-cell subset, or that Lyt-2$^+$ lymphocytes are heterogeneous with respect to their maturation stages, and that in both cases signals different from IL2 are required for their propagation. However, even the admixture of various lymphokine sources and accessory cells to cultures did not result in frequencies greater than 1 in 3 (data not shown) of responding Lyt-2$^+$ precursor cells, thus leaving more than 60% of the lymphocytes incapable of being inducible under "optimal conditions."

Despite the central role of IL2 for the induction process of CTL-P, the data presented suggest that other exogenously added factors distinct from IL2 and present in conventional lymphokine sources can contribute to the generation of CTL. However, our results indicate that in contrast to CDF (RAULET and BEVAN 1982; WAGNER et al. 1982) or to an IL2R-inducing factor recently described by Wagner et al. (this volume), the activity present on Con A-SN and MLC-SN influences the expansion phase rather than the induction phase of CTL-P. A comparison of the different biological activities derived from conventional sources or from cloned T-cell lines is at present difficult, and their significance will only be elucidated when cloned DNA probes for the individual lymphokines become available.

184   M.M. Simon et al.

We showed in the experiments that the addition of rec. mIFN-γ did not significantly alter the CTL responses of IL2-driven lectin-sensitized Lyt-2$^+$ lymphocytes. However, we found that in LD a high proportion of activated CTL-P secreted IFN-γ in the presence of IL2, and that the development of CTL from Lyt-2$^+$ lymphocytes in the presence of lectin and IL2 was inhibited by moAb to IFN-γ. This not only emphasizes the close association between cytotoxic T-cell function and release of IFN-γ (KLEIN and BEVAN 1983), but also suggests that CTL-P produce and respond to their own factor. This may also explain the failure to influence the generation of CTL by adding exogenous IFN-γ. The data extend previous findings on the modulation of mixed lymphocyte reaction by the same monoclonal anti-IFN-γ antibodies (LANDOLFO et al. 1985), and indicate still another immunoregulatory effect of IFN-γ: its direct interaction with CTL-P during their induction.

It has been reported recently that a high proportion of lectin-sensitized cytolytic Lyt-2$^+$ lymphocytes are able to proliferate independently of exogenous help, suggesting that they produce their own IL2 (VON BOEHMER et al. 1984). Together with the finding that CTL-P also secrete IFN-γ after induction by IL2, this would mean that signals delivered by either lectin or antigen can initiate a process of self-perpetuating growth and differentiation of CTL-P. However, we have so far been unable with antigen or lectin alone to directly induce highly purified resting Lyt-2$^+$ lymphocytes to proliferate and to develop into CTL or to produce IL2.

We therefore conclude that two exogenous signals provided by antigen/lectin and IL-2 are necessary for the induction of CTL-P, but that a third independent signal given by endogenously produced IFN-γ is essential for their further development into effector cells.

Acknowledgements. We thank G. Nerz, M. Prester, I. Kutter, and N. Leibrock for excellent technical and secretarial assistance, U. Brugger for operating the Ortho 50-H, Dr. K. Fey who kindly provided the MINCHI programme for calculating precursor frequencies, and Dr. Jean Langhorne for critically reading the manuscript. We are grateful to the Sandoz Forschungsinstitut, Vienna, for the generous gift of human recombinant interleukin 2, and to Boehringer, Ingelheim, for supplying us with mouse recombinant IFN-gamma (produced by Genentech, Inc.). This work was supported by Deutsche Forschungsgemeinschaft, Si 214/5.

References

Altman A, Cohen IR (1975) Cell-free media of mixed lymphocyte cultures augmenting sensitization in vitro of mouse T lymphocyte against allogeneic fibroblasts. Eur J Immunol 5:437–444
Burstone MS (1957) The cytochemical localization of esterase. J Natl Cancer Inst 18:167–172
Cantor H, Boyse EA (1975) Functional subclasses of T lymphocytes bearing different Ly antigens. II. Cooperation between subclasses of Ly+ cells in the generation of killer activity. J Exp Med 141:1390–1399
Ceredig R, Dialynas DP, Fitch FW, MacDonald HR (1983) Precursurs of T cell growth factor producing cells in the thymus: ontogeny, frequency, and quantitative recovery in a subpopulation of phenotypically mature thymocytes defined by monoclonal antibody GK-1.5. J Exp Med 158:1654–1671
Devos R, Plaetinik G, Fiers W (1984) Induction of cytolytic cells by pure recombinant human interleukin 2. Eur J Immunol 14:1057–1060
Erard F, Corthesy P, Nabholz M, Lowenthal JW, Zaech P, Plaetinck G, MacDonald HR (1985) In-

Antigen- and Lectin-Sensitized Murine Cytolytic T Lymphocyte   185

terleukin 2 is both necessary and sufficient for the growth and differentiation of lectin-stimulated cytolytic T lymphocyte precursors. J Immunol 134:1644

Folk W, Männel DN, Dröge W (1983) Activation of CTL requires at least two spleen cell-derived factors besides interleukin 2. J Immunol 130:2214

Gillis S, Ferm MM, Ou W, Smith KA (1978) T cell growth factor: parameters of production and a quantitative microassay for activity. J Immunol 120:2027

Glasebrook AL, Kelso A, Zubler RH, Ely JM, Prystowsky MB, Fitch FW (1982) Lymphokine production by cytolytic and noncytolytic alloreactive T cell clones. In: Fathmann CG, Fitch FW (eds) Isolation, characterization and utilization of T lymphocyte clones. Academic, New York

Gullberg M, Pobor G, Bandeira A, Larsson EL, Coutinho A (1983) Differential requirements for activation and growth of unprimed cytotoxic and helper T lymphocytes. Eur J Immunol 13:719–725

Hochgeschwender U, Simon MM (1985) Signals from mitogen or antigen and interleukin 2 are sufficient for the transition of precursor cells of Lyt-2$^+$ but not of Lyt-2$^-$ lymphocytes into effector cells. XV. Leukozytenkulturen-Konferenz, 1985. Bessler, Tübingen

Hünig T, Loos M, Schimpl A (1983) The role of accessory cells in polyclonal T cell activation. I. Both induction of interleukin 2 production and of interleukin 2 responsiveness by concanavalin A are accessory cell dependent. Eur J Immunol 13:1–6

Kanagawa O (1983) Three different signals are required for the induction of cytolytic T lymphocytes from resting precursors. J Immunol 131:606

Kiessling R, Klein E, Pross H, Wigzell H (1975) Natural killer cells in the mouse. II. Cytotoxic cells with specificity for mouse Moloney leukemia cells. Characteristics of the killer cell. Eur J Immunol 5:117–121

Klein JR, Bevan MJ (1983) Secretion of immune interferon and generation of cytolytic T cell activity in nude mice are dependent on Interleukin 2 : age associated endogenous production of interleukin 2 in nude mice. J Immunol 130:1780–1783

Koch S, Zalcberg JR, McKenzie IFC (1984) Description of a murine B lymphoma tumor-specific antigen. J Immunol 133:1070

Kuppers RC, Simon MM, Eichmann K (1984) The growth of concanavalin-A activated, Lyt selected subsets in IL-2 containing supernatants. Immunobiol 167:365–375

Landolfo S, Cofano F, Giovarelli M, Prat M, Cavallo G, Forni G (1985) Inhibition of interferon-γ suppresses histocompatibility antigen recognition by T-lymphocytes. Science (in press)

Osawa H, Diamantstein T (1984) A rat monoclonal antibody that binds specifically to mouse T lymphoblasts and inhibits IL-2 receptor functions: a putative anti-IL-2 receptor antibody. J Immunol 132 : 2445

Plate JMD (1976) Soluble factors substitue for T-T-cell collaboration in generation of T-killer lymphocytes. Nature 260:329–331

Prat M, Gribaudo G, Comoglio PM, Cavallo G, Landolfo S (1984) Monoclonal antibodies against murine γ interferon. Proc Natl Acad Sci USA 81:4515–4519

Raulet DH, Bevan MJ (1982) A differentiation factor required for the expression of cytotoxic T-cell function. Nature 296:754–764

Simon MM, Edwards AJ, Hämmerling U, McKenzie IFC, Eichmann K, Simpson E (1981) Generation of effector cells from T cell subsets. III. Synergy between Lyt-1 and Lyt-123/23 lymphocytes in the generation of H-2-restricted and alloreactive cytotoxid T cells. Eur J Immunol 11:246–250

Simon MM, Prester M, Nerz G, Kuppers RC (1984) Quantitative studies on T-cell functions in MRL/MP-Ipr/Ipr mice. Clin Immunol Immunopathol 33:39–53

Simon PL, Farrar JJ, King PD (1979) Biochemical relationship between murine immune interferon and a killer cell helper factor. J Immunol 1222:127

Smith KA (1980) T cell growth factor. Immunol Rev 51:336–357

Taswell C (1981) Limiting dilution assays for the determination of immunocompetent cell frequencies. I. Data analysis. J Immunol 126:1614

von Boehmer H, Kisielow P, Leiserson W, Haas W (1984) Lyt-2$^-$ T cell-independent functions of Lyt-2$^+$ cells stimulated with antigen or concanavalin A. J Immunol 133:59

Wagner H, Röllinghoff M (1978) T-T-cell interactions during in vitro cytotoxic allograft responses. I. Soluble products from activated Lyt-1$^+$ cells trigger autonomously antigen-primed Ly23$^+$ T cells to cell proliferation and cytolytic activity. J Exp Med 148:1523

Wagner H, Hardt C, Rouse BT, Röllinghoff M, Scheurich P, Pfizenmaier K (1982) Dissection of the proliferative and differentiative signals controlling murine cytotoxic T lymphocyte responses. J Exp Med 155:1876

Activation Requirements for Resting T Lymphocytes

H.R. MacDonald and F. Erard

1 Introduction 187
2 Polyclonal Activation 188
2.1 Mitogenic Lectins 188
2.2 Antibodies to the T-Cell Antigen Receptor Complex 189
2.3 Other Antibodies 190
3 Antigen-Specific Activation 190
4 The Role of "Differentiation Factors" 191
5 Conclusions 192
References 192

1 Introduction

The growth of T lymphocytes is generally believed to be under dual control (reviewed in Smith 1980). Initially, interaction of specific antigen receptors on the T-cell surface with antigen (or its presumed operational equivalent mitogenic lectin) leads to the expression of receptors for the polypeptide growth hormone interleukin 2 (IL2). Following IL2 receptor expression, subsequent T-cell growth is regulated by the concentration of both IL2-receptors and IL2 itself in a manner similar to that observed for other polypeptide hormones. In the context of such a model, T-cell "activation" can be defined rather narrowly as that series of events which are required to induce IL2 responsiveness (i.e., IL2 receptor expression).

In the present brief review, we will restrict ourselves for the most part to the above definition of T-cell activation. In particular, we will discuss the cellular and molecular (i.e., soluble factor) requirements for the induction of IL2 responsiveness and IL2 receptor expression in resting T cells. In so doing, we will deliberately avoid discussing the multitude of data available on the activation requirements of primed T cells, T-cell clones, and T-T hybridomas, on the grounds that such cells frequently exhibit less stringent activation requirements than resting lymphocytes. Readers interested in a broader definition of T cell activation are referred to a recent review by Larsson (1984).

Ludwig Institute for Cancer Research, Lausanne Branch, and Genetics Unit, Swiss Institute for Experimental Cancer Research, CH-1066 Epalinges

188   H.R. MacDonald and F. Erard

2   Polyclonal Activation

2.1   Mitogenic Lectins

The most extensively studied system for the activation of T lymphocytes is that of mitogenic lectins such as phytohemagglutinin (PHA), concanavalin A (Con A), or leukoagglutinin (LA). Such systems have the advantage (by comparison with antigen-specific systems) of activating a large proportion of cells; however, they suffer from the limitation that the precise nature of the stimulatory structure (presumed to be a glycoprotein) is generally not known.

Lectin stimulation of resting T lymphocytes results in responsiveness to IL2. In early studies, it was demonstrated that Lyt-2$^+$ cells were preferentially induced to grow in crude preparations of IL2 following exposure to Con A (LARSSON et al. 1981; GULLBERG and LARSSON 1983). More recent work from our own laboratory (ERARD et al. 1985a) and others (VOHR and HÜNIG 1985; SIMON et al., this volume) has confirmed this finding using highly purified (positively selected) populations of Lyt-2$^+$ cells and purified sources of IL2 obtained either by affinity chromatography or by recombinant DNA technology. In the latter studies, optimal concentrations of IL2 were found to be sufficient for the growth of lectin-stimulated Lyt-2$^+$ cells, and the addition of other lymphokines did not alter the growth rate.

The question of whether accessory cells and/or cell-cell contact are required for the activation of Lyt-2$^+$ cells remains controversial. Recently HÜNIG (1983) proposed that purified isolated T cells cannot respond to Con A; however, we have been able to induce proliferation of individual (micromanipulated) Lyt-2$^+$

Table 1. Differential IL2 responsiveness of murine T cell subsets activated by lectin, phorbol ester, or monoclonal anti-Thy-1 antibodies

Stimulus	^{3}H-thymidine incorporation (cpm $\times$ 10^{-3})	
	Lyt-2$^+$	L3T4$^+$
Experiment 1		
–	0.8 ± 0.4	0.9 ± 0.2
LA	127 ± 22	2.7 ± 2.7
PMA	139 ± 11	0.7 ± 0.2
LA + PMA	89 ± 6	15 ± 6
Experiment 2		
–	2.4 ± 0.1	1.1 ± 0.1
Thy-1	44 ± 2.3	4.0 ± 0.5
Thy-1 + PMA	84 ± 1.6	50 ± 1.6

LA, leukoagglutinin; PMA, phorbol ester

Purified T cells were stimulated with the indicated combinations of LA (2.5 μg/ml), PMA (1 ng/ml) or monoclonal anti-Thy-1 antibody V8 (10 μg/ml; MACDONALD et al. 1985) in the presence of an excess of recombinant IL2 (200 units/ml). Incorporation of ^{3}H-thymidine was measured either on day 6 (experiment 1) or day 3 (experiment 2) after culture of 2000 or 100000 responding cells, respectively cells in the presence of LA and IL2 (ERARD et al. 1985a), confirming an earlier report by TEH and TEH (1980). Thus it would seem that there is no obligate requirement for cell contact in the activation process.

In contrast to Lyt-2$^+$ cells, purified L3T4$^+$ cells do not proliferate in response to lectin plus IL2. Early studies by GULLBERG et al. (1983) indicated that Lyt-2$^-$ cells responded very poorly to IL2 following Con A stimulation. We have now confirmed these results using highly purified L3T4$^+$ cells stimulated with either Con A or LA (Table 1). Interestingly, the simultaneous addition of lectin plus phorbol ester (PMA) was synergistic in the induction of IL2 responsiveness by L3T4$^+$ cells. Other recent studies by MALEK et al. (1985) have shown that a combination of Con A plus PMA is required to induce high levels of IL2 receptors on enriched populations of L3T4$^+$ cells, whereas Con A alone is sufficient for Lyt-2$^+$ cells. Taken together, these data lead to the conclusion that the activation requirements of L3T4$^+$ cells are considerably more complex than those of Lyt-2$^+$ cells. These complex requirements are presumably related to the results of previous studies which demonstrated a need for so-called "accessory cells" in the activation of L3T4$^+$ cells (HÜNIG et al. 1983; CZITROM et al. 1983).

2.2 Antibodies to the T-Cell Antigen Receptor Complex

Potentially the most direct approach to analysis of the requirements for T-cell activation is by means of antibodies directed against the antigen receptor complex. Unfortunately, at the present time there is no monoclonal antibody (mAb) which reacts with antigen receptors on all T lymphocytes. It has been known for some time, however, that mAbs directed against receptors of T-cell clones are able to induce proliferation (and concomitant IL2 secretion) by those clones (MEUER et al. 1983b). Furthermore, BIGLER et al. (1985) have recently shown that an mAb raised against the antigen receptor of a leukemia cell line reacts with a small proportion (1%–2%) of resting T lymphocytes, thereby activating them to proliferate. In the latter context, it is noteworthy that a rat mAb reacting with antigen receptors on 20% of mouse T cells has been described (HASKINS et al. 1984), but no studies of activation of normal resting T cells have been carried out with this reagent.

In the absence of a universal mAb recognizing antigen receptors on all T cells, several groups have analyzed the mitogenic properties of mAbs directed against the human T3 antigenic complex, which consists of three polypeptide chains which appear to be noncovalently associated in some way with the T cell antigen receptor (MEUER et al. 1983a). Monoclonal antibodies directed against T3 are mitogenic for resting human T lymphocytes (VAN WAUWE et al. 1980; BEVERLY and CALLARD 1982), and this activating property appears to be dependent upon the presence of accessory cells (TAX et al. 1984). Interestingly, the requirement for accessory cells in this system can be replaced by PMA (HARA and FU 1985), in apparent analogy with the lectin stimulation of murine L3T4$^+$ cells mentioned above.

The question of whether antibodies to T3 or to the antigen receptor differentially activate human T-cell subsets has not (to our knowledge) been carefully addressed. It is clear that both T8$^+$ and T4$^+$ clones can be stimulated to proliferation and IL2 secretion by anti-T3 antibodies insolubilized on Sepharose beads (MEUER et al. 1983b), but (as mentioned in Sect. 1) such systems do not necessarily pertain to the activation requirements of resting T lymphocytes.

2.3 Other Antibodies

In addition to antibodies directed against the T-cell antigen receptor or other structures known to be physically associated with the receptor (such as T3), several other antibodies have been found to activate resting T lymphocytes. For example, in the mouse it has been clear for some time that rabbit antisera to mouse brain are able to stimulate T-cell proliferation (NORCROSS and SMITH 1979; LARSSON and COUTINHO 1980; JONES and JANEWAY 1981). A number of lines of evidence suggest that the stimulatory determinant recognized by these polyclonal sera is in fact the cell surface glycoprotein Thy-1. Most convincingly, several investigators have recently raised rat mAbs to Thy-1 which are stimulatory for resting T cells (GUNTER et al. 1984; MACDONALD et al. 1985).

As was previously mentioned for lectins, there appears to be an interesting dissociation of Lyt-2$^+$ and L3T4$^+$ subsets in terms of their response to anti-Thy-1 antibodies. Whereas purified Lyt-2$^+$ cells can be induced to IL2 responsiveness by either polyclonal (GULLBERG et al. 1985) or monoclonal anti-Thy-1 antibodies (Table 1), no such activation of L3T4$^+$ cells can be demonstrated. However, the combination of PMA plus anti-Thy-1 antibodies is able to stimulate IL2-dependent proliferation of the L3T4$^+$ subset (Table 1).

In the human, several other cell surface glycoproteins have been identified as potential activating structures. Thus, mAbs directed against the T11 (MEUER et al. 1984) or Tp44 (HARA et al. 1985) molecules are able to induce polyclonal T lymphocyte proliferation. The case of T11 is of particular interest in the sense that a combination of mAbs (recognizing independent epitopes) is required in order to induce proliferation of resting cells.

The ability of mAbs directed against three apparently unrelated, non-antigen-receptor-associated structures (Thy-1, T11, Tp44) to activate T lymphocytes raises fundamental questions about the specificity of the activation pathways. In this context, it is important to emphasize that the ligands recognized by these molecules (if they exist) have not been identified, and thus it cannot be concluded with certainty that these represent true "alternate pathways" of activation in the physiological sense.

3 Antigen-Specific Activation

The most complex experimental situation in which to study T-cell activation is unfortunately the most physiological one, i.e., antigen-specific activation. The reasons for this complexity are two-fold:

1. Antigen-specific T cells bear clonally distributed receptors and hence (by definition) are present at only a very low frequency in the population.

2. Presentation of antigen is a complicated process involving intracellular processing as well as expression of antigenic determinants in "association" with major histocompatibility complex (MHC) class I or class II molecules.

At the moment there is no system in which these difficulties can be completely overcome. However, the analysis of alloreactive T cells simplifies the situation somewhat, in that a relatively high percentage (1%–2%) of T cells respond to a given set of histocompatibility antigens, and in addition the expression of these antigens is a constitutive property of the stimulating cell. Using such an approach, we have recently investigated the minimal requirements for the induction of growth of purified Lyt-2$^+$ cells responding to MHC class I alloantigens (ERARD et al. 1985b). We observed that IL2 responsiveness could be induced by a variety of cell lines (of different tissue origin) expressing the appropriate antigenic determinants. While falling short of a formal proof, such studies suggest very strongly that no specialized interactions (or factors) are required to induce antigen-specific growth of Lyt-2$^+$ cells.

The situation with antigen-specific activation of L3T4$^+$ cells again appears to be more complex. Previous studies have indicated a role for specialized (Ia$^+$) accessory cells in allospecific stimulation of purified L3T4$^+$ cells (CZITROM et al. 1983). Since stimulating cells in these (and other) experiments were only partially purified, future work should be aimed at defining appropriate Ia$^+$ cell lines which retain this stimulating capacity. Analogous progress has been made in the study of activation of T-T hybrids or clones by protein antigens or peptide fragments via the use of cloned B cell lymphomas as antigen-presenting cells (SHIMONKEVITZ et al. 1983); however, such studies cannot readily address the activation requirements of resting L3T4$^+$ lymphocytes because of the aforementioned low frequency of antigen-specific cells in the unprimed population.

4 The Role of "Differentiation Factors"

This brief review has focussed on the activation and growth requirements of T-cell subsets. It should, however, be noted that a number of investigators have addressed the question of whether or not additional factors may be involved in the acquisition of differentiated function by T cells. The best studied (although still highly controversial) system is the development of cytolytic activity by Lyt-2$^+$ cells stimulated by lectins or alloantigens. Using bulk cultures and lectin stimulation, several groups have reported a requirement for a soluble factor distinct from IL2 (present in Con A supernatant) in the induction of cytolytic activity (RAULET and BEVAN 1982; WAGNER et al. 1982; KANAGAWA 1983; FOLK et al. 1983). Other workers using purified Lyt-2$^+$ cells have been unable to confirm these observations in the sense that IL2 was found to be sufficient for optimal generation of cytolytic activity in low-density microcultures (ERARD et al. 1985a, b; VOHR and HÜNIG 1985). The reasons for these apparent discrepancies remain obscure, but the possibility exists that some factor(s) may increase IL2 concentrations which would otherwise be limiting in the original studies. It cannot of course be ruled out in any of these studies that differentiation factors do exist, but are produced in sufficient quantities by the responding Lyt-2$^+$ cells themselves. A case in point is the study of SIMON et al. (this volume), which indicates that endogenous production of interferon-γ may be necessary for the induction of cytolytic activity in the Lyt-2$^+$ subset.

Another controversial subject is the requirement for a distinct soluble factor in the induction of IL2 receptor expression by Lyt-2$^+$ cells. The existence of such a factor, termed receptor-inducing factor or RIF, has been postulated on the basis of recent studies by HARDT et al. (1985). Although not yet confirmed by other groups, the possibility once again exists that such a putative factor may be produced in an autocrine fashion by Lyt-2$^+$ cells.

5 Conclusions

In this brief review, we have attempted to focus attention on the various ways in which resting T cells can be activated to express IL2 receptors and hence proliferate in response to IL2. In so doing, we have touched upon two major issues:

1. The diversity of stimuli (in addition to antigen) which result in IL2-dependent proliferation (including lectins, PMA, and antibodies to the antigen receptor complex or to other cell surface structures such as T11, Tp44, and Thy-1).

2. The distinct activation requirements (at least in the mouse) for Lyt-2$^+$ and L3T4$^+$ subsets.

With regard to the diversity of stimuli, it remains to be determined whether the multitude of apparently indepedent ligands activate T cells via different pathways or alternatively at different stages of a common pathway. This caveat is also potentially relevant to the dissociation between Lyt-2$^+$ and L3T4$^+$ subsets, since it would appear that certain stimuli which act synergistically in activating the latter (for example, lectin and PMA) are by themselves capable of stimulating the former. Such a finding is difficult to reconcile with models in which the two putative signals are acting at different stages of a common activation pathway; rather, it would seem to suggest the existence of fundamental differences (either qualitative or quantitative) in the activation requirements of the two subsets.

In conclusion, it is difficult at the present time to draw any parallels between the physiological activation of T cells (by specific antigen) and the aforementioned nonspecific stimuli. However, it is apparent that the availability of homogeneous ligands (such as mAbs) and of purified populations of target cells should prove useful for the future elucidation of the molecular mechanisms of T lymphocyte activation.

References

Beverly PCL, Callard RE (1982) Distinctive functional characteristics of human T lymphocytes defined by E-rosetting or a monoclonal anti-T cell antibody. Eur J Immunol 11:329

Bigler RD, Posnett DN, Chiorazzi N (1985) Stimulation of a subset of normal resting T lymphocytes by a monoclonal antibody to a crossreactive determinant of the human T cell antigen receptor. J Exp Med 161:1450

Activation Requirements for Resting T Lymphocytes 193

Czitrom AA, Sunshine GH, Reme T, Ceredig R, Glasebrook AL, Kelso A, MacDonald HR (1983) Stimulator cell requirements for allospecific T cell subsets: specialized accessory cells are required to activate helper but not cytolytic T lymphocyte precursors. J Immunol 130:546

Erard F, Corthésy P, Nabholz M, Lowenthal JW, Zaech P, Plaetinck G, MacDonald HR (1985a) Interleukin 2 is both necessary and sufficient for the growth and differentiation of lectin-stimulated cytolytic T lymphocyte precursors. J Immunol 134:1644

Erard F, Nabholz M, MacDonald HR (1985b) Antigen stimulation of cytolytic T lymphocyte precursors: minimal requirements for growth and acquisition of cytolytic activity. Eur J Immunol 15:798

Folk W, Männel DN, Dröge W (1983) Activation of CTL requires at least two spleen cell-derived factors besides interleukin 2. J Immunol 130:2214

Gullberg M, Larsson EL (1983) Con A-induced TCGF reactivity is selectively acquired by Lyt-2 positive T cell precursors. J Immunol 131:19

Gullberg M, Pobor G, Bandeira A, Larsson EL, Coutinho A (1983) Differential requirements for activation and growth of unprimed cytotoxic and helper T lymphocytes. Eur J Immunol 13:719

Gullberg M, Carlsson SR, Larsson EL (1985) Activation of Lyt-2$^+$ T cells by antibodies towards brain-associated antigens. I. Accessory cell requirement and role of Fc receptors in the induction of reactivity to interleukin 2. Eur J Immunol 15:393

Gunter K, Malek TR, Shevach EM (1984) T cell-activating properties of an anti-Thy-1 monoclonal antibody. Possible analogy to OKT3/LEU-4. J Exp Med 159:716

Hara T, Fu SM (1985) Human T cell activation. I. Monocyte-independent activation and proliferation induced by anti-T3 monoclonal antibodies in the presence of tumor promotor 12-O-tetradecanoyl phorbol-13-acetate. J Exp Med 161:641

Hara T, Fu SM, Hansen JA (1985) Human T cell activation. II. A new activation pathway used by a major T cell population via a disulphide-bonded dimer of a 44 kilodalton polypeptide (9.3 antigen). J Exp Med 161:1513

Hardt C, Diamantstein T, Wagner H (1985) Signal requirements for the in vitro differentiation of cytotoxic T lymphocytes (CTL): distinct soluble mediators promote preactivation of CTL precursors, clonal growth and differentiation into cytotoxic effector cells. Eur J Immunol 15:472

Haskins K, Hannum C, White J, Roehm N, Kubo R, Kappler J, Marrack P (1984) The major histocompatibility complex-restricted antigen receptor on T cells. VI. An antibody to a receptor allotype. J Exp Med 160:452

Hünig T (1983) The role of accessory cells in polyclonal T cell activation. II. Induction of interleukin 2 responsiveness requires cell-cell contact. Eur J Immunol 13:596

Hünig T, Loos M, Schimpl A (1983) The role of accessory cells in polyclonal T cell activation. I. Both induction of interleukin 2 production and of interleukin 2 responsiveness by concanavalin A are accessory cell dependent. Eur J Immunol 13:1

Jones B, Janeway CA (1981) Functional activities of antibodies against brain-associated T cell antigen. I. Induction of T cell proliferation. Eur J Immunol 11:584

Kanagawa O (1983) Three different signals are required for the induction of cytolytic T lymphocytes from resting precursors. J Immunol 131:606

Larsson EL (1984) Activation and growth requirements for cytotoxic and noncytotoxic T lymphocytes. Cell Immunol 89:223

Larsson EL, Coutinho A (1980) Mechanism of T cell activation. I. A screening of "step one" ligands. Eur J Immunol 10:93

Larsson EL, Fischer-Lindahl K, Langhorne J, Coutinho A (1981) Quantitative studies on concanavalin A-induced, TCGF-reactive T cells. I. Correlation between proliferation and lectin-dependent cytolytic activity. J Immunol 127:1081

MacDonald HR, Bron C, Rousseaux M, Horvath C, Cerottini JC (1985) Production and characterization of monoclonal anti-Thy-1 antibodies that stimulate lymphokine production by cytolytic T cell clones. Eur J Immunol 15:495

Malek TR, Schmidt JA, Shevach EM (1985) The murine IL 2 receptor. III. Cellular requirements for the induction of IL 2 receptor expression on T cell subpopulations. J Immunol 134:2405

Meuer SC, Acuto O, Hussey RE, Hodgdon JC, Fitzgerald KA, Schlossman SF, Reinherz EL (1983a) Evidence for the T3-associated 90 KD heterodimer as the T cell antigen receptor. Nature 303:808

Meuer SC, Hodgdon JC, Hussey RE, Protentis JP, Schlossman SF, Reinherz EL (1983b) Antigen-like effects of monoclonal antibodies directed at receptors on human T cell clones. J Exp Med 158:988

Meuer SC, Hussey RE, Fabbi M, Fox D, Acuto O, Fitzgerald KA, Hodgdon JC, Protentis JP, Schlossman SF, Reinherz EL (1984) An alternative pathway of T cell activation: a functional role for the 50 KD T11 sheep erythrocyte receptor protein. Cell 36:897

Norcross MA, Smith RT (1979) Regulation of T cell mitogen activity of anti-lymphocyte serum by a B-helper cell. J Immunol 122:1620

Raulet DH, Bevan MJ (1982) A differentiation factor required for the expression of cytotoxic T-cell function. Nature 196:754

Shimonkevitz R, Kappler J, Marrack P, Grey H (1983) Antigen recognition by H-2-restricted T cells. I. Cell-free antigen processing. J Exp Med 158:303

Smith KA (1980) T cell growth factor. Immunol Rev 51:336

Tax WJM, Hermes FFM, Willems RW, Capel PJA, Koene RAP (1984) Fc receptors for mouse IgG1 on human monocytes: polymorphism and role in antibody-induced T cell proliferation. J Immunol 133:1185

Teh HS, Teh SJ (1980) Direct evidence for a two-signal mechanism of cytotoxic T lymphocyte activation. Nature 285:163

van Wauwe FP, DeMay JR, Goossener JG (1980) OKT3: a monoclonal anti-human T lymphocyte antibody with potent mitogenic properties. J Immunol 124:2708

Vohr HW, Hünig T (1985) Induction of proliferative and cytotoxic responses in resting Lyt-2$^+$ T cells with lectin and recombinant interleukin 2. Eur J Immunol 15:332

Wagner H, Hardt C, Rouse BT, Röllinghoff M, Scheurich P, Pfizenmaier K (1982) Dissection of the proliferative and differentiative signals controlling murine cytotoxic T lymphocyte responses. J Exp Med 155:1876

Part E: Self-Nonself Discrimination in the T-Cell Compartment

Introductory Remarks

M. FELDMANN

A reasonably accurate discrimination between nonself antigens which need to elicit immune responses and self components which must avoid eliciting immune responses is essential for health. It is evident that this discrimination is not always effective, since 'spontaneous' autoimmune diseases of humans or experimental animals are far from rare.

Unlike may areas of immunology which have been dramatically clarified by the use of cell- or gene-cloning technology, the mechanisms underlying self-nonself discrimination remain as ill understood and as hotly disputed as ever. It seems unlikely that a single mechanism could suffice, and many of the postulated mechanisms are discussed in the following chapters, with the consensus favouring the view that an integrated role of multiple mechanisms ensures reasonable accuracy of self-nonself discrimination.

Nossal and his colleagues present their thoughts on T-cell tolerance and the functional deletion or silencing of components of the T lymphocyte repertoire through early contact with antigen plus self-MHC (major histocompatibility complex). This process is akin to the clonal abortion/anergy that his group studied in B lymphocytes, and is complemented by T suppressor cells. The concept is based on four different experimental models analysed by limiting dilution, and is reinforced by an analysis of the quantitative nature of antigen-receptor interactions, which is influenced by many factors such as antigen concentration and receptor-binding avidity.

Kölsch and colleagues discuss the role of suppressor T cells in preventing the rejection of immunogenic tumours. They find that tumour-specific suppressor cells arise very early, and may be protecting the tumour as 'self'. This is clearly an example where the self-nonself discrimination needs to be understood further if we are to be able to modulate it and so favour tumour rejection. The capacity to clone suppressor cells more effectively will facilitate progress in this area.

A topic of fundamental importance in self-/nonself discrimination is the nature of T cell receptors and how they recognise antigen. Despite considerable progress in this field with the cloning of T cell receptor α- and β-chains, this has not yet fully resolved the paradox of '1 or 2' receptors for antigen on T cells, nor how they recognise antigen. This is especially so in view of the finding of a

---

ICRF Tumour Immunology Unit, Zoology Department, University College London, Gower Street, London WC1E 6BT, United Kingdom

Present address: Charing Cross Medical Research Centre, Lurgan Avenue, Hammersmith, London W6 8LW, United Kingdom

198   M. Feldmann: Introductory Remarks

γ-mRNA which may well be translated into a protein. Until solubilized receptors can be evaluated for antigen binding, it will not be clear how receptors recognise antigens in the context of MHC molecules, and new speculation may therefore be useful. Hoffman and his colleagues discuss this issue and its implications in terms of thymus education and autoreactivity.

The capacity of a cell being recognised to suppress the activity of the cell recognising it was termed 'veto' activity by Rick Miller, in terms of alloresponses. This activity is considered to be of importance in self tolerance, and Claësson reviews the evidence that it may play a role in vivo, for example in abrogating GVH (graft vs host) responses. There are still many aspects of this phenomenon which require clarification, such as the full range of cells with veto activity and the exact mechanism of this phenomenon. New findings reported here are the veto activity of noncytotoxic Lyt-2⁻ cells, and the blocking of veto activity by anti-class I antibodies.

The development of tolerance during ontogeny in the thymus is a major component of self-nonself discrimination. Owing to recent developments in organ culture, it has been possible to study this question in a more direct manner. Owen and his colleagues have shown that a single thymic stem cell can colonize a thymic epithelial lobe in vitro and generate phenotypically distinct T-cell populations, suggesting that T-cell diversification takes place intrathymically. In studies in which thymic epithelial lobes were colonized in vitro by stem cells of a different MHC haplotype, they found that thymic epithelial MHC antigens do not induce tolerance in lymphoid progeny of stem cells which are, however, tolerant of their own haplotype. In contrast, grafts of thymic epithelial lobes to nude mice induce nonresponsiveness to epithelial antigens, but this is associated with acquisition of graft MHC antigens by host peripheral cells. This mechanism may therefore involve a form of receptor blockade rather than central inactivation of reactive clones.

Another approach to analysing mechanisms of self tolerance involves the use of IL2-dependent T-cell clones. Feldmann et al. describe an approach in which the conditions which discriminate between induction of immunity or tolerance are determined. High antigen concentrations and lack of antigen-presenting cells favour the latter. However, the signal provided by antigen-presenting cells is not yet known. Autoimmunity may be viewed as a failure of the mechanisms involved in self-nonself discrimination. This may be studied by analysing the nature of the T cell clones which were activated in vivo during the disease. Such analysis may be performed by culturing isolated T cells from autoimmune tissue such as that obtained from patients with Graves' hyperthyroidism, studying the lymphoid cells which are activated in vivo and which express receptors for IL2, and then cloning these cells. Results of the beginnings of such an analysis have been described by Feldmann and colleagues. It was found that there were T cells of helper phenotype which specifically recognise MHC class II positive autologous thyrocytes. Other clones recognised autologous class II positive thyrocytes, but also autologous blood cells. These are autologous mixed lymphocyte reaction (MLR) cells, which have been postulated to be high-rate lymphokine producers, perhaps of importance in autoimmunity. Their function here is not yet understood, as, unlike the thyroid-specific clones, they cannot provide an explanation for the specificity of the disease.

Functional Clonal Deletion and Suppression as Complementary Mechanisms in T Lymphocyte Tolerance

G.J.V. NOSSAL, B.L. PIKE, M.F. GOOD, J.F.A.P. MILLER, and J.R. GAMBLE

1 Introduction 199
2 Functional Clonal Deletion 201
2.1 Immunologic Tolerance to MHC Antigens 201
2.2 Cytotoxic T Lymphocyte Precursors in Chimeric Thymus Produced In Vitro from Embryonic Anlagen 202
2.3 Suppression as a Complementary Mechanism Operative in Adult Hapten-Induced CTL Tolerance 203
3 Induction of Immunologic Tolerance in Newborn Mice by Spleen Cells Differing in H-2K or H-2D but Not "I-J" Genotype 204
4 Conclusions 204
References 205

1 Introduction

Immunology is frequently the prisoner of its own semantics. Evolution designed an immune system equipped to recognize all foreign antigens, the structure of which it cannot know in advance. The solution involves repertoires of unique clonotypes for both B and T lymphocytes, resulting in a heterogeneity of binding avidities with respect to any given epitope. For the B cell, we now know that as many as 1 in 30 B cells can form antibody leading to lysis of haptenated erythrocytes, suggesting that there are many thousands of ways of forming an antihapten, antibody-combining site. So the question frequently is not, does this B cell recognize that antigen?, but, how well does this B cell recognize that antigen? This much our language can cope with, but when we come to issues like antigen-initiated clonal expansion and differentiation, it is too clumsy to say: This antigen in that dose will trigger two rounds of division in that B cell, with its low-affinity receptors, but ten in that other B cell with its high-affinity receptors. Therefore, we will pose the question and our experimental approaches to it in the simpler yes or no format.

Consider now how much more complex the matter becomes when we ponder immunologic tolerance within the B lymphocyte compartment. If indeed tolerance to self-antigens were uniquely due to some repertoire-purging mechanism, it seems obvious that this mechanism could not 'afford' to be complete. If any contact, of however low an affinity, with any number of self-antigen molecules could tolerize an immature B cell, there would soon be no repertoire left, given

---

The Walter and Eliza Hall Institute of Medical Research, Post Office, The Royal Melbourne Hospital, Victoria 3050, Australia

Current Topics in Microbiology and Immunology, Vol. 126
© Springer-Verlag Berlin · Heidelberg 1986

the vast number of self-epitopes. It is easier to think of an anti-albumin or an anti-insulin Ig receptor, as if this were an all-or-none matter. Viewed in this light, any appearance of titratable autoantibody, of no matter how low an avidity or how transient an appearance, can be seen as negating self-tolerance among B cells. The operative question, of course, is whether an animal possesses as many B cells with receptors capable of binding a particular self antigen as it does B cells capable of binding the same molecule from a foreign species, and if so, whether the avidity is of binding parallel, and whether the cells are equally readily triggered when the antigen concerned is offered in immunogenic form. But that question is both subtle and complex, rarely posed rhetorically and virtually never experimentally, yet it is central to any discussion of self-tolerance.

If we have a semantic and experimental dilemma for B-cell tolerance, how much more is this true for T-cell tolerance. The activated B cell at least makes a product which can readily be measured at the single cell and single clone level. In T lymphocyte research, not only do we miss our hemolytic plaque assay, our capacity to study equilibrium dialysis, and all the other tools of immunochemical quantitation; we also have to confront the extra difficulties posed by a cell which sees not foreign antigen, but foreign antigen plus self-MHC (major histocompatibility complex). We therefore labor under more severe experimental constraints, and these color our thinking.

Consider a relatively simple experiment in T-cell physiology: an investigator stimulates a population of T lymphocytes with the mitogen concanavalin A, and arranges circumstances such that proliferation in clonal fashion can proceed without the need for helper cells because exogenous growth factors are added. Some days later, the resulting clone is tested for cytotoxic activity against a given allogeneic target cell population. The experiment succeeds: a frequency x of cytotoxic T lymphocyte precursors (CTL-P) is obtained. But who notes or cares about an enormous heterogeneity in the cytotoxic capacity among positive clones? It is a universal experience that isotope release counts vary considerably. Even though clone size will vary considerably, is it not probable that the chief determinant of differential lytic potential in this system is the avidity of binding between T lymphocyte receptor(s) and target cell class I MHC antigens? In other words, will there not be a great range of degrees of antigen recognition, a problem of degeneracy and redundancy at least equal to, if not greater than, that encountered for the B cell?

Though our knowledge of the v gene repertoires for the T cell β- and α-chains is still rudimentary, it is clear that the numbers are much smaller than for antibody v genes. It therefore seems likely that the total T cell repertoire will be smaller than that for B cells. Perhaps the need for stabilization through linked recognition of self overcomes this less refined diversity of T cell paratopes. Given a smaller repertoire, random cross-reactivities will be even more frequent than among B cells, and the limited analysis of cloned T-cell lines suggests this may indeed be the case. If so, it will be all the more important that any repertoire-purging mechanism underlying tolerance be incomplete. Absolute clonal abortion of anti-self would lead to absence of an immune response even more surely than for B cells.

Avidity thresholds and clone size variability are not the only limiting factors making CTL-P clone enumeration experiments complex to interpret. Inherent lysability of targets represents another, quite important operational variable. Even more significant, however, are limitations imposed by triggering thresholds. Cytotoxic clone frequency values obtained by mitogenic stimulation are higher, perhaps by a factor of 10 or more, than those obtained with appropriate allogeneic stimulator cells. Is it possible that many cells, the receptors of which 'fit' alloantigens well enough to cause cytotoxic lysis if the cell is artificially activated, do not, however, have a sufficient goodness of fit to be stimulated by that same alloantigen? If so, the triggering threshold may be the chief determinant of physiologically meaningful CTL-P frequency, and the frequency determined after mitogenic activation could be frankly misleading.

We are driven, therefore, to the postulate that functional clonal silencing of elements in the T cell repertoire will, because of the degeneracy and redundancy within the immune system, fail to provide a complete mechanism against anti-self T-cell responses. It therefore seems logical that a second or fail-safe mechanism may be required not instead of, but in addition to, clonal abortion/anergy. We therefore see functional clonal deletion and antigen-specific suppressor T cells not as opposing concepts, but as mutually complementary mechanisms in T lymphocyte tolerance.

To substantiate this hypothesis, we now review four separate sets of experimental data, all consistent with functional clonal deletion and some supportive of ancillary suppressor mechanisms.

2 Functional Clonal Deletion

2.1 Immunologic Tolerance to MHC Antigens

NOSSAL and PIKE (1981) studied this problem using a classical model of allotolerance. CBA (H-2^k) mice were rendered tolerant to H-2^d antigens by injection of (CBA × BALB/c)F$_1$ spleen cells at birth. At intervals of 2 days – 12 weeks, the frequencies of anti-H-2^d cytotoxic T lymphocyte precursor cells (CTL-P) in thymus and spleen were determined by a limiting dilution microculture assay system for CTL-P. This assay, utilizing irradiated H-2^d stimulator cells and concanavalin A-induced spleen cell-conditioned medium, was shown to be linear over the range 30 – 100000 responder cells and uninfluenced by IJ-positive cells. A profound and long-lasting deficit in activatable CTL-P, first demonstrable by day 5 of life in the thymus and day 8 – 10 in the spleen, developed in mice which had been rendered tolerant and reached a >95% reduction by 6 weeks. Functional clonal deletion thus seems to be at least as important in the tolerant state as suppressor T cells. Repeated in vivo administration of anti-IJ^k serum partially inhibited clonal deletion, suggesting either that suppressor T cells are actively involved in producing clonal deletion or that IJ^k-bearing cells in the donor inoculum or the host represent an important factor. However, the effects of the anti-IJ

202 G.J.V. Nossal et al.

treatment were not only incomplete but also transient, suggesting that the postulated suppressor cells were not the only factor at work.

The observed CTL clone numbers developing in cultures from normal or tolerant mice did not depart from the linearity expected from the Poisson equation even when the lowest practical number of spleen cells was used. This was 30 spleen cells/well (i.e., ten T cells or three Lyt-2$^+$ T cells) for normal spleen, and 10 times more for tolerant spleen. With such low numbers, antigen-specific suppressor cells could hardly have been active in culture wells, and thus, if active in the system, must have exercised their effects in vivo. While no support for a departure from linearity was given by the data, it must be recalled that the work of COOPER et al. (1984) claiming nonlinearity was performed after mitogenic, not antigenic, probing of the repertoire.

2.2 Cytotoxic T Lymphocyte Precursors in Chimeric Thymus Produced In Vitro from Embryonic Anlagen

One problem with the allotolerance model is that it is somewhat unphysiological. A large bolus of living, MHC antigen-bearing cells is introduced at a single time point, and at a stage in the mouse's ontogeny when a few mature T cells have already been seeded out from the thymus. A situation which might more closely mimic the real life situation, where potential high-avidity anti-self MHC T cells could be dealt with as each arises in the thymus, is therefore required. An experimental system with some desirable features in this regard was devised (GOOD et al. 1983).

Chimeric thymuses, formed by fusing the prelymphoid third pharyngeal pouches of fetal mice with fetal liver, were allowed to develop entirely in vitro. Syngeneic and allogeneic chimeras were prepared, and both types of thymus were shown to contain substantial numbers of functional CTL-P reactive against 'third party' alloantigens. However, alloreactivity specific for H-2 antigens present on either the third pharyngeal pouch or the fetal liver was minimal. In three different allogeneic chimeric thymuses, the frequencies of CTL-P reactive to H-2 antigens present on the third pharyngeal pouches were reduced to 1%, 4%, and 0% of control values, whereas in the one allogeneic chimera tested for alloreactivity to H-2 antigens present on the fetal liver, the CTL-P frequency was reduced to less than 1% of control values. The phenotype of the H-2 tolerance is shown to be one of functional clonal deletion of the CTL-P.

In this system, the absolute frequencies of clonable responder cells in control situations varied from 70 to 400/10^6 cells, broadly comparable to (if not a little higher than) the frequencies encountered at a comparable age in an intact mouse. In this system, no evidence of active suppression was obtained. The system is technically demanding, and does involve some pitfalls. For example, CBA mice could not be used as fetal liver donors, because clonal analyses were uninterpretable, probably because of a greater tendency for CBA T cells to undergo the 'specificity degradation' described by Shortman et al. elsewhere in this volume.

2.3 Suppression as a Complementary Mechanism Operative in Adult Hapten-Induced CTL Tolerance

To broaden the canvas, a well-known model of nonreactivity in the adult, generally believed to be exclusively or chiefly due to suppressor cells, was studied (GOOD and NOSSAL 1983b). Immunologic tolerance to the hapten TNP was induced in adult mice through i.v. injection of reactive TNBS. To probe the cellular basis of the tolerant state, splenic CTL-P were stimulated in vitro with haptenated x-irradiated syngeneic spleen cells in the presence or absence of exogenously added growth factors derived from concanavalin A-stimulated spleen cell-conditioned medium (CAS). The cultures were either conventional bulk cultures or limiting dilution cloning cultures. For the latter, cytotoxicity was assessed through a semiautomated, radioautographic ^{111}In-release assay. Suppressive potential was assessed by mixing spleen cells from tolerant mice with normal spleen cells before culture.

In the absence of CAS, bulk cultures showed profound tolerance, and suppressive capacity was clearly evident. Suppression was dependent on the presence of TNP-self during culture, and affected the generation of CTL from CTL-P, but not the effector function of CTL. Cyclophosphamide treatment did not prevent tolerance induction. In the presence of CAS, bulk cultures still showed marked tolerance, but mixing experiments now yielded no evidence of suppression.

As documented previously (GOOD and NOSSAL 1983a), limiting dilution cultures of tolerant spleen cells in the presence of CAS showed a functional clonal deletion of hapten-specific CTL-P. In the absence of CAS, limiting dilution cultures became dependent on helper T cells as the limiting element. Tolerant populations showed a diminution of activatable helper T lymphocyte precursors (HTL-P), which may have been due to a functional clonal deletion of HTL-P and/or a concomitant activation of suppressor T cells. Adoptive transfer studies showed that cells from tolerant mice did not detectably influence the number of hapten-specific CTL-P in the spleen of host animals. Taken together, the results suggest that both functional clonal deletion of CTL-P and suppression of HTL-P contribute to the tolerant state induced. We draw attention to the fact that, in a system where suppression is pronounced, concomitant functional clonal deletion could very readily be missed unless it is looked for specifically through careful clonal analysis.

Some very interesting experiments on the frequency of antigen-specific suppressor T lymphocyte precursors (STL-P) against alloantigens have been performed by GOOD et al. (1985). This investigation depended on adding limitingly small numbers of activated suppressors to clonal mixed lymphocyte cultures. The indications were that specific STL-P were considerably less frequent than CTL-P, an observation that argues against the criticism that a very frequent (and thus not limiting) suppressor T cell is invalidating the results of limiting dilution analysis for a very readily suppressible subset of CTL-P.

3 Induction of Immunologic Tolerance in Newborn Mice by Spleen Cells Differing in H-2K or H-2D but Not "I-J" Genotype

Because the classical Medawar model of tolerance induced in the newborn by injection of semiallogeneic cells is so widely used, we returned to it to study the role of the controversial "I-J" marker. Newborn mice of various strains belonging to the B10A series of recombinants received injections of spleen cells from adult donors in order to induce immunologic tolerance to antigens of the MHC. Donor-host combinations were chosen so as to provide differences at H-2K or H-2D as well as in various portions of the Ia region. The experiments were predicated on the hypothesis that differences at I-J might be required for activation of suppressor cells, and thus for the induction of the tolerant state. Tolerance was assessed both by skin grafting and by enumeration of antiallogeneic CTL-P through in vitro limiting dilution cloning analysis.

Host mice which differed from the donor strain only at H-2D, or at H-2K and H-2I-A, were rendered tolerant just as readily as those that differed at I-J plus H-2D or I-J plus H-2K and H-2I-A. The hypothesis that I-J differences are essential for tolerance induction was thus clearly negated.

Of course, this does not rule out some role for suppressor cells in the model. It does put a nail in the coffin, (if one were needed) of the hypothesis that an I-J gene product functions as the class II restriction element for the population of STL.

4 Conclusions

We believe that this spectrum of experiments lends credibility to the notion that functional silencing or actual elimination of elements of the T-cell repertoire occurs in T-cell tolerance as it does in B-cell tolerance. We make no claim that it is the only mechanism (quite the reverse). We also have no data bearing on the central question of how it occurs. It seems logical to conclude that the in vivo site is the thymus, and there is some partial but by no means compelling kinetic evidence that this is so. We also cannot say much about the suppressor phenomena encountered in this work. There is nothing to negate the simple notion that these are anti-idiotypic CTL, except the rather fragmentary in vivo anti-I-J experiments.

We are sensitive to the fact that all our allegedly pure clones are derived from wells in which, initially, more than one T cell was present. For this reason, we next intend to probe the anti-allo-MHC tolerance model using Shortman and Wilson's (this volume) high-efficiency mitogen-driven cloning system. We believe this may yield more readily interpretable results than those predicated on the removal from starting populations of anti-idiotypic STL (STOCKINGER 1984).

Acknowledgements. This work was supported by the N.H. and M.R.C. Canberra, Australia, and by grants AI 03958 and AI 18439 from the National Institute for Allergy and Infectious Diseases, United States Public Health Service, and by generous private donations to The Walter and Eliza Hall Institute of Medical Research.

The excellent technical assistance of Leonie Gibson, Angela Milligan, and Andrea Mason is gratefully acknowledged.

References

Cooper J, Eichmann K, Fey K, Melchers J, Simon MM, Weltzien HU (1984) Network regulation among T cells: qualitative and quantitative studies on suppression in the non-immune state. Immunol Rev 79:63–86

Good MF, Nossal GJV (1983a) Characteristics of tolerance induction amongst adult hapten-specific T lymphocyte precursors revealed by clonal analysis. J Immunol 130:78–85

Good MF, Nossal GJV (1983b) Functional clonal deletion and suppression as complementary mechanisms operative in adult hapten-induced cytotoxic T cell tolerance. J Immunol 131:2662–2669

Good MF, Pyke KW, Nossal GJV (1983) Functional clonal deletion of cytotoxic T-lymphocyte precursors in chimeric thymus produced in vitro from embryonic *Anlagen*. Proc Natl Acad Sci USA 80:3045–3049

Good MF, Halliday JW, Powell LW (1985) A method for analysing the clonal precursors of concanavalin-A-induced suppressor cells. J Immunol Methods (in press)

Nossal GJV (1983) Cellular mechanisms of immunological tolerance. Ann Rev Immunol 1:33–62

Nossal GJV, Pike BL (1980) Clonal anergy: persistence in tolerant mice of antigen-binding B lymphocytes incapable of responding to antigen or mitogen. Proc Natl Acad Sci USA 77:1602–1606

Nossal GJV, Pike BL (1981) Function clonal deletion in immunological tolerance to major histocompatibility complex antigens. Proc Natl Acad Sci USA 78:3844–3847

Stockinger B (1984) Cytotoxic T-cell precursors revealed in neonatally tolerant mice. Proc Natl Acad Sci USA 81:220–223

Human T Cell Clones, Tolerance,
and the Analysis of Autoimmunity

M. Feldmann[1], J.R. Lamb[2], and M. Londei[1]

1 Introduction 207
2 Autoreactive T-Cell Clones 208
3 Immunological Tolerance In Vitro 209
References 211

1 Introduction

A vast number of diseases previously considered to be of 'unknown aetiology' are now understood to be due to the pathogenic effects of autoimmunity (reviewed in Smith and Steinberg 1983). Owing to the pivotal role of T cells in the induction of immune responses, we have been interested in the T cells which are present and activated at sites of autoimmune reactions. As thyroid tissue is not infrequently removed at operation from patients with Graves' disease (autoimmune hyperthyroidism), we have been able to study the lymphoid cells which are activated in vivo, express IL2 receptors, and so can be cloned. These represent an image of the disease process as it occurs in vivo (Londei et al. 1985).

High concentrations of antigen induce unresponsiveness in animals or lymphoid cell populations in vitro, which is usually called 'immunological tolerance'. We have been studying a model of T-cell tolerance induced in influenza A haemagglutinin-specific human helper T-cell clones by high concentrations of the appropriate synthetic peptides of the haemagglutinin sequence (reviewed in Feldmann et al. 1985). The salient features of this model will be reviewed in Sect. 3. In view of the fact that loss of tolerance is operationally the key problem in autoimmunity, it would be desirable to be able to study tolerance in T-cell clones which are derived from autoimmune patients and which recognize characterized antigens. Regrettably this is not yet possible, but may become so in the near future.

ICRF Tumour Immunology Unit, Zoology Department, University College London, Gower Street, London WC1E 6BT, United Kingdom

Present addresses:
[1] Charing Cross Medical Research Centre, Lurgan Avenue, Hammersmith, London W6 8LW, United Kingdom
[2] MRC Tuberculosis and Related Infections Unit, Hammersmith Hospital, DuCane Road, London W12 0HS, United Kingdom

Current Topics in Microbiology and Immunology, Vol. 126
© Springer-Verlag Berlin · Heidelberg 1986

2 Autoreactive T-Cell Clones

Thyroid tissue from Graves' disease patients, aseptically removed at surgery, was divided into two parts. One was digested with collagenase in the absence of serum to isolate thyroid epithelial cells, which were then cryopreserved. The other half was teased apart and the lymphoid cell-rich suspension purified on a Ficoll-Hypaque gradient. Lymphocytes were cultured in mitogen-free IL2 for 7 days, enriched in Ficoll-Hypaque, and plated at 0.3 cells/well in Terasaki plates in IL2 with autologous irradiated peripheral blood lymphocytes (PBL) as a source of filler cells. As the cells grew, they were propagated into larger volumes (96-well plates, 24-well plates) and tested for responses to various stimuli.

Over the first six patients analysed, typically around 15% of the cloned T cells responded by proliferation only to autologous thyrocytes, whereas approximately 5%–10% responded to autologous thyroid and blood cells and were thus 'autologous MLR' (mixed lymphocyte reaction) cells. The remainder of the clones did not proliferate in response to autologous thyroid or blood, but did respond to IL2 (LONDEI et al. 1985). Their specificity is not known at present, but these cells could include suppressor T cells, or cytotoxic T cells which do not proliferate readily, possibly because they do not release IL2.

We have focussed our interest on the thyroid-specific T cells. These have been phenotyped, using antibodies to CD3 (UCHT1), CD4 (Leu 3A) and CD8 (UCHT2). All tested so far (12) were CD4$^+$, and thus were of the helper/inducer surface phenotype. The restriction specificity of these cells was tested by blocking experiments, using monoclonal antibodies to major histocompatibility complex (MHC) class II antigens. A presentative experiment is set out in Table 1 and indicates that these cells are restricted by MHC class II antigens, although the restriction element is not yet defined, as the antibodies used are not absolutely specific for any one type of HLA class II (HLA-DR, HLA-DP or HLA-DQ).

Table 1. Inhibition of autoreactive T cell proliferation by anti-class II antibodies

Cells	Serum	Response (cpm ± SE)
Clone 17	–	845 ± 106
Clone 17 + TEC	–	3718 ± 912
Clone 17 + allo-TEC	–	686 ± 115
Clone 17 + TEC	Anti-class II	772 ± 55
Clone 17 + TEC	Anti-T p67	3503 ± 885
Clone 17 + TEC	Anti-B p32	3855 ± 91

Clone 17 (thyroid-specific) T cells, 10^4/well, were stimulated with 10^4 autologous (DR2,3) thyrocytes or allogeneic (DR1,10) thyrocytes in 96-well, flat-bottomed plates for 3 days, in triplicate, before being incubated with 1 μCi of ^{3}H-thymidine, incorporation of which was measured by liquid scintillation spectroscopy. Results are expressed as arithmetic means ± SE. Antibodies used were anti-class II, a mixture of all three specificities: anti-DR, anti-DQ, anti-DP, DA2; H1G78; and DA62.31. Controls were anti-T cell p67 (G19-3.2, T1 antigen) and anti-B cell p32 (TH7, B1 antigen). TEC = Thyrocytes. (Results taken from LONDEI et al. 1985)

There are CD4$^+$ T cells which are cytotoxic; to investigate this possibility, co-culture experiments were performed on coverslips. After 2 days, the coverslips were washed to remove unattached cells. Cloned thyroid-specific T cells adhered to thyroid cells, which were morphologically intact despite contact with T cells for 48 h. Thus these are not killer cells, but helper/inducer cells. Staining of these cells indicated that the T cells express the Tac antigen which is the IL2 receptor, and that both thyroid and T cells express class II antigen. Thyrocyte expression of class II antigen was enhanced on coculture.

These T-cell clones provide a model of a human autoimmune disease in vitro, and further analysis should provide insight into the pathogenesis of Graves' disease. Analogous experiments with other autoimmune diseases should be possible to elucidate the pathogenesis of these diseases, e.g. Hashimoto's thyroiditis, and rheumatoid arthritis, and it should be possible to use this model to investigate therapeutic possibilities.

3 Immunological Tolerance In Vitro

Immunological tolerance is believed to be a major mechanism of the discrimination between self and nonself which is essential for health, and operational loss of 'self-tolerance' results in autoimmunity (SMITH and STEINBERG 1983; NOSSAL 1983). Previous studies in vivo have made it clear that tolerance at the T-cell level correlates more closely with the physiological state than tolerance at the B-cell level (CHILLER and WEIGLE 1972). However, studies on the mechanism of T-cell tolerance have been restricted by the lack of suitable in vitro models in contrast to B-cell tolerance (NOSSAL 1983). Screening of human influenza haemagglutinin-specific T-cell clones revealed that many responded to different concentrations of antigen with a bell-shaped curve, i.e. they responded suboptimally to supraoptimal concentrations of antigen. Preincubation experiments were performed to determine whether a brief (3- to 16-h) exposure to high concentrations of antigen, e.g. of synthetic peptide p20 (amino acids 306-329 of the HA-1 molecule), would abrogate the response to an optimal concentration of p20 (e.g. 1 μg/ml) in the presence of antigen-presenting cells. It was found that concentrations of 10 μg/ml or more abrogated the response (LAMB et al. 1983). The specificity of tolerance induced in a clone is difficult to test, as the usual control, antigen specificity, cannot be used because there are no responsive cells to other antigens. It was found that the response of these tolerant cells to IL2 was normal, so this could be used as a specificity control (LAMB et al. 1983).

Several conclusions may be reached on the basis of these experiments. The first, since *antigen* in the absence of other cells diminished the response to a *helper* clone, was that tolerance need not involve suppressor T cells. Another conclusion, based on the fact that tolerant T cells still responded to IL2 for a week after tolerance induction, was that tolerance did not involve the rapid death of T cells.

It was noted early that tolerance was induced more readily in the absence of antigen-presenting cells. There are several possible reasons for this. One may be

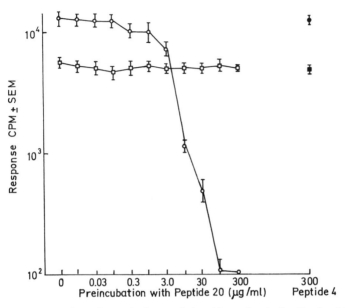

Fig. 1. Dose dependency of tolerance induced by preincubating T cells with specific antigen. Clone HA-1.7 (10^5 cells/ml) was incubated in the presence or absence of varying concentration of specific peptide (peptide 20; 0.01–300 µg/ml). The pretreatment was performed in round-bottomed, 96-well microtiter plates for 16 h at 37 °C. The plates were washed twice and 5×10^3 viable T cells were added to 5×10^3 irradiated antigen-pulsed E⁻ cells. Cells from each group were assayed for their ability to proliferate in the absence of TCGF alone. Proliferation was determined by [³H] TdR incorporation (○), HA-1.7 preincubated with specific antigen (HA peptide 20) and then tested for the response to peptide 20 in the presence of accessory cells. ●, HA-1.7 preincubated with specific antigen (HA peptide 20) and then tested for the response to TCGF in the absence of accessory cells. □, HA-1.7 preincubated with non-cross-reactive antigen (HA peptide 4; 300 µg/ml) and then tested for the response to peptide 20 in the presence of accessory cells. ■, HA-1.7 preincubated with non-cross-reactive antigen (HA peptide 4; 300 µg/ml) and then tested for the response to TCGF in the absence of accessory cells. (From LAMB et al. 1983)

that during tolerance antigen is recognized in the absence of the corecognition of MHC components, as happens most readily in the absence of antigen-presenting cells. However, this was shown not to be the case (LAMB and FELDMANN 1984), so we do not yet know the role of antigen-presenting cells in partially abrogating tolerance. One hypothesis, which we are actively pursuing, is that IL1 may be involved.

We are currently interested in the mechanism of tolerance. What happens to the 'tolerant' T cell to prevent its response to antigen? Surface events have been examined using monoclonal antibodies. It was found that there was an extensive loss of T3 antigen from the cell surface, depending on the antigen concentration to which it was exposed (ZANDERS et al. 1984). Because of the concomitant loss of T3 antigen and antigen-specific receptors, as detected by 'anticlonotype' antibodies (MEUER et al. 1984), we think that the antigen-specific receptors on tolerant cells have also been cleared from the surface during T-cell tolerance. However, this has not yet been proven. We have used antigen-binding assays (based on the binding of T cells to antigen-pulsed monolayers) to determine whether tolerant cells have functional receptors. Preliminary studies have indicated that they do not, but these studies are not yet completed.

Thus, our basic concept is that tolerance involves a loss of antigen-specific receptors, which do not reappear. This would presuppose some switching-off of genes controlling T-cell receptors (T-cell receptor α and β chain, and T3), which we propose to examine.

References

Chiller JM, Weigle WO (1972) Cellular basis of immunological unresponsiveness. Contemp Top Immunobiol 1:119–142

Feldmann M, Zanders ED, Lamb JR (1985) Tolerance in T cell clones. Immunol Today 6:No 2:58–62

Lamb JR, Feldmann M (1984) Essential requirement for major histocompatibility complex recognition in T cell tolerance induction. Nature 308:72–74

Lamb JR, Skidmore BJ, Green N, Chiller JM, Feldmann M (1983) Introduction of tolerance in influenza virus immune T lymphocyte clones with synthetic peptides of influenza haemagglutinin. J Exp Med 157:1434–1447

Londei M, Bottazzo GF, Feldmann M (1985) Human T cell clones from autoimmune thyroid glands: specific recognition of autologous thyroid cells. Science 228:85–89

Meuer S, Acuto O, Hercend T, Schlossman SF, Reinherz EL (1984) The human T cell receptor. Ann Rev Immunol 2:23–50

Nossal GJV (1983) Cellular mechanisms of immunological tolerance. Ann Rev Immunol 1:33–62

Smith HR, Steinberg AD (1983) Autoimmunity – a perspective. Ann Rev Immunol 1:175–210

Zanders ED, Lamb JR, Feldmann M, Green N, Beverley PCL (1983) Tolerance of T cell clones is associated with membrane antigen changes. Nature 303:625–627

Antiself Suppressive (Veto) Activity of Responder Cells in Mixed Lymphocyte Cultures

M.H. CLAËSSON and C. RÖPKE

1   Introduction   213
2   Materials and Methods   214
3   Results   215
3.1   Veto Activity Is Present in Primary MLC Responder Cells   215
3.2   Veto Activity Is Mediated by Both Lyt-2$^+$ and Lyt-2$^-$ MLC Responder Cells   216
3.3   Development of Veto Activity in Allogeneic and Autologous MLC   216
3.4   Veto Activity Is Blocked by Anti-Class I but Not by Anti-Class II Antibodies   217
3.5   Early and Late MLC-Generated Cytotoxic Cells Can Be Suppressed by Veto Activity   218
3.6   MLC Responder Cells of Host Haplotype Inhibit the Development of Allogeneic Acute GVH Reactivity   219
3.7   Cloned CTLs of Host Haplotype Inhibit Development of Chronic Allogeneic GVH Disease   220
4   Discussion   220
References   223

1   Introduction

Self-tolerance is a fundamental property of the immune system. Both autoantigen-specific suppressor lymphocytes (STL) and anti-idiotype-specific STL have been suggested to be important for the maintenance of self-tolerance (VENTO et al. 1984; TAKEMORI and RAJEWSKY 1984). Self-tolerance has also been claimed to be maintained by a number of different lymphocyte populations mainly within the T-cell lineage. Both in vitro and in vivo, these suppressor cells downregulate cytotoxic lymphocyte precursors with reactivity against the H-2 haplotype of the suppressor cell. Suppressor cells with such antiself suppressor activity have been named veto cells (MILLER 1980; MURAOKA and MILLER 1980). Veto cell function appears to be the property of both T lymphocytes and other lymphoid cells at many levels of cell differentiation (MILLER 1980; MURAOKA and MILLER 1980, 1984; RAMMENSEE et al. 1982). Recently, strong veto activity was shown to be present in allospecific cloned cytotoxic T-cell lines (FINK et al. 1984a; CLAËSSON and MILLER 1984). In this study we shall show that the responder cell population of a one-way allogeneic and of an autologous mixed lymphocyte culture (MLC) exhibits strong veto activity. We also present preliminary data showing that cells

---

Institute of Medical Anatomy, Dept. A, University of Copenhagen, The Panum Institute, Blegdamsvej 3, DK-2200 Copenhagen N

with veto activity can inhibit the development of lethal graft vs host (GVH) disease when injected together with allogeneic lymphocytes into irradiated recipients.

2 Materials and Methods

Mice. Inbred strains C57BL/6 (B6, H-2^b), BALB/c (H-2^d), and C3H (H-2^k) were obtained from the Panum Institute stock. SJL/Bom (H-2^s) mice were purchased from Gl. Bomholtgård, Laven, Denmark. B10BR (H-2^k) mice were purchased from The Jackson Laboratory, Bar Harbor, Maine, United States of America.

Concanavalin A (Con A)-Stimulated Rat Spleen Cell-Conditioned Medium (Con A-CM). Spleen cells (5×10^6/ml) from Wistar rats were incubated for 48 h in culture medium (RPMI-1640 plus 10% fetal calf serum) containing 4 μg Con A/ml. The culture medium was harvested and 20 mg α-methylmannoside/ml added. Aliquots of 10 ml were stored at -20 °C until required for use.

Mixed Lymphocyte Reaction (MLR) Cultures. MLC responder cells studied for veto activity were generated in bulk cultures (10 ml) with 10^6 responder cells and 10^6 mitomycin-treated stimulator cells per milliliter. Assay cultures for veto activity were set up in 12×75-mm plastic tubes (Falcon, Oxnard, USA) or in 24-well culture plates (Nunc, Roskilde, Denmark) in a final volume of 1 ml, using 5×10^5 responder cells and 1×10^6 mitomycin-treated stimulator spleen cells, or 1×10^6 each of two types of stimulator cells mixed where indicated as described by FINK et al. (1984a). In most experiments, 20% Con A-CM was added initially to the assay MLC.

Cytotoxic T Lymphocyte (CTL) Clone. The CTL clone (4B3) studied in the present work was obtained from Dr. R.G. Miller, Ontario Cancer Institute, Toronto, Canada. It was derived by limiting dilution from secondary MLC culture of B6 spleen cells stimulated with irradiated BALB/c spleen cells by methods described by CLAËSSON and MILLER (1985). CTLs were cloned by limiting dilution in the presence of irradiated allostimulator cells and 30% supernatant from secondary MLC cultures. The CTL clone, 4B3, was maintained by weekly reculturing of 10^5 CTLs with 10^7 irradiated or mitomycin-treated spleen cells.

Antibodies. Monoclonal anti-H-2^b antibody was obtained from hybridoma clone 20-8-4S (American Type Culture Collection, Rockville, USA). Removal of H-2^b positive cells from the MLC cultures was done exactly as described by CLAËSSON and MILLER (1984). Monoclonal anti-H-2^k and fluorescein-labeled anti-Lyt-2 antibodies were purchased from Becton Dickinson, Mountain View, United States of America. Labeling and sorting of cells on fluorescence-activated cell sorter (FACS) were performed as described by RÖPKE (1984).

Cytotoxic Assay. Cytotoxic activity of MLR cultures was determined after 5–6 days of culture in a 4-h ^{51}Cr release assay using day 2 Con A-induced spleen cells or tumor cell lines (P815, RBL-5) maintained in vitro as target cells. Labeling procedure and calculation of specific cytotoxic activity were performed as described by CLAËSSON and MILLER (1984).

3 Results

3.1 Veto Activity Is Present in Primary MLC Responder Cells

The results in Fig. 1 demonstrate the ability of day 5 B6 anti-SJL (H-2^b anti-H-2^s) responder cells to inhibit the development of cytotoxic activity against the H-2^b haplotype when assayed in a C3H anti-B6 and C3H anti-BALB/c MLC. No inhibition of cytotoxic activity against the third party (H-2^d) haplotype was seen. The inhibitory activity of a cloned allospecific cytotoxic CTL line (4B3, H-2^b; CLAËSSON and MILLER 1984) is included for comparison. The specificity pattern of the inhibition shown in Fig. 1 is of the so-called veto type, i.e., the CTL is downregulated by recognition of the regulator (veto) cell (MILLER 1980).

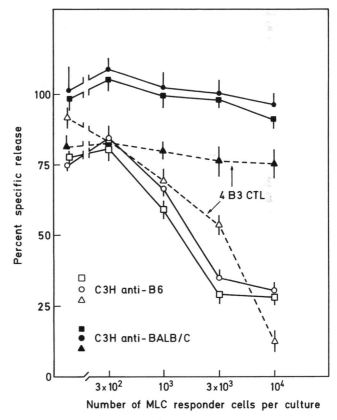

Fig. 1. Specific suppression of CTL generation in H-2^k anti-(H-2^b + H-2^d) MLC by day 5 MLC (B6 anti-SJL) responder cells. Each *point* represents the mean cytotoxic activity obtained from three replicate cultures. *Bars* are 2 × SD. Target cells were RBL-5 (H-2^b), and P815 (H-2^d). Total and spontaneous ^{51}Cr release were 1067 and 371 cpm for RBL5 and 1457 and 268 cpm for P815. ■ ●, □ ○, two separate experiments. ▲ △, experiment with a cloned CTL shown for comparison

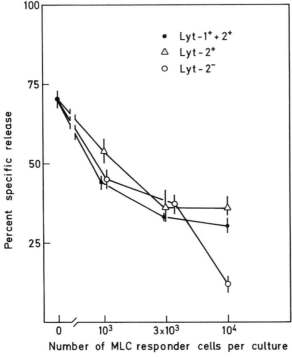

Fig. 2. Suppression of CTL generation in an $H-2^k$ anti-$H-2^b$ MLC by day 5 MLC (B6 anti-SJL) responder cells. Responder cells were labeled with a fluorescein-conjugated anti-Lyt-2 antibody and sorted on FACS into Lyt-2^+ and Lyt-2^- subsets. Each *point* represents the mean cytotoxic activity of three replicate cultures. Target cells were RBL-5 tumor cells

3.2 Veto Activity Is Mediated by Both Lyt-2^+ and Lyt-2^- MLC Responder Cells

Day 5 B6 anti-SJL MLC responder cells were separated into Lyt-2^+ cells (approximately 80% of the responder cells) and Lyt-2^- cells, using a FACS. The sorted cells were assayed for veto activity in a C3H anti-B6 MLC. Figure 2 shows that both cell subsets exhibited a level of veto activity comparable to the inhibitory activity of unseparated cells.

3.3 Development of Veto Activity in Allogeneic and Autologous MLC

MLC cultures of the types B6 anti-SJL and B6 anti-B6 were set up. In the case of the autologous B6 MLC, the same individual mouse spleen was used as the source of both responder cells and mitomycin-treated stimulator cells. Responder cells were recovered from day 2 to day 5 of culture and assayed for veto activity in a C3H anti-B6 and C3H anti-BALB/c MLC and for cytotoxic activity on appropriate Con A blast cells. Figure 3 shows the results. Strong veto activity was present in both the allogeneic and the autologous responder cell popula-

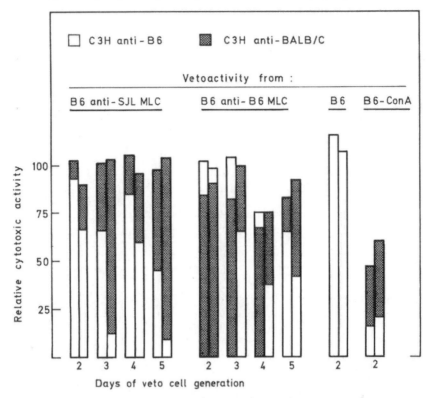

Fig. 3. Suppression of CTL generation in an H-2^k anti-(H-2^b + H-2^d) MLC by day 2–5 MLC (B6 anti-SJL or B6 anti-B6) responder cells. Each *column* represents mean cytotoxic activity from four replicate cultures after addition of 10^3 (*first column*) and 10^4 (*second column*) responder "veto" cells per milliliter of culture. Suppression by 10^3 and 10^4 normal spleen cells (*B6*) and day 2 Con A-activated spleen cells is also sown

tions from day 3 to day 5 of culture. However, the autologous responder cells were less specific and appeared to inhibit cytotoxic activity against third-party stimulator cells to some extent. As shown in Fig. 3, normal spleen cells completely lacked inhibitory activity, whereas day 2 Con A-activated spleen cells strongly inhibited cytotoxic activity against both self and third-party haplotype. No cytotoxic activity developed in the autologous MLC, whereas such activity was present in allogeneic MLC from day 3 of culture (data not included).

3.4 Veto Activity Is Blocked by Anti-Class I but Not by Anti-Class II Antibodies

Monoclonal antibodies against class I MHC antigens (K^k and K^bD^b) and class II antigen (Ia^k) were added to veto-assay MLC (see Table 1) at a wide range of concentrations. The development of cytotoxic activity was then studied in the absence and presence of MLC responder cells (H-2^b or H-2^k) with veto activity.

218   M.H. Claësson and C. Röpke

Table 1. Percentage of specific cytotoxic activity generated in 5 days in MLR[A] after addition of appropriate MLC responder cells with veto activity and different concentrations of monoclonal antibodies against class I and II MHC antigens of the veto cells. Each value represents mean specific ^{51}Cr release by triplicate cultures

Antibody specificity	Veto cells[B]		Antibody dilution in assay MLC					
	Haplotype	Addition	0	0.01 %	0.1 %	1 %	2 %	4 %
Anti-H-2K^{b}D^b	H-2^b	+	28	27	30	40	51	nt
		−	71	76	76	63	55	nt
			% inhibition[C] of veto:	−5 %	0 %	40 %	88 %	
Anti-H-2K^k	H-2^k	+	18	18	21	37	37	36
		−	59	57	76	65	66	54
			% inhibition of veto:	−2 %	−5 %	38 %	36 %	52 %
Anti-H-2 Ia^k	H-2^k	+	23	18	16	18	3	−4
		−	65	61	64	37	7	3
			% inhibition of veto:	−8 %	−15 %	21 %	22 %	
Anti-H-2K^{b}D^b	H-2^k	+	22	15	11	13	25	18
		−	67	63	53	52	53	37
			% inhibition of veto:	−14 %	−13 %	−12 %	21 %	23 %

nt, no test

[A] MLC assays were set up in 1 ml culture medium with 4×10^5 responder cells and 1×10^6 mitomycin-treated stimulator cells per culture and 20 % Con A-SN. Cultures were washed once prior to cytotoxic assay

[B] Responder cells from day 5 MLC cultures; $\pm 10^4$ cells were added to each assay MLC

[C] Inhibition of veto (%) was calculated as: $\dfrac{\text{\% inhibition in the presence of veto + antibody}}{\text{\% inhibition in the presence of veto only}} \times 100 \%$;

Numbers in boxes represent inhibition of veto activity greater than 30 %

It is seen in Table 1 that anti-class I antibodies do not influence generation of cytotoxic activity when added to the MLC at 0.1 %−1 %. Above this concentration an inhibitory effect is observed. Surprisingly, the anti-Ia^k antibody inhibited the BALB/c anti-C3H MLC in spite of the presence of 20 % Con A-SN (supernatant) in all cultures. Data in Table 1 show that anti-K^{b}D^b and anti-K^k antibodies at concentrations of 1 %−4 % inhibit veto activity of B6 (H-2^b) and C3H (H-2^k) MLC responder cells, respectively. An irrelevant antibody, anti-H-2^b, tested against veto cells of H-2^k haplotype, did not influence veto activity. Also, the anti-Ia^k antibody appeared without veto-inhibitory activity.

3.5 Early and Late MLC-Generated Cytotoxic Cells Can Be Suppressed by Veto Activity

A cloned allospecific CTL line (4B3) known to express veto activity (Fig. 1, CLAËSSON and MILLER 1984) was used. The 4B3 cells were added to the assay

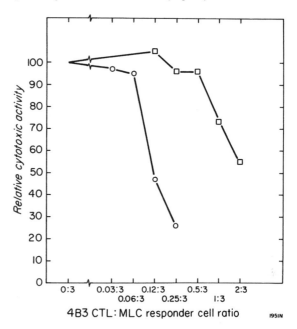

Fig. 4. 4B3 CTL-mediated veto activity in BR anti-B6 MLR culture when added at 24 h (○) and 72 h (□) at different cell numbers to assay MLC and removed from the MLC at 48 h (○) and 96 h (□) of MLR culture. MLC were set up with 3×10^5 responder and 1.5×10^6 stimulator cells. At day 5 of MLR each culture was split into three replicates and assayed for cytotoxicity against B6 Con A blast cells. Relative cytotoxic activity was calculated as cytotoxic response of MLC with added CTL × 100/cytotoxic response of MLC without added CTL

MLC (BR anti-B6) at 24 h and 72 h of culture, and subsequently removed after 24 h, using anti-H-2^b plus complement treatment. The MLC was assayed for cytotoxic activity at day 5 of culture. Figure 4 shows the results from one set of experiments. It is seen that generation of cytotoxic cells (anti-H-2^b CTLs), was inhibited by 4B3 CTL cells added both early and late in culture. Approximately 20 times as many 4B3 cells were needed to suppress the development of cytotoxic cells by 50% at 72–96 h as compared to 24–48 h. Similar results were obtained in a second set of experiments using another allospecific H-2^b CTL clone.

3.6 MLC Responder Cells of Host Haplotype Inhibit the Development of Allogeneic Acute GVH Reactivity

Groups of BALB/c mice were irradiated with 500 rad and injected i.v. with 10^7 B6 spleen cells. They all died of acute GVH disease within 6–8 days after injection (Fig. 5). When irradiated BALB/c mice were injected with a mixture of 10^7 B6 spleen cells and 5×10^6 day 5 BALB/c anti-SJL MLC responder (veto) cells, very few mice died and death occurred later (day 10–12), at a time interval where some irradiated, noninjected mice also died, probably because of lack of hemopoietic reconstitution. A certain dose dependency exists in this system, since no protection against GVH disease was seen when groups of mice were injected with 10^7 B6 spleen cells mixed with low numbers (10^6) of BALB/c anti-SJL MLC responder cells (data not shown). Likewise, normal BALB/c spleen cells did not inhibit development of acute GVH disease (Fig. 5).

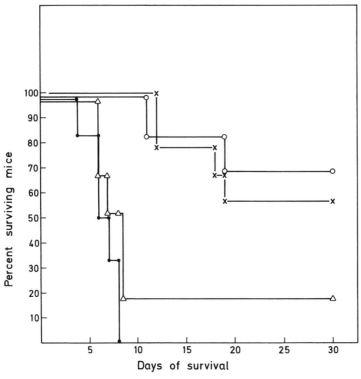

Fig. 5. Survival of BALB/c mice treated with 500 rad and left uninjected (*crosses*), or injected i.v. with 10^7 B6 (allogeneic) spleen cells (●); a mixture of 10^7 B6 spleen cells and 5×10^6 day 5 BALB/c anti-SJL MLC responder (veto) cells (○); or a mixture of 10^7 B6 spleen cells and 5×10^6 BALB/c spleen cells (△). There were six animals in each group

3.7 Cloned CTLs of Host Haplotype Inhibit Development of Chronic Allogeneic GVH Disease

Figure 6 shows the survival curves for three groups of ten B6 mice treated with 900 rad and left uninjected, or injected with allogeneic cells (a mixture of 3.5×10^6 bone marrow cells and 1.5×10^6 lymph node cells), plus or minus 2.5×10^5 syngeneic allospecific (anti-$H-2^d$) 4B3 CTL cells known to exert strong veto activity (Fig. 1, CLAËSSON and MILLER 1984). Seven out of ten mice in the CTL-protected group of mice did not develop GVH disease, whereas nine out of ten mice receiving only allogeneic cells developed and died of typical chronic GVH disease.

4 Discussion

The major findings of the present study were:

1. Responder cells from day 3 to day 5 of autologous or allogeneic MLC, regardless of their Lyt phenotype, exert powerful antiself suppressive activity. In

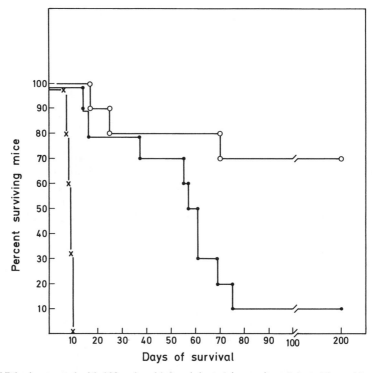

Fig. 6. Survival of B6 mice treated with 900 rad and left uninjected (*crosses*), or injected i.v. with a mixture of $3.5 \times 10^6 + 1.5 \times 10^6$ allogeneic bone marrow and lymph node cells (●); or injected with a mixture of allogeneic cells mentioned above and 2.5×10^5 syngeneic allospecific CTL clone cells (○)

the autologous situation this activity appeared to be less specific (inhibition of reactivity against third party) than in the allogeneic MLC.

2. Veto activity can be specifically inhibited by anti-class I MHC antibodies, whereas an anti-class II antibody did not show this effect.

3. Both early and late developing CTLs are capable of being suppressed by veto activity.

4. Allogeneic GVH reactivity can be prevented by coinjection of recipient-type cells with veto activity.

The veto activity of day 5 MLC responder cells appeared on a cell per cell basis to equal that of allospecific CTL clones previously shown to exert such activity (Fig. 1, CLAËSSON and MILLER 1984). Although we have demonstrated that when present in very high numbers CTL clones with veto activity can kill the CTL precursors which recognize them, the exact mechanism behind veto suppression is largely unknown. The demonstration of veto activity already present in day 3 MLC responder cells and in the Lyt-2⁻ day 5 MLC responder cell population strongly suggests that killing is not the major mechanism behind veto suppression. The finding of strong veto activity during the development of an autologous MLC, where no cytotoxic activity could be demonstrated, also points to a noncytotoxic veto mechanism, and further suggests that this activity is of importance for the maintenance of self-tolerance. Similarly, the strong veto activity in allospecific CTL clones (FINK et al. 1984a; CLAËSSON and MILLER 1984) may reflect an intraclonal regulatory activity, the aim of which is to downregulate potential autoaggression. Such autokilling has in fact recently been shown to develop in allospecific CTL clones in the absence of an appropriate alloantigen stimulation (CLAËSSON and MILLER 1985). The demonstration that the presence of anti-MHC class I but not class II antibodies in the assay MLC inhibits veto activity suggests that class I antigens or some unknown molecules associated with class I antigens are directly involved in the mechanism of suppression. Normal spleen cells, or spleen cells activated with Con A for 2 days, do not possess specific veto activity (Fig. 3) but express high densities of MHC class I antigens. Thus, it is most reasonable to assume that the target structure on veto cells recognized by CTLs is an association between class I antigen and a hitherto unknown structure in the cell membrane. We are currently investigating this possibility.

Data from our group and other groups (CLAËSSON and MILLER 1984; FINK et al. 1984b) suggested that early CTL precursors are the most sensitive targets for veto activity. However, the present veto cell-dose titration experiments using an allospecific CTL clone as the source of veto activity (Fig. 4) showed that generation of early and late CTLs was inhibited by approximately 50% after addition at 24 h and 72 h of assay MLC culture of 10^4 and 2×10^5 veto cells, respectively. Since the number of specific MLC responder cells probably increases by a factor of 20, i.e., five divisions from day 2–4 of culture, these results strongly suggest that on a cell per cell basis early and late responder cells are equally sensitive to veto cell suppression.

Early work by MILLER and PHILLIPS (1976) and later by other groups (RAMMENSEE et al. 1982, 1984) showed that i.v. injected allogeneic lymphocytes induced a specific suppression of CTL generation against the donor haplotype in vitro, when recipient spleen cells were tested as responder cells against donor stimulator cells in an MLC. This kind of experiment has been taken as evidence for the performance of veto activity in vivo by the injected allogeneic cells. A more direct attempt to demonstrate veto activity in vivo was undertaken in the present study using an adult allogeneic GVH model. We found that coinjection of allogeneic spleen cells and syngeneic MLC responder cells with veto activity into 500-rad treated mice effectively protected the animals against an acute fatal GVH disease, whereas normal syngeneic spleen cells had no protective effect. Similarly, we observed a protective effect of syngeneic allospecific CTL cells against the development of chronic, lethal GVH: injection of as few as 2.5×10^5 syngeneic allospecific 4B3 CTL cells (with veto activity) into mice receiving 900 rad and a mixture of 5×10^6 allogeneic bone marrow and lymph node cells protected seven out of ten mice against GVH disease. In the light of these results showing veto activity in vivo it appears that autologous cell preparations with veto activity might be a valuable tool in the attempt to prevent the development of GVH reactivity in human recipients of allogeneic bone marrow transplants.

Acknowledgement. This work was supported by grants from the Danish Medical Research Council and the Danish Cancer Foundation.

References

Claësson MH, Miller RG (1984) Functional heterogeneity in allospecific cytotoxic T cell clones. I. CTL clones express strong anti-self suppressive activity. J Exp Med 160:1702–1716

Claësson MH, Miller RG (1985) Functional heterogeneity in allospecific cytotoxic T lymphocyte clones. II. Development of syngeneic cytotoxicity in the absence of specific antigenic stimulation. J Immunol 134:684–690

Fink PJ, Rammensee HG, Bevan MJ (1984a) Cloned cytolytic T cells can suppress primary cytotoxic responses directed against them. J Immunol 133:1775–1781

Fink PJ, Rammensee HG, Benedetto JD, Staerz UD, Lefrancois L, Bevan MJ (1984b) Studies on the mechanism of suppression of primary cytotoxic responses by cloned cytotoxic T lymphocytes. J Immunol 133:1769–1774

Miller RG (1980) An immunological suppressor cell inactivating cytotoxic T lymphocyte precursor cells recognizing it. Nature 287:544–546

Miller RG, Phillips RA (1976) Reduction of the in vitro cytotoxic lymphocyte response produced by in vivo exposure to semiallogeneic cells: Recruitment or active suppression? J Immunol 117:1913–1921

Muraoka S, Miller RG (1980) Cells in bone marrow and in T cell colonies grown from bone marrow can suppress generation of cytotoxic T lymphocytes directed against their self-antigens. J Exp Med 152:54–71

Muraoka S, Miller RG (1984) Cells in murine fetal liver and in lymphoid colonies grown from fetal liver can suppress generation of cytotoxic T lymphocytes directed against their self-antigens. J Immunol 131:45–49

Rammensee HG, Nagy ZA, Klein J (1982) Suppression of cell-mediated lymphocytotoxicity against minor histocompatibility antigens mediated by Lyt-1$^+$ T cells of stimulator-strain origin. Eur J Immunol 12:930–934

Rammensee HG, Fink RJ, Bevan MJ (1984) Functional clonal deletion of class I specific cytotoxic T lymphocytes by veto cells that express antigen. J Immunol 133:2390–2396

Röpke C (1984) Characterization of T lymphocyte colony-forming cells in the mouse. J Immunol 132:1625–1631

Takemori T, Rajewsky K (1984) Mechanism of neonatally induced idiotypic suppression and its relevance for the acquisition of self-tolerance. Immunol Rev 79:103–117

Vento S, Hegarty JE, Bottasso G, Macchia E, Williams R, Eddleston ALWF (1984) Antigen specific suppressor cell function in autoimmune chronic active hepatitis. Lancet i:1200–1204

Analysis of T Suppressor Cell Mediated Tumor Escape Mechanisms

H.-D. HAUBECK, O. KLOKE[1], and E. KÖLSCH

1 Introduction 225
2 Induction of Specific Ts Cells at Early Stages of Tumorigenesis 225
3 Clonal Analysis of Ts Cells 226
3.1 In Vitro Function of the Tumor-Specific Ts Clone A12-D11 226
3.2 In Vivo Function of the Tumor-Specific Ts Clone A12-D11/t 227
4 Use of a Self Antigenic Determinant in a Ts Cell Mediated Tumor Escape Mechanism 228
5 Conclusion 229
References 230

1 Introduction

Although T suppressor (Ts) cells have been described in a number of experimental tumor systems (FUJIMOTO et al. 1976; BERENDT and NORTH 1980; HAUBECK and KÖLSCH 1982; NAOR 1983; ROBERTS et al. 1983; TILKIN et al. 1984; ULLRICH and KRIPKE 1984) the question remains whether activation of Ts cells is the primary cause for the progressive growth of immunogenic tumors or a secondary phenomenon induced during late stages of tumorigenesis. If specific Ts cells indeed prevent a protective immune response against the tumor, then it is most likely that these Ts cells are activated in early stages of tumorigenesis. To test this hypothesis we have used a model simulating the increase of antigenic load during early stages of tumorigenesis in order to analyze the immune response of BALB/c mice against the syngeneic plasmacytoma ADJ-PC-5 (HAUBECK and KÖLSCH 1982). In this system we were able to demonstrate that tumor-specific Ts cells were indeed activated at very early stages of tumor growth when the cell burden is in the range of 10^3–10^4 tumor cells. The further analysis of Ts cells in tumorigenesis and of the antigens involved in their induction will now be facilitated by the isolation of a tumor-specific Ts clone.

2 Induction of Specific Ts Cells at Early Stages of Tumorigenesis

Initial stages of tumor growth are not easily accessible to investigation. Therefore an experimental protocol was developed to mimic tumorigenesis as closely

Department of Immunology, University of Münster, Domagkstrasse 3, D-4400 Münster

[1] *Present address:* Department of Internal Medicine (Cancer Research), West German Tumor Center, University of Essen, Hufelandstrasse 55, D-4300 Essen

as possible (HAUBECK and KÖLSCH 1982). BALB/c mice were injected intraperitoneally with exponentially increasing numbers of irradiated syngeneic ADJ-PC-5 plasmacytoma cells. The nonsecretor variant of the ADJ-PC-5 plasmacytoma was used throughout the study. The initial injection began with two cells per mouse, and according to the generation time of this tumor, subsequent doses were doubled until mice had received up to 10^5 tumor cells. At various stages of treatment, peritoneal exudate cells (PEC) and spleen cells (SC) were tested for either cytotoxicity or specific suppression of the induction of a primary in vitro cytotoxic T-cell response (MLTC) of BALB/c SC against ADJ-PC-5 plasmacytoma cells. PEC had no cytotoxic activity. Instead, PEC from mice in which the final tumor cell number had reached or exceeded 10^3 irradiated ADJ-PC-5 cells induced complete specific suppression of the primary cytotoxic T-cell response (MLTC) against ADJ-PC-5. The specificity of these Ts cells was tested in a primary MLC against allogeneic stimulator cells as well as in primary MLTC against a panel of syngeneic tumor cells (HAUBECK and KÖLSCH, Immunobiology, in press). The phenotype of these Ts cells was Thy-1.2$^+$, Lyt-1.2$^-$, Lyt-2.2$^+$, I-A^{d-}. Only the induction phase of the cytotoxic T-cell response is susceptible to suppression by these Ts cells. Differentiated cytotoxic T cells as well as tumor-specific cytotoxic T-cell clones cannot be suppressed.

3 Clonal Analysis of Ts Cells

3.1 In Vitro Function of the Tumor-Specific Ts Clone A12-D11

In order to analyze further the role of Ts cells in tumorigenesis we have attempted to establish tumor-specific Ts clones. We have now isolated a tumor-specific Ts clone from the draining lymphnode of an ADJ-PC-5 tumor-bearing BALB/c mouse (HAUBECK and KÖLSCH 1985). The clone A12 and the subclone A12-D11 (which was selected for further analysis) suppress specifically a primary cytotoxic BALB/c anti-ADJ-PC-5 response. They have themselves no cytotoxic activity against ADJ-PC-5. The phenotype of the Ts clone A12-D11 is Thy-1.2$^+$, Lyt-1.2$^-$, Lyt-2.2$^+$, I-A^{d-}.

For the biochemical analysis of possible Ts factors as well as for the tests of the in vivo function of Ts clones, large quantities of cloned cells are needed. Experiments of that type were hampered by the fact that the clone A12-D11 did not grow very well. This disadvantage was overcome by the spontaneous generation of a transformed subline of A12-D11. This subline A12-D11/t (t for transformed) now grows tumorlike, e.g., independent of antigen, IL-2, and feeder cells, but retains the specific suppressive activity and the phenotype of the original A12-D11 Ts clone. Specific suppression of a primary cytotoxic BALB/c anti-ADJ-PC-5 response by A12-D11/t cells is shown in Fig. 1. As A12-D11/t has been derived from A12-D11 and has the same specific function and phenotype, we believe that A12-D11/t is a true representative of ADJ-PC-5 specific Ts cells found in early stages of tumorigenesis.

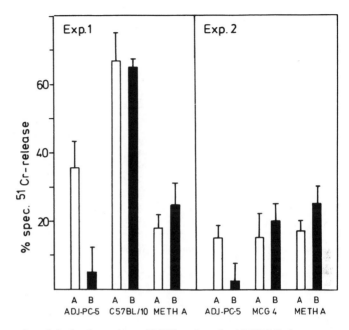

Fig. 1. Specificity of suppression of the in vitro primary MLTC against the ADJ-PC-5 plasmacytoma. 10^4 mitomycin-treated A12-D11/t Ts cells were added to primary MLTC of BALB/c SC against ADJ-PC-5 and other stimulator cells as indicated. *A*, Control response in absence of A12-D11/t cells; *B*, response in presence of A12-D11/t cells. Means % specific ^{51}Cr-release (±SD) of triplicates in a 6-h assay at E:T ratios of 30:1 (*Exp. 1*) and 40:1 (*Exp. 2*)

3.2 In Vivo Function of the Tumor-Specific Ts Clone A12-D11/t

A major problem when working with T-cell clones lies in the fact that results obtained in vitro are difficult to transpose into an in vivo situation. In order to test the in vivo function of A12-D11/t cells mitomycin-treated A12-D11/t cells were injected i.p. into BALB/c mice. One week later spleen cells from these animals were tested for their ability to mount a primary MLC or MLTC against different targets. Whereas the response against ADJ-PC-5 was completely abolished, the reactivity against the BALB/c fibrosarcoma Meth A was only slightly affected. The response against the BALB/c lymphoma ULMC and the BALB/c fibrosarcoma WEHI 164, as well as an alloresponse against C57BL/10 remained unaffected (Table 1). Ts cells mediating this specific unresponsiveness against ADJ-PC-5 cells can be recovered from the spleens of the animals injected intraperitoneally with A12-D11/t. Whether these cells are A12-D11/t cells which have migrated into the spleen or are second-set Ts cells induced by A12-D11/t cells has yet to be analyzed.

228   H.-D. Haubeck et al.

Table 1. Specific in vivo suppression of the BALB/c anti ADJ-PC-5 cytotoxic T-cell response by A12-D11/t Ts cells

| Responder[a] | % Specific release | | | | |
| | Stimulator cells and targets | | | | |
	ADJ-PC-5	Meth A	ULMC	WEHI 164	C57BL/10[b]
Experiment 1[c]					
BALB/c (nil)	nd	29 ± 5	34 ± 2	20 ± 4	60 ± 5
BALB/c (A12-D11/t)	10 ± 4	19 ± 4	33 ± 7	17 ± 3	70 ± 1
BALB/c (A12-D11/t1)	40 ± 4	36 ± 6	40 ± 11	nd	75 ± 5
Experiment 2[d]					
BALB/c (nil)	57 ± 8	61 ± 4	nd	nd	47 ± 15
BALB/c (A12-D11/t)	0 ± 5	26 ± 5	nd	nd	56 ± 5
BALB/c (A12-D11/t1)	14 ± 12	43 ± 3	nd	nd	55 ± 14

[a] In brackets, treatment of the animals providing the responder cells is indicated
[b] EL4 was used as target
[c] Animals were injected with 5×10^5 Ts cells (ratio E:T = 20:1)
[d] Animals were injected with 2×10^6 Ts cells (ratio E:T = 30:1)

4   Use of a Self Antigenic Determinant in a Ts Cell Mediated Tumor Escape Mechanism

In an attempt to apply the concept of early induction of Ts cells in neoplasia (as outlined in Sect. 2) to the induction of tolerance to allografts we have tried to induce Ts cells against alloantigens. However, the repeated injection of initially small but exponentially increasing numbers of allogeneic spleen cells in various strain combinations failed to induce specific Ts cells. This was found in allogeneic combinations (e.g., C57BL/6 mice injected with DBA/2 SC) as well as in two syngeneic combinations using SC with minor H-Y antigens or TNP-modified self-determinants.

In order to explain the apparent discrepancy between these and the tumor cell data, and in order to test the hypothesis that the suppression is a tumor-associated phenomenon, we tried to induce by the same protocol specific Ts cells in CBA/J ($H-2^k$) mice with the tumor ADJ-PC-5 ($H-2^d$). Ts cells from these animals were indeed able to suppress the induction of a primary in vitro CBA/J anti-BALB/c cytotoxic T-cell response (Fig. 2). This suppression was specific since CBA/J anti-C57BL/10, CBA/J anti-C57BL/6, and CBA/J anti-B10.D2 cytotoxic responses remained unaffected. The interaction of Ts cells from CBA/J mice with CBA/J responder cells is restricted because a C57BL/10 anti-BALB/c MLC is not suppressed. The Ts cells had no cytotoxic activity against ADJ-PC-5 cells or BALB/c Con A blasts. In addition they had no NK activity as tested against YAC-1 cells.

The finding that a CBA/J ($H-2^k$) anti-BALB/c ($H-2^d$) response is suppressed whereas a CBA/J anti-B10.D2 ($H-2^d$) is not, rules out the possibility that $H-2^d$ encoded molecules are recognized as the target-antigen by the Ts cells. The responder cells, e.g., T helper or cytotoxic T-cell precursors, in the CBA/J anti-BALB/c ($H-2^d$) and the CBA/J anti-B10.D2 ($H-2^d$) MLC are presumably the

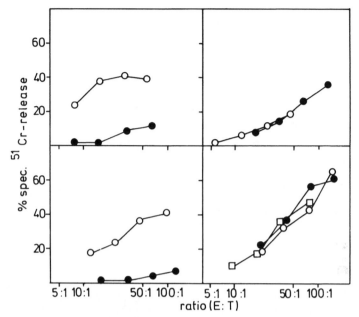

Fig. 2. Specific suppression of a CBA/J anti-BALB/c cytotoxic T-cell response by Ts cells induced in CBA/J mice by injection of graded numbers of ADJ-PC-5 plasmacytoma cells. ADJ-PC-5 cells were injected into CBA/J mice according to a protocol outlined in Sect. 2. Ts cells generated by this protocol were tested for their effect on the induction of various allo MLC. 5×10^6 PEC as source of Ts cells were added at the beginning of a primary MLC with 2×10^7 responder cells and 1×10^7 irradiated stimulator cells. Six days later cells were harvested and tested for specific cytotoxic T-cell activity in a 6-h ^{51}Cr-release assay against the appropriate Con A-blast target cells. *Lower left*, a CBA/J (H-2^k) anti-BALB/c (H-2^d) response is suppressed in presence (●–●) but not in absence (○–○) of Ts cells. *Upper left*, the same result is found when (BALB/c × C57BL/6) F1 SC were used as stimulator cells. In contrast a CBA/J (H-2^k) anti-B10.D2 (H-2^d) response cannot be suppressed by these Ts cells (*lower right*). An additional control was used by adding PEC from CBA/J mice repeatedly injected with saline instead of tumor cells (□–□); likewise no suppression of a CBA/J (H-2^k) anti-C57BL/10 (H-2^b) response can be found (*upper right*)

same, e.g., directed against H-2^d encoded molecules. This indicates that the Ts cells involved in the suppression of the CBA/J anti-BALB/c response have to be restimulated in vitro to exhibit their suppressive function, apparently by an antigen which is not H-2^d encoded but is expressed by normal BALB/c SC. Nevertheless the suppression can only be seen if the Ts cells are induced in vivo by ADJ-PC-5 cells. The data strongly suggest that the antigen shared by ADJ-PC-5 tumor cells and normal BALB/c spleen cells is not a tumor-specific neoantigen but a self antigen also present on normal lymphoid cells. Biochemical studies are under way to clarify why it is more potent in its tumor-associated form.

5 Conclusion

The plasmacytoma ADJ-PC-5, despite its immunogenicity, grows progressively in the syngeneic BALB/c host. It induces in low cell doses, e.g., at very early stages of tumorigenesis, specific Ts cells which are able to prevent a strong cytotoxic T-cell response against the tumor. We have now isolated an ADJ-PC-5 specific Ts-clone and analyzed its in vitro and in vivo functions. The study of antigens involved in Ts cell activation has led to a concept according to which the Ts cell inducing antigens in this tumor system are not neoantigens, but rather self antigens, which are used normally for the maintenance of self-tolerance. However, there might be a different regulation of the expression of such "self" Ts cell-inducing antigens on normal cells and on tumor cells, favoring the escape of tumor cells which express such "self" antigens at a high level.

Acknowledgement. This work was supported by the Deutsche Forschungsgemeinschaft through grant Ko 379/13-1 and SFB 310 and by the Ministerium für Wissenschaft und Forschung des Landes Nordrhein-Westfalen Az. IV B 5 – 9357.

References

Berendt MJ, North NJ (1980) T-cell-mediated suppression of anti-tumor immunity. An explanation for progressive growth of an immunogenic tumor. J Exp Med 151:69–80

Fujimoto S, Greene MI, Sehon AH (1976) Regulation of the immune response to tumor antigens. I. Immunosuppressor cells in tumor-bearing hosts. J Immunol 116:791–799

Haubeck HD, Kölsch E (1982) Regulation of immune responses against the syngeneic ADJ-PC-5 plasmacytoma in BALB/c mice. III. Induction of specific T suppressor cells to the BALB/c plasmacytoma ADJ-PC-5 during early stages of tumorigenesis. Immunology 47:503–510

Haubeck HD, Kölsch E (1985) Isolation and characterization of in vitro and in vivo functions of a tumor-specific T suppressor cell clone from a BALB/c mouse bearing the syngeneic ADJ-PC-5 plasmacytoma. J Immunol 135:4297–4302

Naor D (1983) Coexistence of immunogenic and suppressogenic epitopes in tumor cells and various types of macromolecules. Cancer Immunol Immunother 16:1–10

Roberts LK, Spellmann CW, Warner NL (1983) Establishment of a continuous T cell line capable of suppressing anti-tumor immune responses in vivo. J Immunol 131:514–519

Tilkin AF, Gomard E, Begue B, Levy JP (1984) T cells from naive mice suppress the in vitro cytotoxic response against endogenous gross virus-induced tumor cells. J Immunol 132:520–526

Ullrich SE, Kripke ML (1984) Mechanisms in the suppression of tumor rejection produced in mice by repeated UV irradiation. J Immunol 133:2786–2790

The T-Cell Receptor Recognizes Nominal and Self Antigen Independently. A Theoretical Alternative to the Modified Self Concept

M.K. Hoffmann, M. Chun, J.A. Hirst, and U. Hämmerling

1 Introduction 231
2 Dual Specificity of the T-Cell Receptor 232
3 The Function of the T-Cell Receptor 232
4 Why Does Self MHC Antigen Not Initiate T-Cell Activation? 233
5 The Allogeneic Effect and Genetically Determined Nonresponder Strains 234
6 Is This Concept Testable? 235
References 237

1 Introduction

We explore the thesis that the T-cell receptor (TCR) interacts with nominal antigen and MHC antigen separately rather than with a complex formed by both antigens (Hoffmann 1984). The TCR has an innate specificity for MHC and its autoreactive potential is exercised during the maturation of the T cell in the thymus. We propose that mature T cells retain this reactivity for self.

It has been shown that effective interaction between the TCR and MHC antigen (leading to T-cell activation) requires simultaneous expression of nominal and MHC antigen on the surface of antigen-presenting cells (Zinkernagel and Doherty 1975; Kappler and Marrack 1977; Matzinger 1981). This has been interpreted to mean that the TCR recognizes a complex of both antigens, neither of which it would recognize alone (Matzinger 1981). We prefer to think that the mature T cell recognizes the very same unmodified MHC determinant which controlled its recruitment in the thymic environment (Hoffmann 1984). This, of course, must not happen spontaneously. Spontaneous interaction between the TCR and MHC antigen in the periphery would lead to uncontrolled autoaggression. Therefore the activation threshold of T cells must be appropriately adjusted. We propose that nominal antigen synergizes with MHC antigen to overcome such threshold barriers in a clonal fashion. In this concept the T cell has a dual specificity for nominal and for MHC antigen. Its receptor recognizes either antigen but not both simultaneously.

Memorial Sloan-Kettering Cancer Center, 1275 York Avenue, New York, NY 10021, USA

Current Topics in Microbiology and Immunology, Vol. 126
© Springer-Verlag Berlin · Heidelberg 1986

2 Dual Specificity of the T-Cell Receptor

The MHC is part of the larger T/t complex in the mouse. Cell surface molecules encoded by this gene complex determine the correct differentiation sequence in the developing organism (BENETT 1981). The MHC K, I, or D region encodes cell surface molecules which specifically control maturation and function of the immune system. In order to serve as communication molecules it is essential that these surface structures recognize (or be recognized by) complementary molecules on other cells with which interaction must occur. T cells recognize K, I, or D region-encoded molecules with the T-cell receptor.

The TCR genes of one mouse (strain) encode receptors diverse enough to recognize MHC antigens from other mice and presumably those of any mouse. (This has been learned from experiments with bone marrow chimeras [LONGO et al. 1981].) Selection for T-cell clones which recognize MHC antigens of the individual animal in which the T cells mature occurs in the thymus. The selection process is thought to be based on the ability of a given T cell to recognize self MHC antigen (JANEWAY et al. 1976). It follows from this that all recruited T cells are autoreactive. This "selected" population of T cells exhibits, nevertheless, still ample diversity, a diversity in the magnitude perhaps of that of B cells; among these T cells, some recognize a determinant on a given nominal antigen in addition to the selecting MHC antigenic determinant. This cross-reactivity is stochastic and a function of the diversity of MHC-antigen reactive T-cell clones.

3 The Function of the T-Cell Receptor

While an interaction between the TCR on T cells and MHC antigen on presenting cells must have occurred in the thymic environment during the T-cell selection process, it is evident that unprovoked interaction must not occur between mature peripheral T cells and MHC-presenting cells. Interaction is elicited, however, by nominal antigen. How can nominal antigen facilitate such a reaction?

The effective strength of interaction between the T cell and cell-bound MHC antigen depends not only on the affinity of the T-cell receptor for MHC but also on the density of the receptor on the T-cell surface. While the nominal antigen is unlikely to modify the affinity of the TCR for MHC antigen, it may modify the density. When foreign antigen is presented to the T cell on the surface of antigen-bearing cells it will interfere with the free movement of the receptor on the T-cell surface and cause accumulation of T-cell receptors in the vicinity. Due to its affinity it will encourage movement towards it and impede movement away from it. Once the aggregation has proceeded to a certain critical point the TCR will begin to interact with MHC-antigen and the process of T-cell activation will commence. Our view on this process is illustrated in Fig. 1. The process results not only in the polymerization of the TCR but also in the polymerization of MHC antigen, which could also have functional significance for the antigen-presenting cells. MHC antigen aggregation may facilitate IL-1 release by macrophages and Ig synthesis by B cells.

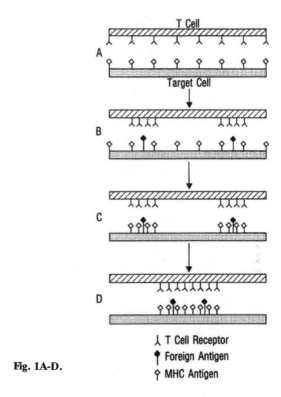

Fig. 1A-D.

Experimental evidence suggesting that aggregation of the T-cell receptor activates T cells has been presented: an antibody directed against the T-cell receptor stimulates T cells in the absence of MHC-presenting cells. In one instance this was achieved with free clonotypic antibody (KAYE and JANEWAY 1984); in other cases it was necessary to link the antireceptor antibody to Sepharose beads (MEUER et al. 1983; KAPPLER et al. 1983).

4 Why Does Self MHC Antigen Not Initiate T Cell Activation?

If the TCR recognizes nominal and MHC antigen independently, one may wonder why nominal but not MHC antigen initiates the process of T-cell activation. This question must be addressed in the context of the mechanism of T-cell selection. While T cells are recruited to enter the T-cell pool based on their ability to recognize auto-MHC antigen, there may be clones among them which have an autoaffinity so high that they would, as mature peripheral T cells, spontaneously interact with MHC-bearing cells. These clones would be harmful for the organism and it seems mandatory that they be prevented from entering the pool of mature cells (JANEWAY et al. 1976). The result of selection is therefore a pool of T-cell clones whose range of affinity for MHC falls between a lower and an upper bound.

234   M.K. Hoffmann et al.

This process does not, however, establish bounds for the affinity of the TCR for nominal antigen, so it is conceivable that the TCR has a higher affinity for nominal antigen than for MHC antigen.

5   The Allogeneic Effect and Genetically Determined Nonresponder Strains

The allogeneic effect and genetically determined responder/nonresponder status are two fundamental aspects of the immunoregulatory role of the MHC (LONGO et al. 1981). When lymphoid cells from one individual are transferred to another individual of the same species they attack the allo-MHC antigen-bearing cells in the host immediately, much in the way they interact with syngeneic cells which express nominal antigen in association with auto-MHC antigen (allogeneic effect). Certain mouse or guinea pig strains have been found to be unresponsive to certain antigens and genetic analysis revealed that the nonresponder status is linked to genes in the MHC. Furthermore, it is the genotype of MHC-antigen bearing cells in the environment rather than the genotype of responding lymphocytes which is the determining factor (LONGO et al. 1981). This suggests that the responder/nonresponder status is determined at the level of T-cell selection, which, as we indicated above, is a function of the T-cell's autoreactivity; only those T-cell clones will be recruited into the T-cell compartment which recognize autoantigenic MHC determinants in the thymic environment. Since specificity for foreign antigen is linked in our concept to specificity for autoantigen, a clone recognizing foreign antigen will only enter the T-cell repertoire if its autoaffinity falls in the correct range.

Our thoughts on this are illustrated in Fig. 2 which schematically describes the influx of prethymic lymphocytes from the bone marrow into the thymus. The cells are numbered to emphasize that they represent distinct clones which differ in their affinity for MHC antigen. In the illustration, the cells may enter one of two thymuses whose environments represent two different MHCs, $H-2^a$ or $H-2^b$. In order to be recruited a T-cell clone must exhibit a minimal degree of autoaffinity below which it would not be selected. On the other hand, if the autoaffinity is too high, clones will be deleted to avoid spontaneous autoaggression. In the example, clone 1 entering thymus $H-2^a$ (left side) exhibits adequate autoreactivity and will be recruited. The same is true for clone 2, while clone 3 will not be recruited due to insufficient autoaffinity. Clone 4 also will not appear in the mature T-cell population since its autoaffinity is too high. If we follow the fate of the very same T-cell clones growing in a different environment (thymus $H-2^b$, right side) the result will be quite different. Clone 1 exhibits insufficient autoaffinity and will not be represented in the mature T-cell population. If this clone happens to be a critical clone for the immune response to a given antigenic determinant (i.e., cross-reacts with that determinant), the $H-2^b$ individual will be a nonresponder, while the $H-2^a$ individual will be a responder. Clone 2 would mature in both environments. Clone 3, not recruited in the $H-2^a$ environment, will be recruited in the $H-2^b$ thymus. Clone 4 is of particular interest because this clone is deleted in $H-2^a$ individuals because of its excessive autoaffinity there; its affinity for $H-2^b$ MHC encoded antigens facilitates its recruitment in this en-

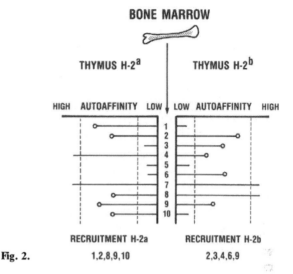

Fig. 2.

vironment and the clone will be represented in H-2^b individuals. One can predict what would happen if mature lymphoid cells of an H-2^b individual were mixed with mature lymphoid cells of an H-2^a individual. Clone 4 would interact with H-2^a MHC antigen with an alloaffinity identical to the autoaffinity which the same clone would have had, hat it been allowed to mature in an H-2^a individual. It is the same clone. Viewed in this way, the allogeneic effect is the consequence of the activity of T-cell clones which are screened out during the selection procedure in the individual which is exposed to allogeneic lymphoid cells.

6 Is This Concept Testable?

While the flow of discoveries has ruled out some hypotheses on the role of the MHC in T-cell activation, it has not been possible to prove any theory on this subject. This is also true for the concept proposed here. Our concept makes certain predictions, however, which may be testable. Key predictions are:
 1. The T-cell receptor recognizes nominal antigen.
 2. The T-cell receptor interacts with unmodified self MHC antigen.
 3. Nominal antigen initiates and, together with MHC antigen, effects aggregation of the TCR. The aggregation process contributes the critical signal for the T-cell activation.

We attempted to collect information about the role of cell surface molecule aggregation in T-cell activation using the T-cell mitogen concanavalin A (Con A) as activation stimulus. Con A is a tetrameric lectin which binds and presumably crosslinks carbohydrate moeties of cell surface glycoprotein (WANG et al. 1978). Con A was found to stimulate isolated normal T cells and T-cell hybridomas when the mitogen dose was high (6–8 μg/ml), but interaction of T cells with accessory cells (AC) was found to be required when lower, commonly used Con A doses (1–2 μg/ml) were employed (HOFFMANN et al. 1985). The AC-dependent response was inhibitable with antibody against Ia molecules indicating that recognition by T cells of Ia molecules on accessory cells is a component of the response. One might expect that if the TCR were the only Ia-recognizing molecule on the T-cell surface the interaction would be genetically restricted. We (HOFFMANN et al. 1985) and others before us (ROSENSTREICH and OPPENHEIM 1976) found no evidence for such a restriction. It would appear therefore that in the nonspecific stimulation of T cells with mitogen, recognition of AC by T cells is not restricted to polymorphic Ia determinants. Nonpolymorphic Ia determinants have been reported to be recognized by the T-cell surface molecule L3T4 (DIALYNAS et al. 1983; WATTS et al. 1984). Antibody against this marker inhibits the Con A response, indicating that this molecule participates in the Con A response too (HOFFMANN et al. 1985). Other investigators produced evidence that AC cell surface components unrelated to the MHC also participate in the mitogenic T-cell activation (HÜNIG 1984; BEKOFF et al. 1985). Using T-cell hybridomas we found that their stimulation with Con A or neuraminidase/galactose/oxidase was inhibitable with antibody against the clonotypic T-cell receptor, antibody against the allotypic TCR (KJ16), and antibody against the LFA antigen (unpublished results).

While these studies have not so far answered the basic questions, they suggest the following considerations. The T-cell receptor for nominal and MHC antigen may be one member in a group of cell surface molecules – perhaps best called communication molecules – which become engaged during the process of T-cell activation. These molecules recognize complementary molecules on opposing cell membranes when cellular interactions occur. They have in common that they do not initiate spontaneous interactions between cells (to an extent that would lead to cellular activation), but when one of them is forced into action all of them follow. For example, when T-cell (hybridoma) activation is initiated with nominal antigen, not only the TCR but also the L3T4 (MARRACK et al. 1983) and the LFA (GOLDE et al. 1985) receptors of the T cell react with their respective counterparts on the surface of the antigen-presenting cell. When the same T cell is stimulated with mitogen in the presence of AC, nonspecific receptors react as well as the TCR (unpublished observation). T-cell activation in such a process will be genetically restricted to polymorphic Ia determinants when the TCR takes the first step and will be unrestricted when initated by other molecules. The initiation process may follow the rules laid out by BELL (1974) for the interaction between cell-bound immunoglobulin receptors on B cells and cross-linked antigen in which the first interaction is most critical to facilitate subsequent ones.

In contrast to B lymphocytes, T cells do not readily bind nominal antigen. This might be considered a contradiction to our concept which states that the TCR recognizes unmodified antigen. We should emphasize, however, that we propose that nominal antigen merely influences the free movement of the TCR on the T-cell surface causing, through its affinity, the aggregation of TCRs. Only a modest affinity is required for this to occur, and in fact high binding affinity would defeat the purpose because a lasting bond would neutralize the aggregate forming force of antigen (Fig. 3). We propose indeed that the T-cell activation

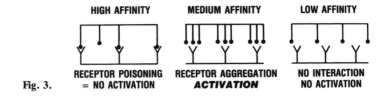

Fig. 3.

process selects against highest TCR affinities in contrast to B-cell activation, where the activation process selects for highest Ig affinity. Despite this down regulation of T-cell affinity for nominal antigen there should be enough affinity of the TCR for nominal antigen to achieve binding when antigenic determinants are densely cross-linked. Binding of densely haptenated carriers to hapten-specific T cells has in fact been demonstrated (RAO et al. 1984; SILICIANO et al. 1985).

The claim of T-cell autoreactivity is not a conceptional novelty. The existence of autoreactive T cells is an established fact. Autoreactivity was first observed in the autologous mixed lymphocyte reaction (VON BOEHMER and ADAMS 1973; GLIMCHER et al. 1981). Autoreactive T cells have been recognized as a byproduct of specific T-cell stimulation (ZAUDERER et al. 1984) and the thymus has been identified as a particularly rich source of autoreactive T cells (ROCK and BENACERRAF 1984). Not known is whether these autoreactive T cells represent a subgroup of T cells, perhaps with certain regulatory functions or whether, as we propose, autoreactivity is a general feature of all T cells, with some T cells more autoreactive than others. To answer this question decisively it would be necessary to show that any antigen-specific T-cell clone can be made autoreactive without the help of nominal antigen. In its minimal requirements one may define autoreactivity as the interaction of the TCR with unmodified MHC antigen. Experimental findings suggest that this requirement is fulfilled in the mitogen-induced interaction of T cells with accessory cells (our unpublished results) and in the activation of T cells by Mls-mismatched accessory cells (KATZ and JANEWAY 1985). The TCR seems to be functionally involved in both reactions since both responses can be blocked with clonotypic antibody. The TCR is known to recognize polymorphic Ia determinants and it would be difficult to imagine that in these responses the receptor recognizes a different molecule.

References

Bekoff M, Kakiuchi T, Grey H (1985) Accessory cell function in the Con A response: role of Ia-positive and Ia-negative accessory cells. J Immunol 184:1337

Bell GI (1974) Model for the binding of multivalent antigen to cells. Nature 248:430

Benett D (1981) T/t locus, its role in embryogeneism and its relations to classical histocompatibility systems. Prog Allergy 29:35

Dialynas DP, Wilde DB, Marrack P, Pierrez A, Wall KA, Harvan W, Otten G, Token MR, Pierre M, Kappler J, Fitch FW (1983) Characterization of the murine antigenic determinant, designated L3T4, recognized by monoclonal antibody GK 1.5: expression of L3T4 functional T-cell clones appears to correlate primarily with class II MHC antigen reactivity. Immunological Rev 74:29

238   M.K. Hoffmann et al.

Glimcher LM, Longo DL, Green I, Schwarz RH (1981) Murine syngeneic mixed lymphocyte response. I. Target antigens are self Ia molecules. J Exp Med 154:1652

Golde WT, Kappler JW, Greenstein JJ, Malissen B, Hood L, Marrack P (1985) Major histocompatibility complex-restricted antigen receptor on T cells. VIII. Role of one LFA-1 molecule. J Exp Med 161:635

Hoffmann MK (1984) T cell antigen receptor function: the concept of autoaggression. Immunol Today 5:10

Hoffmann MK, Chun M, Hirst JA (1986) Accessory cells enhance the sensitivity of T cells to the mitogen concanavalin A. Lymphokine Research, 5; I.

Hünig T (1984) The role of accessory cells in polyclonal T cell activation. III. No requirement for recognition of H-2 encoded antigens or accessory cells. Eur J Immunol 14:483

Janeway CA Jr, Wigzell H, Binz H (1976) Two different V_H gene products make up the T cell receptors. Scand J Immunol 5:993

Kappler J, Marrack P (1977) The role of H-2 linked genes in helper T cell function. I. In vitro expression in B cells of immune response genes controlling helper T cell activity. J Exp Med 146:1748

Kappler JR, Kubo R, Horkin K, White J, Marrack P (1983) The mouse T cell receptor: comparison of MHC-restricted receptors on two T cell hybridomas. Cell 34:727

Katz ME, Janeway CA Jr (1985) The immunology of T cell responses to Mls locus disparate stimulator cells. J Immunol 134:2064

Kaye J, Janeway CA Jr (1984) Induction of receptors for interleukin 2 requires T cell ag:Ia receptor crosslinking and interleukin 1. Lymphokine Res 3:175

Longo DL, Matis LA, Schwarz RH (1981) Insights into immune response gene function from experiments with chimeric animals. CRC Crit Rev Immunol 5:83

Marrack P, Endres R, Shimonkrevitz R, Zlotnik A, Dialynar D, Fitch F, Kappler J (1983) The major histocompatibility complex-restricted antigen receptor on T cells. J Exp Med 158:1077

Matzinger P (1981) A one-receptor view of T-cell behavior. Nature 292:497

Meuer SC, Hodgdon JC, Hussey RE, Rotentin JP, Schlossman SF, Reinherz EL (1983) Antigen-like effects of monoclonal antibodies directed at receptors on human T cell clones. J Exp Med 158:988

Rao A, Ko WW, Faas SJ, Cantor H (1984) Binding of antigen in the absence of histocompatibility proteins by arsenate-reactive T cell clones. Cell 36:879

Rock KL, Benacerraf B (1984) Thymic T cells are driven to expand upon interaction with self class II major histocompatibility complex gene products on accessory cells. Proc Natl Acad Sci USA 81:1221

Rosenstreich DL, Oppenheim J (1976) The role of macrophages in the activation of T and B lymphocytes in vitro. In: Nelson DJ (ed) Immunology of the macrophage. Academic, New York, p 162

Siliciano R, Dintzis R, Dintzis H, Shin H (1985) The binding of nominal antigen to T cell clones. Fed Proc (Abstract) 6524

von Boehmer H, Adams PB (1973) Syngeneic mixed lymphocyte reaction between thymocytes and peripheral lymphoid cells in mice: strain specificity and nature of the target cells. J Immunol 110:376

Watts TH, Brian AA, Kappler JW, Marrack P (1984) Antigen presentation by supported planar membrane containing affinity-purified I-A^d. Proc Natl Acad Sci USA 81:7564

Zauderer M, Campell H, Johnson DR, Seman M (1984) Helper function of antigen-induced specific and autoreactive T cell colonies. J Mol Cell Immunol 2:65

Zinkernagel RM, Doherty PC (1975) H-2 compatibility requirement for T-cell-mediated lysis of target cells, infected with lymphocytic choriomeningitis virus. Different cytotoxic T-cell specificities are associated with structures coded for in H-2K or H-2D. J Exp Med 141:1427

Part F: T-Cell Mediated Autoreactivity

Introductory Remarks

R.G. Miller

There is almost universal agreement about one factor which distinguishes the T-cell repertoire from the B-cell repertoire: T-cell recognition shows MHC restriction. T cells do not recognize free antigen but only antigen on the surface of another cell. They then recognize not only the antigen but part of the cell presenting it, in particular molecules coded for within the MHC. Specificity is then for the (foreign) antigen and the (self) MHC structure. Specificity is further restricted in that private, allelically distributed epitopes of MHC molecules form part of the structure recognized.

Most thinking about repertoire structure starts from the assumption that the repertoire is fixed prior to exposure to antigen and that an immune response consists of the activation and clonal expansion of a precursor cell bearing a receptor of the appropriate specificity. Several of the chapters in this volume cast doubt on this assumption. The extreme opposite view would be that the repertoire develops entirely as part of an ongoing response under the control of the local environment in which this response is occurring. This view is almost certainly too extreme, but reality may well contain elements of it.

Although much of the literature claims that the T-cell repertoire has a higher representation of T cells reactive against antigen plus self MHC than antigen plus allo MHC, results presented here cast this in doubt. If self MHC preference exists, it strengthens the argument of reactivity against environmental MHC during T-cell development being an important force in repertoire development. If one admits the possibility of repertoire development continuing during an ongoing response then the model can be modified to allow for allo MHC preference if allo MHC is present during the response. Evidence consistent with this point of view is presented here.

There is no question that one can detect T cells with reactivity against self MHC. The argument is over its significance. On the one hand, it could be an in vitro artefact; on the other, biologically significant. If biologically significant, the self reactivity could represent either the starting point for repertoire development from which other specificities develop or could be a mechanism for regulating an ongoing response. Several arguments favoring the former, particularly the simultaneous existence of syngeneic cytotoxicity and (anti-self) veto activity in thymic lymphoid colonies reported here, are given here but the latter cannot be excluded. See, for example, the report here of a self-I-A reactive T-cell clone

---

Ontario Cancer Institute and Department of Immunology, University of Toronto, 500 Sherbourne St., Toronto, Ontario M4X 1K9, Canada

which preferentially stimulates activated B cells. It is possible that responses against self class I and self class II MHC determinants are qualitatively different. Anti-self class I might be involved only in ontogeny and be kept under control by the veto phenomenon whereas anti-self class II might not be under veto control and play an active role in regulation.

The papers presented here raise as many questions as they answer: significant progress in resolving these issues is probably dependent upon a better understanding of the molecular mechanisms underlying T-cell recognition. Fortunately, molecular probes for the various molecules involved in T-cell recognition (e.g., T_i, T_3, T_4, T_8 in man) are now becoming available. The challenge now is to develop the methodology to enable us to use these probes to analyze small clones of T lymphocytes involved in different kinds of immune responses and at different stages of these responses.

T-Cell Reactivity to Polymorphic MHC Determinants
I. MHC-Guided T-Cell Reactivity

J. REIMANN[1], K. HEEG[1], D. KABELITZ[1], H. WAGNER[1], and R.G. MILLER[2]

1 The Problem of MHC Gene Product Function(s)   243
2 Polymorphism of MHC Molecules   244
3 The Organization of T-Cell Recognition   245
4 Diversity of the T-Cell Repertoire   249
5 The Generation of Diversity of the T-Cell Repertoire: A Speculative View   250
6 Somatic Diversification of the T-Cell Repertoire: The Problems   251
7 The Type of Effector Function Expressed by T-Cells Correlates with the Class of MHC Molecules It Recognizes   253
8 Perspectives   254
References   255

1 The Problem of MHC Gene Product Function(s)

The function of major histocompatibility complex (MHC) molecules remains elusive. Our detailed knowledge of their structural (genetic and biochemical) features contrasts sharply with our essentially speculative ideas concerning their function(s), which furthermore seem at present to be locked into sets of mutually exclusive hypotheses.

MHC molecules seem to be involved in various recognition processes of non-lymphoid cells, and different interpretations of the biological role of MHC molecules in these cellular functions have been suggested. MHC molecules might be related to the "primordial need for a mechanism of self-recognition of all (unicellular and pluricellular) organisms" (DAUSSET and CONTU 1980). Derived from allorecognition systems in tunicates (SCOFIELD et al. 1982), MHC gene products have been proposed to "intervene in (a) non-immunological self-recognition between cells in obviously non-immunological situations, and (b) in immunological-like self-recognition which can be interpreted as a simple extension of the preceding non-immunological self-recognition" (DAUSSET and CONTU 1980). Apparently of a different nature are suggestions that link MHC molecules to cell positioning and homing (BODMER 1972; LENGEROVA et al. 1977; CURTIS 1979) or cell-cell adhesion phenomena (BARTLETT and EDIDIN 1977). A novel view on nonimmune MHC molecule function was generated by the observation of interac-

---

[1] Institute of Medical Microbiology and Immunology, University of Ulm, D-7900 Ulm
[2] Ontario Cancer Institute, Toronto, Ontario, Canada

Current Topics in Microbiology and Immunology, Vol. 126
© Springer-Verlag Berlin · Heidelberg 1986

tions at the cell surface of HLA molecules with many kinds of ligands, e.g., antibiotic, γ-endorphin, glucagon, insulin, somatostatin, or epidermal growth factor (reviewed in EDIDIN 1983; SIMONSEN and OLSSON 1983). These distinct points of view have not yet converged to the point at which it would be possible to conceive the immune system as a particular form of extremely diversified specific recognition evolved within the framework of a more ancient cell-to-cell interaction process. We hence have to restrict the discussion on the involvement of MHC molecules in antigen-mediated lymphocyte interactions.

The influence of MHC molecules on T-cell function is evident in four apparently distinct phenomena (reviewed in COHN 1983):

1. MHC molecules are involved in restrictive recognition of antigen by T cells, i.e., the allele-specific recognition of a polymorphic determinant of a MHC glycoprotein on the surface of a cell bearing a nonself antigen.

2. The type of effector function a T-cell subset expresses correlates with the biochemically and genetically distinct class of MHC molecules that it recognizes (SWAIN 1980).

3. MHC molecules are target structures for T-cell-mediated alloreactivity, i.e., the easily detectable reactivity of peripheral T-cell populations towards nonself allelic determinants on MHC-encoded molecules of different members of the same species.

4. The capacity of the antigen-specific receptor repertoire of T cells to discriminate self and nonself determinants, i.e., the establishment of self-tolerance, is MHC-restricted (DOS REIS and SHEVACH 1983; MATZINGER et al. 1984; RAMMENSEE and BEVAN 1984).

These four MHC-dependent T-cell functions are distinct, but it has often been suggested that they might be closely interrelated.

In this series of three papers, we do not aim at "new" hypothetical constructs on how MHC molecules work. We describe strictly at the cellular level various phenomena of anti-MHC T-cell reactivity (and related questions of the T-cell receptor repertoire). We ask for the experimental evidence of some of the (often implicit) a priori assumptions on which many models of the T-cell system are based, and whenever possible we try to discern alternative terms in interpreting the data.

2 Polymorphism of MHC Molecules

Interactions involving MHC molecules can occur between many different non-immune and immune cell types in the presence of an extensive polymorphism of these molecules. Polymorphism is thus compatible with any putative function of MHC molecules, the phenotypic expression of which has been maintained during evolution on all metazoan cells beyond a certain early stage of ontogeny. But polymorphism of MHC molecules is a species-specific trait: two phylogenetically related species (i.e., the hamster and the mouse) illustrate extremes of MHC polymorphism. While the mouse has probably as many as 100 different allelic forms at each class I H-2 locus (KLEIN and FIGUEROA 1981), the hamster appears to express only a single class I MHC phenotype (STREILIN 1981). We have described elsewhere how the reproductive ecology of the mouse would allow the establishment of MHC polymorphism by genetic drift, while that of the hamster would not (REIMANN and MILLER 1983c). We concluded that polymorphism is compatible with, though neither of constitutive necessity nor of evolutionary advantage for any putative role of MHC molecules. At the same time, STREILIN and DUNCAN (1983) derived an alternative interpretation from similar considerations, in which they suggested different functional roles for polymorphic and nonpolymorphic MHC gene products.

This view of extensive polymorphism as a compatible though nonessential condition for MHC molecule function suggested to us that one polymorphic MHC determinant should be as "functional" as its allelic counterpart. This idea was at the origin of an experimental approach that compared clonally in vitro developing T-cell populations reactive to syngeneic MHC determinants with those reactive to allogeneic MHC determinants (see the following papers). These experiments have revealed unexpected analogies.

3 The Organization of T-Cell Recognition

The fundamental difference in antigen recognition of T cells and B cells (i.e., antibodies) came as a surprise. While antibodies bind free antigen, T cells recognize only cell-bound antigen in the context of a polymorphic MHC determinant. This might indicate that the T-cell system was evolved as a mechanism to direct a (protective) effector function towards a cellular target, or that the low avidity of this type of antigen-receptor interaction required assembly of antigenic determinants in two (rather than three) dimensions. Irrespective of these interpretations, it has made the experimental analysis of T-cell recognition desparately complex: it requires the dissection of the process of communication between two cells over "synaptic" distances via membrane-associated and/or humoral signals and receptors.

T-cell recognition is only detectable as "(nonself) antigen associated with a polymorphic epitope on (self) MHC molecules." This allele-specific "restriction" is apparent in the specificity phenotype of the antigen-receptor expressed by functional T cells, and it is only apparent because MHC-encoded restriction determinants are polymorphic. Hence, MHC-restricted recognition by T cells was discovered in the mouse, and not in the hamster. Although the structural integrity of the third (nonpolymorphic) external domain of class I MHC molecules seems to be required for restricted T-cell recognition to occur, this monomorphic reactivity of the involved T-cell receptor does not emerge in its specificity pattern (POTTER et al. 1983). A similar case can be made for membrane-associated Lyt-2 glycoproteins which are somehow involved in T-cell recognition (MACDONALD ét al. 1982). In the following brief outline we attempt to delineate different levels of the hierarchically organized regulation of T-cell recognition by allele-specific MHC determinants which do appear, or do not appear, in the specificity phenotype of the T-cell receptor involved.

246   J. Reimann et al.

Table 1. MHC molecules influence the mode of recognition of T cells

Group	T cells sensitized to antigen X in the context of (semi)syngeneic cells expressing varying sets of class I MHC haplotypes[a]		Lysis of targets expressing antigen X plus particular MHC haplotype (combinations)
A		A1+X	+
		A2+X	−
		A3+X	+
B	B1	A1+X	+
	B2	A1+X	−
C	B1	A1+X(s)	−
	−	A1+X(s)	+

[a] T-cell populations from naive mice or in vivo sensitized mice are (re)stimulated with cell-associated antigen (X) under bulk culture conditions. After 5–7 days, the generation of specific cytolytic effector cells is assayed in standard short term readouts.
   Representative examples (to facilitate comparison between the actual H-2 restriction determinants and the symbols used in the text and tables, the symbols are referred to in parentheses):

Group A: TNP stimulates a cytotoxic response in the context of D^d and D^b (A1), but not D^k (A2) (SHEARER et al. 1975).
   Murine sarcoma virus MSV antigens are recognized in the context of D^b or K^d (A1), but not K^b or D^d (A2) (GOMARD et al. 1977).
   Influenza virus antigens are recognized in the context of K^k (A1), but not K^b (A2) (DOHERTY et al. 1978).
   H-Y antigens are recognized in the context of K^d and D^b (A1), but not K^k or D^d (A2) (SIMPSON 1982).

Group B: The cytotoxic response to TNP in the context of D^k (A1) is "allowed" in the presence of K^d (B1), but "suppressed" in the presence of K^k (B2) (FUJIWARA et al. 1982).
   The cytotoxic response to vaccinia/sendai virus antigens in the context of D^b (A1) is "allowed" in the presence of K^b (B1), but "suppressed" in the presence of K^k (B2) (ZINKERNAGEL et al. 1978).

Group C: This group has similarity to group B. F1 (1 × 2) effector cells are activated by parental cells expressing the minor H autoantigen X(s) in the context of parental class I restriction determinant A1 (e.g., K^b in the F1 (B6D2)-anti-B6 semi-syngeneic MLR), and lyse targets expressing A1+X(s) only if the class I gene products of the other parent (i.e., A2, B2 or K^dD^d) are not expressed on the same target (ISHIKAWA and DUTTON 1979; NAKANO et al. 1981)

   T cells recognize antigen X in association with MHC molecule A1; the (class I or class II) MHC molecule A1 is said to function as a "restriction" element. In many (but not all) species, the genetic locus, of which A1 is the product, has many allelic forms, e.g., A1, A2, A3. Of these, some are able to function as restriction elements for X, while others (e.g., A2) are not and are designated "nonresponder" alleles for X (SHEARER et al. 1975; FORMAN 1975; GOMARD et al. 1977; DOHERTY et al. 1978; SIMPSON 1982) (Table 1, group A). At this level, the function of the MHC molecules as a restriction element for X for an autologous T cell is thus dependent on the allele-specific determinant(s) of the molecule.
   But this is only effective when other conditions are met. Within the MHC, another duplicated locus B (with the allelic forms B1, B2, B3, ...) encodes mole-

Table 2. The interference of two ongoing immune responses

T cells are stimulated with antigen(s) X and/or Y on		Lysis of targets expressing	
Syngeneic A1, B1 cells		A1+X	B1+Y
B1	A1+X	+	−
B1+Y	A1	−	+
B1+Y	A1+X	+	−
Syngeneic A2, B2 cells		A2+X	B2+Y
B2	A2+X	+	−
B2+Y	A2	−	+
B2+Y	A2+X	−	+

H-Y (X) incompatible skin grafts specifically inhibit the rejection of concurrently applied H-1, H-34, H-36 (Y) incompatible grafts, but not the rejection of concurrently applied H-23 incompatible grafts (JOHNSON et al. 1981)

More than 40 minor H determinants (X, Y) display allotypic differences between C57B1/6 and BALB/c mice. Cross-immunizations of C57B1/6 and BALB.B mice (H-2b), or BALB/c and B6.C mice (H-2d), the MHC class I haplotypes b or d determine which of the minor H antigens are immunodominant target structures, and which are immunosilent (WETTSTEIN and BAILEY 1982)

cules of the same type (e.g., class I), which are codominantly expressed on the cell surface and influence the ability of A1 to function as a restriction element for antigen X. The ability of the responder A1 allele to transform X into a state recognizable by autologous T cells is allowed for in the presence of, e.g., the allelic form B1, but suppressed in the presence of, e.g., the allelic form B2 (ZIN-KERNAGEL et al. 1978; FUJIWARA et al. 1982) (Table 1, group B). Thus, the function of A1 MHC molecules as restriction elements for X is expressed/allowed for in the presence of B1 MHC molecules, but is not expressed/suppressed in the presence of the allelic MHC molecule B2. It is therefore apparent that recognition of X by T cells depends on (or is regulated by) MHC molecules at two levels, i.e., T-cell recognition functions through a hierarchically organized set of relationships: X seen in association with A1, (X+A1) seen in association with B1.

If two antigens X and Y are present on the same cell surface, the following restricted T-cell responses are expected (depending on the presence of the particular combination of allelic forms of A and B): (1) exclusively anti-X; (2) exclusively anti-Y; (3) anti-X and anti-Y; and (4) none. But X and Y are very rarely recognized in the same T-cell response (JOHNSON et al. 1981; WETTSTEIN and BAILEY 1982) (Table 2). This can be explained in the terms developed above. The response to (X+A1), allowed for in the presence of B1, exerts an inhibitory influence on the response to (Y+B1), which would be allowed in the presence of A1 (and takes place in the absence of X). As, in the absence of X, the response to (Y+B1) is allowed in the presence of A1, but not allowed in the presence of A2, we have to conclude that (X+A1) "looks functionally like" A2. The simultaneous presentation of two different antigens introduces therefore a type of regulation into the response which depends on antigen-induced polymorphism of MHC molecules. (It should be noted that this seriously questions the validity of a popular type of experiment to discriminate MHC molecule function from "background" molecule function, in which the function of different allogeneic MHCs on the same background is assayed with congenic mice; as MHC molecules organize the immunodominance hierarchies of background gene products, the same backgrounds are expected to "look" very different, i.e., are organized in a very different way for recognition by T cells.)

F1 antiparent mixed lymphocyte cultures can be viewed in a similar way. In the F1 (A1, B1 × A2, B2) antiparent (A1, B1) mixed lymphocyte culture, MLC (Ishikawa and Dutton 1979; Nakano et al. 1981; Nakamura and Cudkowicz 1982), F1 hybrid effector cells specifically lyse only parental (A1, B1) targets although they recognize (conjugate with) F1-self (A1, B1 × A2, B2) targets (Table 1, group C). Hence, the presence of (A2, B2) MHC molecules codominantly expressed on the surface of F1 hybrid stimulator/target cells does not allow a functional (lytic) interaction.

Three main points of interest emerge from this analysis.

1. Allele-specific MHC determinants are involved in different hierarchically organized levels in the regulation of T-cell recognition/activation. They restrict recognition of foreign antigens by T cells, but in addition, they "restrict" restricted antigen recognition by T cells. A particular spectrum of specific T-cell reactivities in the repertoire of an individual mouse can therefore not be traced back to a particular allelic form of the particular MHC gene product (that would confer responder or nonresponder status to this individual mouse for these particular antigenic determinants, as proposed by the determinant selection hypothesis), but the T-cell repertoire is shaped by a "common action" of all allelic MHC gene products expressed in the particular mouse (Sherman 1980, 1982a, b, 1985).

2. If individual allelic forms of MHC gene products are selectively added to or removed from the system, regulatory disturbance results. Thus, in the F1-antiparent MLR, removal of one parental set of allelic MHC gene products from the stimulator cells leads to an unusual form of antiself T-cell reactivity towards the set of allelic MHC determinants of the other parent. Or, self-tolerance is broken by stimulating the T-cell system with cells bearing a foreign allogeneic MHC gene product in addition to a complete set of self MHC molecules, even if the organism had been neonatally tolerized to this particular allogeneic MHC molecule (Streilin 1979). Somewhat similar are our own observations that neonatally tolerized mice can be specifically sensitized to the tolerogen by challenge with cells bearing in addition to the tolerizing allogeneic MHC molecule a third party allogeneic MHC determinant (K. Heeg, unpublished).

3. In most readout systems, we actually assay a functional parameter expressed by a given T-cell population in response to binding to cell-associated antigen. We do not know at which stage of the activation pathway that leads from T-cell recognition to the expression of function the described levels of regulation operate. Specific recognition of T cells can take place without activation of the respective T-effector function: as mentioned above, self-reactive CTL generated

in the F1 (A × B)-antiparent (A or B) MLC specifically conjugate with syngeneic F1 targets but do not lyse F1 targets (while they form conjugates and lyse the respective parental targets).

4 Diversity of the T-Cell Repertoire

The peripheral T-cell population of a mouse is presumably able to specifically react to $>10^4$ different epitopes because of the large diversity of clonally distributed antigen-recognizing receptors (SHERMAN 1980, 1982a, b). The B-cell system seems "complete" in its ability to recognize antigens, i.e., the antibody molecules produced by the B cells of an individual can recognize any (foreign or self) epitope (COUTINHO 1980). We have presented comparable data for the T-cell system: every MHC-bearing target cell tested had an equal and high chance to be specifically recognized by a CTL population that clonally developed from mitogen-activated T blasts under limiting dilution conditions (HEEG et al. 1985). The only difference seems to be that T-cell recognition is MHC restricted while B-cell (antibody) recognition is not, although exceptions to this rule have been reported (SHERMAN et al. 1983).

When T cells are polyclonally activated, clonally expanded under limiting dilution conditions, and their specific reactivity read out against a panel of targets, about 1 out of 100 T-cell clones is found to be specifically reactive towards one of the tested targets (EICHMANN et al. 1983; HEEG et al. 1985). Similar data have been obtained in systems in which T cells were specifically induced to clonal development under limiting dilution conditions by antigenic stimulation (REIMANN et al. 1985a, b). This seems to suggest that the T-cell repertoire is very restricted in its ability to discriminate between two different antigenic determinants.

The notion of T-cell recognition "specificity" needs some comment. In a common type of specific readout, lytic reactivity is screened against a restricted panel of target cells which express many different potentially antigenic determinants on the cell surface. It could thus be argued that this type of specificity analysis only provides very "crude" estimates of T-cell receptor diversity and probably underestimates the magnitude of diversity. In contrast, a "fine" specificity analysis of T-cell recognition, such as the extensive and convincing studies of L. SHERMAN (1980, 1982a, b), would analyze lysis patterns of alloreactive monoclonal CTL populations read out against a large panel of mutant MHC-bearing targets. But these data can be taken as evidence for fine specificity of the T-cell receptor phenotype only if allorecognition is assumed nonrestricted. The alternative "altered self" view of T-cell recognition (MATZINGER and BEVAN 1977; MATZINGER 1981) would propose that a mutant allo MHC determinant reorganizes the visibility of many background determinants for T cells and thus introduces allorestricted polyspecificity into the system. We do not yet have a system available in which the T-cell response can be read out against a panel of targets bearing different mutant variants of a background gene product which is recognized in the context of an identical MHC restriction determinant. We thus do not know how to distinguish crude estimates of T-cell receptor diversity from fine specificity analysis. All systems might, in fact, be crude.

It is noteworthy that a similar paradox appeared in the B-cell system. It has been unequivocally shown that antibodies discriminate $>10^5$ different epitopes. But one out of three splenic B cells are driven by lipopolysaccharide into clonal expansion under limiting dilution conditions; one out of 100 of these mitogen-stimulated B-cell clones produced antibodies that bound trinitrophenyl-modified sheep red blood cells (ANDERSSON et al. 1977). In contrast to the T-cell system, there is overwhelming evidence for somatic diversification of antibody specificity during clonal B-cell development induced by antigenic stimulation (see Sect. 5).

The discrepancies in repertoire estimates may indicate that the different systems used to derive estimates of the diversity of the T-cell repertoire are not comparable. The estimate of $>10^4$ specificities within the T-cell repertoire was deduced from the analysis of lytic patterns expressed by cloned T-cell lines established in long term culture (SHERMAN 1980, 1982a, b); the estimate of 10^2 specificities within the T-cell repertoire was deduced from limiting dilution analysis (LDA). Although the fascination of LDA is to define the receptor specificity of freshly isolated lymphocytes at the clonal level, the "input" into the system (e.g., the receptor specificity of a given precursor lymphocyte that is going to be expanded) is never controlled. It is therefore uncertain whether the measured "output" was present at the initiation of the system (i.e., was just quantitatively expanded to render it detectable by current assay methods), or whether it was generated during the days of in vitro incubation that were necessary for the system to yield a measurable answer. If somatic diversification of the T-cell receptor specificity in the course of clonal expansion in vitro could be demonstrated, it would resolve the apparent contradiction.

5 The Generation of Diversity of the T-Cell Repertoire: A Speculative View

A hypothesis on somatic diversification could envision T cells engaged in a lifelong differentiation pathway, that – although transiently interrupted by resting states – proceeds in successive (antigen/mitogen-induced) bursts of development, in the course of which diversification of the repertoire of receptor specificities occurs. Environmental constraints channel this discontinuous "stream" of newly generated specificities into prevalent directions, sidelines of which are constantly trimmed off by diversion, suppression, and/or cytotoxic interactions. As often proposed (VON BOEHMER et al. 1978; REIMANN and MILLER 1983a, b), the diversification process may originate from self-reactive receptor phenotypes. Once the process of diversification of receptor specificities is en route away from self-reactivity, the question of how is it directed arises. Obvious candidates for this guiding role in diversification are MHC molecules. The MHC haplotypes (A1, B1) and (A2, B2) lead to different T-cell repertoires in two congenic mice, but an F1 (A1, B1 × A2, B2) mouse has a repertoire different again from the sum of the two parental (A1, B1 and A2, B2) repertoires (SHERMAN 1980). Hence the repertoire is not a mosaic of independent parts that are developed in association with individual allele-specific determinants on MHC molecules, but is shaped by a "common action" of all allele-specific determinants present on MHC molecules of the particular individual.

This view is obviously not in line with clonal selection theory, which postulates (BURNET 1959): (1) each individual T and B lymphocyte is irreversibly committed to a particular monospecific receptor phenotype early in its development, i.e., the diversity of the repertoire is present before antigenic stimulation drives lymphocyte differentiation into effector and/or memory lineages; (2) antigenic stimulation induces clonal expansion of monospecific effector and/or memory immune cells; and (3) throughout this clonal expansion, receptor phenotypes remain unchanged.

6 Somatic Diversification of the T-Cell Repertoire: The Problems

Somatic diversification of the antibody repertoire is now well established. The first unambiguous experimental evidence for changing specificities in clonal B-cell development was presented by A. Cunningham and coworkers more than 10 years ago (CUNNINGHAM 1974; CUNNINGHAM and PILARSKI 1974a, b; CUNNINGHAM and FORDHAM 1974). In an extensive series of experiments he demonstrated at the single cell level that B-cell daughters can produce antibodies of different specificity than their parent cell. This was confirmed at the molecular level when appropriate technologies became available: the approach of molecular genetics has demonstrated one point mutation per B-cell division (MCKEAN et al. 1984; SABLITZKY and RAJEWSKI 1984), presumably resulting from the expression of an active site-specific hypermutational process at the DNA level (BALTIMORE 1981; KIM et al. 1981; TONEGAWA 1983).

The evidence for somatic diversification during clonal T-cell development is preliminary. We have shown that about 10% of cytotoxic T-cell populations clonally developing under limiting dilution conditions can change their specific lytic reactivity pattern within 2–4 days (REIMANN and MILLER 1985). This is in contrast to the stable expression of a given receptor specificity by clonal populations of T cells established in long term culture or T-T hybridomas, although occasionaal changes in the specific reactivity pattern of T-cell clones have been reported (GUIMEZANES et al. 1982; WRAITH 1984). More definitive evidence was provided by AUGUSTIN and SIM (1984), who have shown at the molecular (protein) level that changing specific reactivity patterns of T-T hybridomas correlate with changes in the amino acid composition of the respective T-cell receptor.

There are four areas in which we see problems arising for the concept of somatic diversification of the T-cell repertoire.

1. The accumulation of point mutations in clonal B-cell development requires cell proliferation. If a mouse is immunized with sheep red blood cells, the number of detectable splenic sheep red blood cell-specific plaque-forming cells rises about 10^4-fold, and it is assumed that this reflects antigen-driven clonal expansion of B cells in vivo. T cells stimulated by mitogen or antigen under limiting dilution conditions clonally expand in vitro; under these conditions, a single T cell can give rise to 10^4–10^5 progeny cells. At first glance, the T-cell system and

252   J. Reimann et al.

the B-cell system thus seem to obey the same rules. A major difference arises when the expansion in numbers of specifically reactive immune cells after sensitization in vivo is compared. In contrast to the dramatic increase in the number of B blasts that produce antibodies binding the immunizing antigen, no increase in the number of specifically reactive (cytotoxic and helper) T cells is found in vivo after immunization with allo MHC bearing cells (KIMURA and WIGZELL 1983), allogeneic minor H bearing cells (MITCHISON and PETTERSON 1983), or hapten-modified syngeneic cells (HAMAN et al. 1983), or after virus infection (K. Heeg, unpublished). There is therefore no experimental evidence for clonal expansion of T cells in the course of a cell-mediated immune response in vivo. Thus, when/where does somatic diversification occur in the functional T-cell system in vivo?

2. T cells recognize antigen in the context of polymorphic MHC determinants; the T-cell receptor thus has two nonoverlapping recognitive sites, it is dual recognitive. If the T-cell receptor specificity is somatically diversifying while T-cell recognition remains restricted to the same MHC determinant, only one part of the receptor (or one receptor) can change its recognition specificity, but not the other of the receptor (or the second receptor). In essence, this model has been proposed by von Boehmer, Haas, and Jerne (VON BOEHMER et al. (1978). We would thus expect that there are two separate recognition sites on one receptor or two separate receptors on T cells, and that somatic diversification would be restricted to only one of these (i.e., the antigen recognizing receptor). This is implied in hypotheses that propose self-reactivity as the origin for the generation of the T-cell receptor repertoire, and the persistence of this self-reactive recognition specificity in form of the (self) restriction specificity in the functional T-cell receptor phenotype.

Alternative hypotheses (MATZINGER and BEVAN 1977) have suggested a one-receptor view of T-cell behavior. Somatic diversification of one receptor would change antigen specificity and restriction specificity, either at the same time or independent of each other. This would be expected to produce many T-cell receptor phenotypes not recognizing available (self) restriction determinants plus antigen, and would thus generate a large pool of nonfunctional T cells. The latter are nonfunctional in a syngeneic environment, but could be functional in an allogeneic environment, as the changed receptor specificity would be expected to react with various allogeneic restriction determinants plus antigen. This could be proposed as an explanation for alloreactive and allorestricted T-cell recognition specificities.

3. A continuously ongoing diversification of the T-cell (and antibody) repertoire is expected to produce an abundance of autoreactive receptor phenotypes. It has been demonstrated that one point mutation within the variable region of an antibody molecule can convert its original specific reactivity to a foreign antigenic determinant into a specific reactivity towards a defined autoantigen (DIAMOND and SCHARFF 1984). Hence the control mechanism for autoreactivity can not be restricted to a particular (early) stage in T-cell development, but must operate continuously. Although a multitude of possible mechanisms has been proposed, definitive evidence is lacking at present.

4. Three somatic mutational mechanisms are employed by B cells to generate immunoglobulin diversity: junctional variability arising from the flexibility in the endpoints at which V, D and J segments may be joined, N-region diversity arising from the apparently random trimming and repair of sequences on either side of the D gene segments during joining, and somatic hypermutation (KIM et al. 1981; ALT and BALTIMORE 1982). T cells may equally employ all three mechanisms to somatically generate diversity (AUGUSTIN and SIM 1984; GOVERMAN et al. 1985). In view of this apparent similarity in the antigen-driven generation of diversity of antigen receptors in B and T cells, it remains enigmatic how the restriction specificities are maintained in the developing specificity repertoire of T-cell populations.

7 The Type of Effector Function Expressed by T-Cells Correlates with the Class of MHC Molecules It Recognizes

There are two classes of MHC molecules. T cells that recognize class I restriction determinants are usually of the cytotoxic/suppressor lineage; T cells that recognize class II restriction determinants are usually of the helper/amplifier lineage. This correlation could indicate that:

1. A functionally defined T-cell subset is committed through the type of antigen receptor it expresses to interact selectively with only one of the two available classes of MHC molecules; i.e., a T-cell receptor "isotype" is a marker for a particular type of effector function and binds only to one of the two classes of MHC molecules.

2. The MHC molecule "imprints" a particular functional phenotype on the T cell recognizing it; i.e., interaction of the T cell with one class of MHC molecules triggers one of different alternative activation pathways in T cells which all lead to the phenotypic expression of different types of effector functions.

3. An intercellular regulation interferes with the recognition of the (class of MHC molecule plus antigen) entity by a particular T-cell subset; i.e., a regulatory cell would only allow functional interactions between certain T-cell subsets and one class of MHC molecules and/or suppress the respective alternative interactions.

There is very scarce experimental evidence for/against any of these alternative interpretations. The (biochemical and genetic) identification of the α- and β-chain of the T-cell receptor for antigen has not revealed different "isotypes" specific for helper or cytotoxic T cells. Possible changes in the functional phenotype of T-cell clones reacting to antigen X in the context of a class I MHC molecule, and cross-reacting to antigen Y in the context of a class II MHC molecule have not yet been described. There is evidence that T cells of the cytotoxic/suppressor lineage inhibit the activation of helper T cells that recognize antigen in the context of class I MHC molecules (VIDOVIC et al. 1984). We have therefore to conclude that this correlation between class of MHC molecule recognized and type of effector function expressed does unfortunately not elucidate the function of MHC molecules.

8 Perspectives

We have discussed various themes that reflect aspects of the relationship between T-cell receptor specificities, polymorphic MHC determinants, and functional T-cell phenotypes. We have explored alternative interpretations which might offer the possibility to understand some phenomena, some of which are described in the accompanying papers.

The repertoire of normal unprimed peripheral cytotoxic T cells seems "complete", as self-reactive, self-restricted, alloreactive, and allorestricted receptor phenotypes are present in equally high frequencies (HEEG et al. 1985). Some indirect evidence and preliminary direct evidence has indicated a major role for somatic diversification in the development of the T-cell receptor repertoire (see Sect. 6). The allelic determinants of MHC gene products seem to guide this somatic diversification process, the outcome of which is a bias of the repertoire for self-restricted and/or alloreactive receptor phenotypes. This guiding role seems to operate at different hierarchically organized levels in T-cell recognition/activation, and only one of the many involved allele-specific determinants becomes apparent in the receptor phenotype of the developing T-cell clone as restriction specificity (see Sect. 3). The T-cell system in an advanced stage of repertoire development (e.g., in an adult mouse) seems to depend on the continuous presence of the complete set of allelic MHC determinants for maintaining its functional integrity, as omissions of syngeneic MHC determinants (as in the F1-antiparent MLR) or addition of allogeneic MHC determinants result in self-reactive and/or alloreactive phenomena. The rules which polymorphic MHC determinants employ to unravel the T-cell repertoire have not yet been defined. Nor do we know if this process ever reaches a stable differentiated end stage, or if it continuously progresses with the persisting risk of autodestruction through dysregulated antiself reactivity.

The problem of repertoire development should be further considered with respect to another set of newly emerged questions about the definition and the stability of the functional phenotype expressed by clonally developing T cells. Major difficulties are encountered in the attempt to define the helper or cytotoxic T-cell lineages. The helper phenotype could be characterized by the secretion of a heterogenous pattern of various lymphokines, but many T-cell clones of the cytotoxic lineage secrete the same lymphokines of the postulated T helper cell type. It might therefore be more appropriate to think of discrete functional "cassettes" (e.g., cytolytic activity, suppressor activity, lymphokine secretion) instead of distinct developmental lineages programmed to express a complex and stable functional phenotype. The "functional phenotype" of a particular T blast stimulated in a particular environment through one of many alternative activation pathways may thus represent a mosaic of selected functional cassettes. This mosaic may depend on the mode of activation of this T blast (i.e., its environment) and/or its developmental history (i.e., its lineage). Allele-specific recognition of MHC determinants may interfere with this process of selecting the appropriate functional cassette.

In a sense, this view of T-cell behavior is the exact opposite of the model proposed by the clonal selection theory of the immune system. It emphasizes change and flexibility in the clonal T-cell response, in terms of discrete components of the functional repertoire as well as of the receptor repertoire. A particular functional and receptor phenotype of a developing T-cell clone which is actually realized at a particular point in time of the immune response is not programmed to remain stable but adapted to change. It might be helpful to attempt to interpret many experimental data in view of both extreme hypotheses.

References

Alt B, Baltimore D (1982) Joining of immunoglobulin heavy chain gene segments: implications from a chromosome with evidence of three D-J(H) fusions. Proc Natl Acad Sci USA 78:5812

Andersson J, Coutinho A, Melchers F (1977) Frequencies of mitogen-reactive B cells in the mouse. II. Frequencies of B cells producing antibodies which lyse sheep or horse erythrocytes and trinitrophenylated or nitroiodophenylated sheep erythrocytes. J Exp Med 145:1520

Augustin AA, Sim GK (1984) T-cell receptors generated via mutations are specific for various major histocompatibility antigens. Cell 39:5

Baltimore D (1981) Somatic mutation gains its place among the generators of diversity. Cell 26:295

Bartlett PF, Edidin M (1977) Effect of the H-2 gene complex on rates of fibroblast intercellular adhesion. J Cell Biol 77:377

Bodmer WF (1972) Evolutionary significance of the HLA system. Nature 237:139

Burnet FM (1959) The clonal selection theory of acquired immunity. Vanderbilt, Nashville, TN

Cohn M (1983) The T-cell receptor mediating restrictive recognition of antigen. Cell 33:657

Coutinho A (1980) The self-non-self discrimination and the nature and acquisition of the antibody repertoire. Ann Immunol (Inst Pasteur) 131D:235

Cunningham AJ (1974) The generation of antibody diversity: its dependence on antigenic stimulation. Contemp Top Immunol 3:1

Cunningham AJ, Fordham SA (1974) Antibody cell daughters can produce antibody of different specificities. Nature 250:669

Cunningham AJ, Pilarski LM (1974a) The generation of antibody diversity. I. Kinetics of production of different antibody specificities during the course of an immune response. Eur J Immunol 4:319

Cunningham AJ, Pilarski LM (1974b) The generation of antibody diversity. II. Plaque morphology as a simple marker for antibody specificity at the single cell level. Eur J Immunol 4:757

Curtis ASG (1979) Histocompatibility systems, recognition and cell positioning. Dev Comp Immunol 3:379

Dausset J, Contu L (1980) Is the MHC a general self-recognition system playing a major unifying role in organisms? Hum Immunol 1:5

Diamond B, Scharff MD (1984) Somatic mutation of the T15 heavy chain gives rise to an antibody with autoantibody specificity. Proc Natl Acad Sci USA 81:5841

Doherty PC, Biddison WE, Bennink JR, Knowles BB (1978) Cytotoxic T cell responses in mice infected with influenza and vaccinia viruses vary in magnitude with H-2 genotype. J Exp Med 148:534

Dos Reis GA, Shevach EM (1983) Antigen-presenting cells from nonresponder strain 2 guinea pigs are fully competent to present bovine insulin B chain to responder strain 2 T cells. Evidence against a determinant selection model and in favor of a clonal deletion model of immune response gene function. J Exp Med 157:1287

Edidin M (1983) MHC antigens and non-immune functions. Immunol Today 4:269

Eichmann K, Fey K, Kuppers K, Melchers I, Simon MM, Weltzien HU (1983) Network regulation among T-cells: conclusions from limiting dilution experiments. Springer Semin Immunopathol 6:7

Forman J (1975) On the role of the H-2 histocompatibility complex in determining the specificity of cytotoxic effector cells sensitized against syngeneic trinitrophenyl-modified targets. J Exp Med 142:403

256   J. Reimann et al.

Fujiwara H, Tsuchida T, Levy RB, Shearer GM (1982) H-2Kk can influence whether cytotoxic T lymphocytes recognize trinitrophenyl in assocation with H-2Dk unique or H-2Kk and H-2Dk shared self determinants. J Immunol 129:1189

Gomard E, Duprez V, Reme T, Colombani MJ, Levy JP (1977) Exclusive involvement of H-2Db or H-2Kd product in the interaction between T-killer lymphocytes and syngeneic H-2b or H-2d viral lymphomas. J Exp Med 146:909

Goverman J, Minard K, Shastri N, Hunkapiller T, Hansburg D, Sercarz E, Hood L (1985) Rearranged T cell receptor genes in a helper T cell clone specific for lysozyme: no correlation between V and MHC restriction. Cell 40:859

Guimezanes A, Albert F, Schmitt-Verhulst AM (1982) I region-restricted T cell line stimulated with hapten-treated syngeneic cells: selection of clones with reactivity for both allogeneic Ia determinants and self-I-A plus hapten. Eur J Immunol 12:195

Haman U, Eichmann K, Krammer PH (1983) Frequencies and regulation of trinitrophenyl-specific cytotoxic T-precursor cells: immunization results in release from suppression. J Immunol 130:7

Heeg K, Zielinski I, Kabelitz D, Wagner H, Reimann J (1985) Anti-MHC reactive T-cells. II. Clonal specificity of mitogen activated cytotoxic T-lymphoblasts. (Submitted)

Ishikawa H, Dutton RW (1979) Primary in vitro cytotoxic response of F1 T lymphocytes against parental antigens. J Immunol 122:529

Johnson LL, Bailey DW, Mobraaten LE (1981) Antigenic competition between minor non-H-2 histocompatibility antigens. Immunogenetics 13:451

Kim S, Davis M, Sinn E, Patten P, Hood L (1981) Antibody diversity: somatic hypermutation of rearranged Vh genes. Cell 27:573

Kimura AK, Wigzell H (1983) Development and function of cytotoxic T lymphocytes (CTL). I. In vivo maturation of CTL precursors in the absence of detectable proliferation results as a normal consequence of alloimmunization. J Immunol 130:2058

Klein J, Figueroa F (1981) Polymorphism of the mouse H-2 loci. Immunol Rev 60:23

Lengerova A, Zeleny V, Haskovec C, Hilgert I (1977) Search for the physiological function of H-2 gene products. Eur J Immunol 7:62

MacDonald HR, Glasebrook AL, Bron C, Kelsoe A, Cerottini JC (1982) Clonal heterogeneity in the functional requirement for Lyt-2/3 molecules on cytolytic T lymphocytes (CTL): possible implications for the affinity of CTL antigen receptors. Immunol Rev 68:89

Matzinger P (1981) A one-receptor view of T-cell behavior. Nature 292:497

Matzinger P, Bevan MJ (1977) Hypothesis. Why do so many lymphocytes respond to major histocompatibility antigens? Cell Immunol 29:1

Matzinger P, Zamoyska R, Waldmann H (1984) Self-tolerance is H-2 restricted. Nature 308:738

McKean D, Huppi K, Bell M, Staudt L, Gerhardt W, Weigert M (1984) Generation of antibody diversity in the immune response of BALB/c mice to influenza virus hemagglutinin. Proc Natl Acad Sci USA 81:3180

Mitchison NA, Petterson S (1983) Does clonal selection occur among T-cells? Ann Immun (Inst Pasteur) 134D:37

Nakamura I, Cudkowicz G (1982) Fine specificity of auto- and allo-reactive cytotoxic T lymphocytes: heteroclitic cross-reactions between mutant and original H-2 antigens. Curr Top Microbiol 99:51

Nakano K, Nakamura I, Cudkowicz G (1981) Generation of F1 hybrid cytotoxic T lymphocytes specific for self H-2. Nature 289:559

Potter TA, Palladino MA, Wilson DB, Rajan TV (1983) Epitopes on H-2D^d somatic cell mutants recognized by cytotoxic T cells. J Exp Med 158:1061

Rammensee HG, Bevan MJ (1984) Evidence from in vitro studies that tolerance to self antigens is MHC restricted. Nature 308:741

Reimann J, Miller RG (1983a) Differentiation from precursors in athymic nude mouse bone marrow of unusual spontaneously cytolytic cells showing anti-self H-2 specificity and bearing T cell markers. J Exp Med 158:1672

Reimann J, Miller RG (1983b) Generation of autoreactive cytotoxic T lymphocytes under limiting dilution conditions. J Immunol 131:2128

Reimann J, Miller RG (1983c) Polymorphism and MHC gene function. Dev Comp Immunol 7:403

Reimann J, Miller RG (1985) Rapid changes in specificity within single clones of cytolytic effector cells. Cell 40:571

T-Cell Reactivity to Polymorphic MHC Determinants. I   257

Reimann J, Heeg K, Miller RG, Wagner H (1985a) Allorective T-cells. I. Alloreactive and allorestricted cytotoxic T-cells. Eur J Immunol 15:387

Reimann J, Kabelitz D, Heeg K, Wagner H (1985b) Allorestricted cytotoxic T-cells. Large numbers of allo-H-2Kb-restricted anti-hapten and anti-viral cytotoxic T-cell populations clonally develop in vitro from murine splenic precursor T-cells. J Exp Med 162:592

Sablitzky F, Rajewsky K (1984) Molecular basis of an isogenic anti-idiotypic response. EMBO J 3:3005

Scofield VL, Schlumpberger JM, West LA, Weissman I (1982) Protochordate allorecognition is controlled by a MHC-like gene system. Nature 295:499

Shearer GM, Rehn TG, Garbarino CA (1975) Cell-mediated lympholysis of trinitrophenyl-modified autologous lymphocytes. J Exp Med 141:1348

Sherman LA (1980) Dissection of the B10.D2 anti-H-2K^b cytolytic T lymphocyte receptor repertoire. J Exp Med 151:1386

Sherman LA (1982a) Genetic and regulatory contributions of the major histocompatibility complex to the developing cytolytic T lymphocyte repertoire. J Immunol 128:1849

Sherman LA (1982b) Influence of the major histocompatibility complex on the repertoire of allospecific cytolytic T lymphocytes. J Exp Med 154:987

Sherman L (1985) The cytolytic T lymphocyte receptor repertoire of H-2 disparate cells obtained from double parental chimeras. J Immunol 1:63

Sherman LA, Vitiello A, Klinman NR (1983) T-cell and B-cell responses to viral antigens at the clonal level Ann Rev Immunol 1:63

Simonsen M, Olsson L (1983) Possible roles of compound membrane receptors in immune system. Ann Immun (Inst Pasteur) 134D:85

Simpson E (1982) The role of H-Y as a minor transplantation antigen. Immunol Today 3:97

Streilin JW (1979) Neonatal tolerance: towards an immunological definition of self. Immunol Rev 46:125

Streilin JW (1981) Hamster immune responsiveness and experimental models of infectious and oncologic diseases. Fed Proc 40:2343

Streilin JW, Duncan WR (1983) On the anomalous nature of the major histocompatibility complex in Syrian hamsters, Hm-1. Transplant Proc 15:1540

Swain SL (1980) Association of Ly phenotypes, T cell function and MHC recognition. Fed Proc 39:3110

Tonegawa S (1983) Somatic generation of antibody diversity. Nature 302:575

Vidovic D, Klein J, Nagy ZA (1984) The role of T cell subsets in the generation of secondary cytolytic responses in vitro against class I and class II major histocompatibility complex antigens. J Immunol 132:1113

von Boehmer H, Haas W, Jerne NK (1978) Major histocompatibility complex-linked immune responsiveness is acquired by lymphocytes of low responder mice differentiating in thymus of high responder mice. Proc Natl Acad Sci USA 75:2439

Wettstein PJ, Bailey DW (1982) Immunodominance in the immune response to "multiple" histocompatibility antigens. Immunogenetics 16:47

Wraith DC (1984) D^k-restricted antiinfluenza cytotoxic T-cell clone loses one of its two alloreactivities. Immunogenetics 20:131

Zinkernagel RM, Althage A, Cooper S, Kreeb G, Klein PA, Sefton B, Flaherty L, Stimpfling J, Shreffler D, Klein J (1978) Ir-genes in H-2 regulate generation of anti-viral cytotoxic T cells. Mapping to K or D and dominants of responsiveness. J Exp Med 148:592

T-Cell Reactivity to Polymorphic MHC Determinants
II. Self-reactive and Self-restricted T Cells

K. HEEG, D. KABELITZ, H. WAGNER, and J. REIMANN

1   Self-reactivity: The Unsolved Issue 259
2   Experimental Systems Detecting Self-reactive T Cells 260
2.1   The Autologous/Syngeneic Mixed Leukocyte Reaction (AMLR/SMLR) 260
2.2   Self-reactivity Expressed by Progenitor Cells of the T-Lineage 262
2.3   Self-reactive T Cells in the Early Cell-Mediated Immune Response In Vivo 262
2.4   Self-reactive T-Cell Clones Under Limiting Dilution Conditions 263
2.5   Self-reactive T Cells Activated Under Bulk Culture Conditions 263
2.6   Interclonal T-T Self-reactivity 263
3   Our Own Experimental Data on Self-reactive T Cells 264
3.1   Systems That Investigate Early Stages of T-Cell Development 264
3.2   Two Experimental Systems Reflecting Late or Mature Stages of Murine T Cells 267
3.3   Experimental Systems Indicating Regulatory Influences on Self-reactivity 268
4   The Physiological Role of Self-reactivity 271
References 271

1 Self-reactivity: The Unsolved Issue

The clonal selection approach is simple and direct: "(1) It is necessary for survival that neither immunocytes nor antibodies should exist in the body which are reactive to more than a minimal degree with any accessible body component. (2) Since immune pattern is generated by a random process, a mechanism must exist by which any 'self-reactive' cells which may emerge can be eliminated or functionally inhibited. More than one mechanism may be needed to establish and maintain this intrinsic immunological tolerance toward self components" (BURNET 1972). Failure of this censorship mechanism to eliminate a "forbidden" self-reactive lymphocyte clone is autoimmune disease.

Network theorists are complex and indirect: "In the opinion of many immunologists, the sets of V genes, encoding antibody structures, have evolved under the influence of a selection pressure exercised by invasive pathogenic micro-organisms. I have never liked this facile idea. I have always believed that a fundamental insight is most likely to emerge if we assume the exact opposite of what seems to be true… As for self-nonself, I, thus, assume that the genes of the immune system have evolved so as to encode antibodies that recognize the self-antigens of the species" (JERNE 1984). The immune system reflects first the universe of autologous epitopes, then produces a reflection of this reflection, and then …

Department of Medical Microbiology and Immunology, University of Ulm, D-7900 Ulm

The issue is anti-MHC directed T-cell reactivity. In this paper we discuss self-reactivity. We try to order the available data on T-cell-mediated reactivity to autologous MHC determinants into groups with underlying common themes. To these, we try to relate our own findings.

2 Experimental Systems Detecting Self-reactive T Cells

Self-reactive T cells with different functional phenotypes have been investigated in a variety of *in vivo* and *in vitro* experimental systems, either at the level of heterogenous populations of T-lymphocytes, or at the level of homogenous cloned T-cell populations. These studies have placed major emphasis on the questions: do self-reactive T cells really exist in the intact peripheral immune system of a normal individual? What functions do self-reactive T cells mediate? What might be their physiological role *in vivo*?

2.1 The Autologous/Syngeneic Mixed Leukocyte Reaction (AMLR/SMLR)

A proliferative response of (thymic, splenic, and lymph node) T cells to autologous or syngeneic non-T cells has been described in an in vitro system, designated AMLR (in man) or SMLR (in mouse, rat, and guinea pig) (reviewed in BATTISTO and PONZIO 1981; WECKSLER et al. 1981). T cells activated in this type of MLR exhibit two basic characteristics of an immune response, i.e., memory and specificity for autologous determinants (WECKSLER and KOZAK 1977). Antigens encoded by genes of the MHC of the respective species play a central role in this antigen-independent T-cell activation process. The functional significance of T cells activated in response to autologous non-T cells in vitro is not clear, as these selfreactive T-cell populations express a multitude of helper, suppressor, and cytolytic activities.

The responder T cell in the AMLR/SMLR is of the helper/inducer class, i.e., displays the Lyt-1$^+$ phenotype in the mouse and the OKT4$^+$ phenotype in man (LATTIME et al. 1980; SMOLEN et al. 1981). This self-reactive T cell is distinct from alloreactive responder T cells, as demonstrated by serologically defined marker expression (HAUSMAN et al. 1983; ELLIS and MOKANAKUMAR 1983) and selective depletion experiments (DOS REIS and SHEVACH 1981; SOPORI et al. 1984). T cells responding in the AMLR/SMLR seem to represent a polyclonally activated population of antigen-specific T-lymphocytes with receptors for self-Ia antigens (HAUSMAN et al. 1980; YAMASHITA and SHEVACH 1980; HAUSMAN et al. 1981; DOS REIS and SHEVACH 1981).

The non-T stimulator cells of this type of MLR can be peritoneal exudate cells (YAMASHITA and SHEVACH 1980), monocytes/macrophages (HAUSMAN et al. 1981), B-lymphocytes (OPELZ et al. 1975), lymphoblastoid cell lines (WECKSLER et al. 1981), dendritic cells (NUSSENZWEIG and STEINMAN 1980), or "null" cells

(WECKSLER et al. 1981). The target structures are class II MHC-encoded molecules, as shown by blocking experiments with monoclonal anti-Ia antibodies, mapping studies, and chimera experiments (YAMASHITA and SHEVACH 1980; HAUSMAN et al. 1981; GLIMCHER et al. 1981, 1982, 1985).

The proliferative response of self-reactive T cells is seen either if fractionated T cells are cocultured with non-T cells (obtained through various separation procedures), or if nonfractionated spleen cell populations are cultured in vitro with antiprostaglandins and/or lymphokine preparations (ZUBERI and KATZ 1984).

Activated self-reactive T cells express a wide spectrum of effector functions. They facilitate the generation of cytotoxic T-lymphocytes (WOLOS and SMITH 1982, 1984; ZUBERI and ALTMAN 1982) and enhance B-cell proliferation and immunoglobulin secretion in a T-dependent humoral immune response in vitro (JAMES et al. 1981; GATENBY et al. 1984, 1985; ZAUDERER et al. 1984; FOLKES and SELL 1984; CLAYBERGER et al. 1984, 1985; KIMOTO et al. 1984; FINNEGAN et al. 1984). Under different experimental conditions, they suppress immunoglobulin secretion by B cells (JAMES et al. 1981; GATENBY et al. 1981; CLAYBERGER et al. 1984) and block responsiveness of cytotoxic T cells to interleukin 2 (STOUT 1984). Some self-reactive T-cell populations, generated in the human AMLR or in the mouse SMLR systems, display cytotoxic activity which is either specific for syngeneic LPS-blast targets (MILLER and KAPLAN 1978), or "NK-like" (TOMONARI 1980) or "lymphocyte activated killer"-like (GOTO and ZWAIFLER 1983).

The SMLR is compromised in strains of mice with autoimmune disease, such as NZB or MRL mice (GLIMCHER et al. 1980); and the AMLR in man is defective in diseases associated with immunological abnormalities. It is suppressed, e.g., in systemic lupus erythematosus, Sjögren syndrome, infectious mononucleosis, and rheumatoid arthritis (WECKSLER et al. 1981), but enhanced in myasthenia gravis (GREENBERG et al. 1984).

There is an ongoing controversy about the involvement of "foreign" constituents (such as heterologous serum components, polyethylene glycol, environmental pathogens, xenogenic red blood cell constituents) in the induction and/or in the expression of self-reactive T cell responses (HUBER et al. 1982; KAGAN and CHOI 1983; HAYWARD and MORI 1984). Although this remains a possibility in some systems, it is definitely excluded in others (YAMASHITA and SHEVACH 1980). The overall conclusion seems to be that self-reactive T cells are in fact generated in these systems.

The biological significance of self-reactive T cells with respect to these MLR systems is discussed as follows. (1) The described phenomena represent in vitro artefacts: T-cell activation in the AMLR/SMLR proceeds through low affinity antiself receptors. This activation pathway is not stimulated in vivo by Ia-antigens alone, but functions only in response to Ia plus foreign antigen. (2) The described phenomena reflect a physiological role of self-reactive T cells. They might be immunoregulatory elements in the normal immune response, or, alternatively, the AMLR/SMLR might reproduce in vitro an early differentiation state of T-lymphocytes in which interaction with Ia alone is sufficient to stimulate T cells in vivo. The latter two themes are recurring in other experimental systems describing self-reactive T cells which will now be discussed.

2.2 Self-reactivity Expressed by Progenitor Cells of the T-Lineage

Thy-1$^+$, Lyt-1$^+$2$^-$ responder cells interact with Ia+ stimulator cells in the thymus in an autochthonous SMLR-like proliferative reaction in the absence of exogenous antigen (BORN and WECKERLE 1982; ROCK and BENACERRAF 1984a). Murine thymocytes induce the monokine interleukin 1 upon in vitro coculture with accessory cells bearing autologous Ia molecules; in the presence of interleukin 1, purified thymic T cells with specificity for self class II MHC antigens expand in a proliferative reaction in vitro (ROCK and BENACERRAF 1984b). This reaction was considered unique to the thymic stage of T-cell development, and it was suggested that this SMLR reflects a key role of the thymus in the selection of a T-cell repertoire with specificity for the restricted recognition of antigen in association with self-MHC gene products. This is incompatible with many reports of self-reactive T cells isolated in the course of a cell-mediated immune response in vivo.

2.3 Self-reactive T Cells in the Early Cell-Mediated Immune Response In Vivo

Increasing amounts of experimental evidence for the appearance of self-reactive T cells in the early course of a cell-mediated immune response in vivo is being published. Self-reactive cytotoxic T-lymphocytes were detected in vivo in the early course of a murine virus infection (PFIZENMAIER et al. 1975). Autoreactive T-cell hybridomas were isolated from draining lymph nodes of mice primed with protein antigens, such as key hole limpet hemocyanin (KIMOTO et al. 1984), ovalbumin (FOLKES and SELL 1984), synthetic peptides (ENDRES et al. 1983), or heterologous insulins (GLIMCHER and SHEVACH 1982) in adjuvant. Stable T-cell lines specific for autologous class II MHC determinants have been established from rats immunized with autologous thyroglobulin in adjuvant (ZANETTI et al. 1984). Autoreactive T-cell clones have been generated from lethally irradiated, immunized, and thymocyte-reconstituted mice (CLAYBERGER et al. 1984, 1985). Intriguing is the observation that long term murine allospecific cytotoxic T-lymphocyte clones can develop high levels of cytotoxicity against syngeneic targets when cultured under appropriate conditions. These clones maintained strict allospecificity as long as they were cultured with the appropriate allogeneic stimulator cells and growth factor(s), but antiself rapidly developed when the allogeneic stimulator cells were replaced by syngeneic or third party allogeneic stimulator cells (CLAESSON and MILLER 1985). This might suggest that even a cloned T-cell population needs a self-reactive precursor pool from which antigenic stimulation can persistently recruit specifically reactive self-restricted T cells.

Common features of the appearance of self-reactive T cells in the course of an immune response in vivo are: (1) an early and transient appearance in the course of the response; (2) most self-reactive T hybridomas were isolated after immunization with protein antigen emulsified in adjuvant; and (3) most self-reactive T-cell hybridomas and clones mediate helper activities for B-cell development.

What is the relationship between self-reactive and self-restricted antigen-specific T-cell populations? Are self-reactive T cells an "activation byproduct" of an

T-Cell Reactivity to Polymorphic MHC Determinants. II   263

(adjuvant-amplified?) T-cell response in vivo, the transient appearance of which would indicate that it is rapidly eliminated? Or, alternatively, is there a precursor/product relationship between self-reactive and self-restricted T cells, in which T cells initially activated in an antigen-independent manner by the MHC determinants through high affinity receptors for self MHC determinants further "mature" to self-restricted receptor phenotypes from the originally self-reactive receptor phenotypes. The latter interpretation implies that self-reactive T hybridomas represent an arrested early maturation stage. In a panel of T-T hybridomas obtained at an early time point after immunization, self-reactive and self-restricted as well as many intermediate receptor phenotypes were found which could represent the different developmental stages of this process (ROCK and BENACERRAF 1983).

2.4 Self-reactive T-Cell Clones Under Limiting Dilution Conditions

Self-reactive cytotoxic T-cell clones are generated "spontaneously" at high frequency from murine T-cell populations cultured under limiting dilution conditions, as shown orginally by J. Marbrook and coworkers (CHING et al. 1977a-d). Self-reactive cytotoxic T-cell clones are detected besides antigen-specific T-cell clones in antigen-induced T-cell responses under limiting dilution conditions (GOOD et al. 1983). There is thus a striking analogy to the systems described above: self-reactive T cells are either "spontaneously" activated (possibly because some regulatory mechanism is diluted out) as in the SMLR, or are "byproducts" in an antigen-driven T-cell response. These systems indicate that self-reactive T cells are clonally expanded under certain conditions, which might offer the chance to observe the intraclonal generation of self-restricted receptor phenotypes in initially self-reactive clonal T-cell populations.

2.5 Self-reactive T Cells Activated Under Bulk Culture Conditions

In bulk cultures of nonfractionated murine spleen cells, self-reactive cytotoxic T cells can be generated by stimulation with fetal calf serum (PECK et al. 1977) or the lymphokine allogeneic effect factor (AEF) (ALTMAN and KATZ 1980). The AEF-induced T cells were effective in serving as effector cells of graft-versus-host reactions in vivo in syngeneic recipients (ALTMAN and KATZ 1980). These data further confirm the existence of self-reactive T cells in the functional cellular immune of normal mice.

2.6 Interclonal T-T Self-reactivity

Human autoreactive T-cell clones are described as expressing immunoregulatory amplifier function (BENSUSSAN et al. 1984). These $T4^+$ T-cell clones are generated in response to autologous antigen-specific self-restricted inducer T-cell clones. In this interclonal interaction, only self class II MHC determinants were specifically recognized by autoreactive T-cell clones in an antigen-independent

264   K. Heeg et al.

manner. These clones induced autologous B cells to produce high levels of immunoglobulin in the absence of exogenous antigen, and could synergize with antigen-specific self-restricted T-helper cells.

From this brief outline, it is evident that in the immune system of normal individuals, there exist T cells manifesting self-reactivity indistinguishable from alloreactivity. As self-reactive T cells have been generated in vivo or their functional activity read out in vivo, it is unlikely that they represent mere in vitro artefacts. Unresolved is the question of the biological significance of self-reactive T cells in the immune system. One recurrent theme proposes their involvement in the immunoregulation of T-cell-dependent immune responses in vivo. An alternative theme is centered around the idea that self-reactive T cells represent the precursor pool from which self-restricted antigen-specific helper and cytotoxic T cells are recruited. The latter idea implies somatic diversification of T-cell receptor phenotypes which might only be initiated after antigen has been introduced into the system.

3   Our Own Experimental Data on Self-reactive T Cells

In various in vitro systems, we have investigated the generation of self-reactive cytotoxic T-cell populations under limiting dilution conditions. The T-cell system was analyzed at early developmental stages as well as at "mature" stages. Emphasis was placed on the questions: (1) are self-reactive cytotoxic T cells detectable in various lymphoid cell populations, and what are the estimated frequencies for precursors of self-reactive cytotoxic T-cell clones; (2) are self-reactive cytotoxic T cells more frequent in early stages of the T-lineage or in the "immature" immune systems; (3) is the expression of a self-reactive T-cell receptor phenotype stable, or does it represent a transient stage during clonal T-cell development in vitro; and (4) do these systems show evidence for a regulatory influence that controls the functional expression of self-reactive cytotoxic T cells.

3.1   Systems That Investigate Early Stages of T-Cell Development

The three experimental systems now described reflect, as we assume, early or "immature" stages of the murine T-cell system.

1. In an in vitro microsystem, we cultured nylon-wool nonadherent nude marrow cells in the presence of conditioned medium under limiting dilution conditions (5–120 cells per 20 μl well) (REIMANN and MILLER 1983a). The system supported the growth and differentiation of about one out of 150 seeded marrow cells in the absence of feeder/filler cells or mitogens. A fraction of the clonally expanding cell populations contained Thy-1$^+$, Lyt-1$^+$ and/or Lyt-2$^+$ lymphoid cells, and of these clonal populations, a large fraction contained cells that expressed spontaneous cytolytic activity against syngeneic or semisyngeneic Con A-blast or tumor cell targets. H-2 incompatible Con A-blast or tumor cell targets were seldom lysed. These lytic cell populations were generated from Thy-1$^-$,

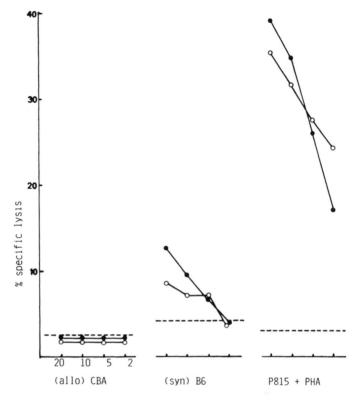

Fig. 1. Bone marrow-derived cytotoxic T-cell lines from normal (euthymic) B6 mice display self-reactivity. Long term lines (O–O line 1, ●–● line 2) of nylon wool nonadherent bone marrow cells were established as described (REIMANN and MILLER 1983a). Cells were grown in the presence of IL-2 containing conditioned medium and syngeneic irradiated splenic filler cells. Of these cells, >98% were Thy-1⁺ and about 50% were Lyt-2⁺. The cell population displayed lytic activity in a lectin-facilitated assay; showed low but reproducible levels of lysis of syngeneic (B6) Con A- or LPS-blast targets; and no lytic reactivity against allogeneic CBA blast targets, BALB/c blast targets, or P815 targets (in the absence of lectin)

Lyt-1⁻, Lyt-2⁻ medullary precursor cells. Short term lines established from these cytolytic cell populations expressed T-cell markers and showed the same autoreactive lytic activity. We have established similar lines from marrow cells of euthymic normal mice in long term cultures (>6 month). These cells are >98% Thy 1⁺, and about 50% Lyt 2⁺. They grow in the presence of syngeneic but not allogeneic irradiated splenic filler cells. Their replating efficiency is about 1/8. They display reproducible though moderate autoreactive, but no alloreactive lytic activity and lyse targets efficiently in a lectin-facilitated assay (Fig. 1).

2. In an analysis of the F1 (AxB)-antiparent (A or B) mixed lymphocyte reaction under limiting dilution conditions, we have detected many cytotoxic clones that lysed self F1 targets (REIMANN and MILLER 1983b). In this system, precursors of cytolytic T-cell clones were not lysed by treatment with anti-Thy-1 monoclonal antibody plus complement, whereas the cytolytic effector cells were

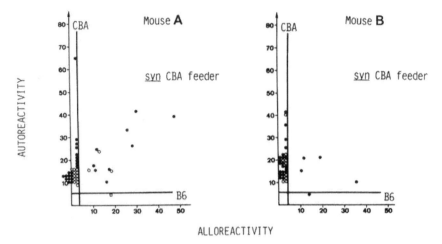

Fig. 2. Generation of autoreactive CTL clones from spleens of germfree CBA mice. Nylon-wool nonadherent splenic responder cells were cocultured with syngeneic irradiated filler cells and IL2 containing conditioned medium under limiting dilution conditions. The cytolytic reactivity of individual microcultures was read out at day 9 (●) and day 12 (○) of in vitro incubation against a panel of targets comprised of syngeneic (*CBA*) and allogeneic (B6 and BALB/c) Con A-blast targets. The lytic reactivity against BALB/c targets (data not shown) was comparable to that against B6 targets. Two representative experiments with two individual mice (A and B) are shown. The frequency estimates for precursors of self-reactive CTL clones was in the range of 1/200 to 1/300

Thy-1^+, Lyt-2^+. The patterns of lysis expressed by individual microcultures against the panel of F1 and both parental targets were unusual; some patterns were consistent with predictions of classic immunogenetic rules (i.e., lysis of F1 targets plus one/both parental targets), but "anomalous" patterns (i.e., lysis of F1 targets on one/both parental targets exclusively) were also seen. When individual microcultures were tested at two different time points, changes in their lytic patterns were routinely seen. While many clones expressed self-reactive anti-F1 lysis at early time points of in vitro incubation, "self-tolerant" patterns of lysis of exclusively one/both parental targets predominated at late time points of culture (REIMANN and MILLER 1985a). This was the first indication that in the course of clonal T-cell development self-reactive receptor phenotypes may shift towards self-tolerant specificities. Attempts to convert self-reactive lytic patterns expressed by in vitro (under limiting dilution conditions) developing cytotoxic T-cell clones into self-tolerant, self-restricted and antigen-specific receptor phenotypes have failed up to now (J.R., unpublished observation).

3. From splenic T cells of normal mice cultured with autologous/syngeneic splenic filler cells and conditioned medium under limiting dilution conditions, about 1/5000 to 1/10000 T cells will give rise to a self-reactive cytotoxic T-cell clone, the mean lysis value of which is low, and the fine specificity of which is ill-defined. In splenic T-cell populations from syngeneic age-matched germ-free mice, about 1/200 to 1/600 cells will give rise to a self-reactive cytotoxic T-cell clone under identical conditions, the mean lysis value of which is high, and the specificity of which is almost exclusively antiself (Fig. 2). One interpretation of

these results is that an "immature" T-cell system exposed to limited antigenic challenges contains a considerable pool of self-reactive T cells, while the reverse is true for a mature T-cell system, which is constantly challenged by antigenic stimuli.

3.2 Two Experimental Systems Reflecting Late or Mature Stages of Murine T Cells

We have analyzed the specificity repertoire of unprimed murine CLP in a limiting dilution culture system, in which one out of two mitogen-activated murine splenic Lyt-2^+ T-blasts clonally expands in the presence of conditioned medium and syngeneic filler cells into a CTL population (HEEG et al. 1985). The specific lytic reactivity of these cultures tested by split well analysis against a panel of Con A-blast targets indicated the following: (a) about one out of hundered tested CTL clones specifically lysed one of the tested targets; and (b) self-reactive CTL receptor phenotypes were as frequent as self-restricted receptor specificities (Fig. 3). This approach thus gave us high numbers of self-reactive T cells inducible from peripheral T-cell populations.

We observed self-reactive patterns of lysis in the course of primary in vitro induced herpes simplex virus (HSV)-specific self-restricted CTL responses under limiting dilution conditions. LDA of this response revealed 1/1000 to 1/2000 splenic T cells that could be induced to specific lytic reactivity against HSV-infected syngeneic B-blast targets in vitro. When microwells were set up with high responder cell numbers (4000–8000/well) we observed predominantly self-reactive lytic patterns (i.e., infected and uninfected syngeneic blast targets were lysed equally well, infected allogeneic blasts were not lysed). Cultures set up with decreasing numbers of responder cells per well showed an increasing fraction of cultures expressing specific self-restricted lysis (i.e., lysed only the infected syngeneic targets); many CTL populations with a high probability of clonality

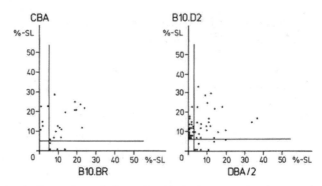

Fig. 3. Self-reactive, self-restricted, alloreactive and allorestricted lytic phenotypes in mitogen-activated splenic T-blasts. Nonfractionated spleen cells from a CBA mouse were activated with Con A as described (HEEG et al. 1985). T-blasts were then seeded at 20 cells/well and cultured for 5 days in the presence of syngeneic peritoneal exudate filler cells, conditioned medium, and recombinant IL2. The cultures were split and read out against the indicated target cells

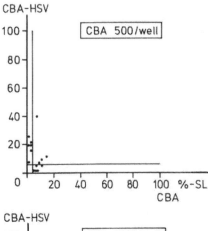

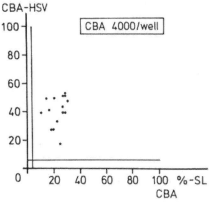

Fig. 4. Self-reactive lytic patterns in the course of primary in vitro HSV-specific self-restricted responses. Nylon-wool nonadherent CBA spleen cells were cultured under LD conditions with herpes simplex virus (HSV)-infected syngeneic splenic stimulator cells. After 7 days, the cultures were split and tested against HSV-infected or noninfected syngeneic B-blast targets. The lytic patterns of individual microcultures seeded at different responder cell concentrations are plotted

(i.e., wells set up with low responder cell numbers [<500/well]) expressed almost exclusively self-restricted lytic patterns (Fig. 4). The manifestation of self-reactivity in the course of a primary immune response in vitro resembles similar observations in EBV-specific HLA-restricted cytolytic responses in the human system (D. Kabelitz, unpublished observations).

3.3 Experimental Systems Indicating Regulatory Influences on Self-reactivity

In two experimental systems we have found evidence that self-reactive CTL populations are subjected to cellular control mechanisms. Both systems were designed according to concepts developed in models of neonatally induced tolerance.

1. We have analyzed primary self-restricted CTL responses under LD conditions in young adult mice injected neonatally with recombinant IL2. It has been reported that the neonatal induction of tolerance can be prevented by the simultaneous injection of IL2 into newborn mice in the first 24 h after birth (MALKOVSKY et al. 1985). We therefore speculated that the establishment of self-tolerance

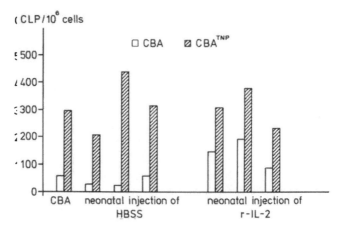

Fig. 5. Neonatal IL2 injection influences the induction of self-tolerance. Newborn CBA mice received a single dose of recombinant IL2 (100000 U) or solvent (HBSS) during the first 24 h after birth. After 6 weeks, splenic T cells from three individual experimental mice and three individual control mice (as well as a noninjected syngeneic control mouse, *CBA*) were cultured under LD conditions with TNP-modified syngeneic stimulator cells for 7 days. Individual cultures were tested by split well analysis against TNP-modified or unmodified syngeneic blast targets. Estimates of the number of CLP/10^6 cells were obtained by LDA

might be partially blocked by neonatal IL2 injection. As compared to their syngeneic litter mates, IL2-injected mice generated more self-reactive CTL clones if cocultured with TNP-modified syngeneic stimulator cells under LD conditions (Fig. 5). This indicated that experimental manipulations known to downregulate tolerance induction can increase the number of self-reactive clones.

2. The model of neonatally induced tolerance to allo MHC antigens is often used to gain insight into the establishment of self-tolerance (STREILEIN 1979). This concept implies that self-reactive CTL clones should be comparable to tolerogen-reactive CTL clones. We studied neonatally induced tolerance in CBA mice (H-2^k) to a class I alloantigen (H-$2D^d$), as a model for self-tolerance.

(a) The splenic tolerogen-inducible CTL pool of neonatally tolerized mice showed a more than 10-fold reduction under LD conditions as compared to spleen cells from nontolerized mice. In contrast, when mitogen-activated splenic T-blasts were clonally expanded under LD conditions in the absence of tolerogen stimulation, the measured frequencies of tolerogen-reactive CTL clones was equal in tolerized and normal mice. This indicated a large pool of tolerogen-reactive CLP in tolerant mice that was not inducible by tolerogen stimulation under LD conditions (HEEG and WAGNER 1985).

(b) The number of tolerogen-reactive CLP that could be induced in a LD system increased significantly when spleen cells from tolerant mice were cultured with stimulator cells bearing allo class II MHC determinants in addition to the tolerogen (Table 1).

(c) Regulatory cells could be absorbed out of a tolerant spleen cell population on monolayers of irradiated antitolerogen-induced MLC blasts from normal nontolerized syngeneic mice. This increased the frequency of tolerogen-induc-

Table 1. A large number of tolerogen-reactive CLP is inducible by stimulator cells bearing allo class II MHC antigens in addition to the tolerogen

Responder	Stimulator cells		
	CBA × A (kkkk × kkkd) D^d	ATL (skkd) $K^s + D^d$	B10.S(7R) (sssd) $K^s + I^s + D^d$
CBA	639[a]	nd	941
CBA_{Tol}[b]	60400	29306	7290

[a] 1/frequency: read out against CBA × A blast targets.
[b] CBA neonatally tolerized to CBA × A cells
nd, not done

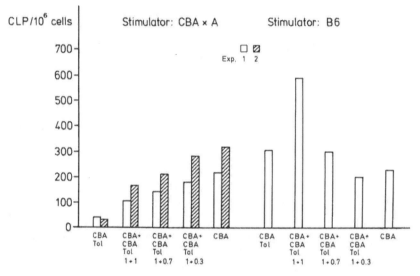

Fig. 6. Cells from tolerant spleen cell populations suppress the induction of tolerogen-reactive CLP in normal nontolerized cell populations. Spleen cells from CBA mice neonatally tolerized to CBA × A (H-$2D^d$) cells were mixed with a constant number of normal nontolerized CBA spleen cells. These mixtures were cultured under LD conditions either with tolerogen-bearing (CBA × A) or third party (B6)-bearing stimulator cells. After 7 days the cultures were tested against the respective blast target cell. The number of CLP/10^6 cells was calculated by LDA

ible CTL clones in tolerant mice 3–6 fold as detected in a tolerogen-stimulated limiting dilution system (STOCKINGER 1984; HEEG and WAGNER 1985).

(d) In some, but not all, tolerized mice a transferable suppressive activity was found. In mixing experiments, cells from these mice decreased the measurable number of tolerogen-inducible T cells of normal nontolerized cell populations while the number of third-party reactive cells was not affected (Fig. 6, HEEG and WAGNER 1985).

Assuming that tolerance induced to allo MHC antigens is a model for self-tolerance, this series of experiments indicated that antitolerogen (antiself) T-cell reactivity is regulated in vivo and in vitro; i.e., self- or tolerogen-reactive T cells do not seem to be clonally deleted during ontogeny.

4 The Physiological Role of Self-reactivity

We have attempted to give a brief outline of the published experimental evidence on self-reactive T cells, and have described our own experimental results. Increasing experimental evidence suggests that activation of self-reactive T cells is obligatory in the initiation of a T-cell mediated response in vivo and in vitro. What are the possible interpretations?

Self-reactive T cells might represent some essential regulatory component in the early immune response. Some experimental systems seem to support this assumption: a clonally expanding inducer T-cell population stimulates clonal expansion of a self-reactive T-cell clone which "helps" in a positive feedback amplification to get the immune response started (see Sect. 2.6). Alternatively, we could assume that the restricted antigen-specific inducer T-cell clone is recruiting self-reactive T cells into the response. If diversification of the T-cell receptor repertoire has its point of origin in anti-MHC reactivity, and if clonal expansion of T cells in vivo is limited, it would be of vital importance to get as many T cells as possible started for this race for a self-restricted receptor specificity which has to lead to a receptor phenotype that reacts with reasonable affinity with the offending antigen. This was the second common theme in the discussion of T-cell mediated self-reactivity: anti-MHC reactivity as the point of origin from which the MHC-restricted repertoire is generated. In this case, repertoire development would always be unidirectional, i.e., away from self-MHC, but it would not explain self-tolerance to non-MHC self constituents. It would furthermore deprive the thymus of its proposed function as restriction specificity-determining site. The experimental data available up to now are not conclusive. But we would consider the generation of self-restricted T-cell receptor phenotypes from self-reactive T-cell receptor phenotypes in the course of a peripheral T-cell response in vivo an attractive alternative interpretation for many of the described self-reactive phenomena.

Acknowledgement. We thank Christiane Steeg, Astrid Bellan, Anja Otterbein, and Claudia Zanker for their excellent technical assistance.

References

Altman A, Katz DH (1980) The induction of autoreactive T lymphocytes by allogeneic effect factor (AEF): relevance to normal pathways of lymphocyte differentiation. Immunol Rev 51:3

Battisto JR, Ponzio NM (1981) Autologous and syngeneic mixed lymphocyte reactions and their immunological significance. Prog Allergy 28:160

272   K. Heeg et al.

Bensusson A, Meuer SC, Schlossman SF, Reinherz EL (1984) Delineation of an immunoregulatory amplifier population recognizing autologous Ia molecules. Analysis with human T cell clones. J Exp Med 159:559

Born W, Weckerle H (1982) Lympho-stromal interactions in the thymus: medullary thymocytes react with I-A determinants on autochthonous thymic stimulator cells. Eur J Immunol 12:51

Burnet MF (1972) Auto-immunity and auto-immune disease. Medical and Technical, Lancaster, UK, p 4

Ching LM, Marbrook J, Walker KZ (1977a) Spontaneous clones of cytotoxic T cells in culture. I. Characteristics of the response. Cell Immunol 31:284

Ching LM, Marbrook J, Walker KZ (1977b) Spontaneous clones of cytotoxic T cells in culture. II. Specificity of the response. Cell Immunol 31:293

Ching LM, Walker KZ, Marbrook J (1977c) Spontaneous clones of cytotoxic T cells in culture. III. Discriminatory lysis of pairs of syngeneic blasts induced by different mitogens. Eur J Immunol 7:850

Ching LM, Walker KZ, Marbrook J (1977d) Clones of cytotoxic lymphocytes in culture: The difference in specificity between stimulated and nonstimulated cytotoxic lymphocytes. Eur J Immunol 7:846

Claësson MH, Miller RG (1985) Functional heterogeneity in allospecific cytotoxic T lymphocyte clones. II. Development of syngeneic cytotoxicity in the absence of specific antigenic stimulation. J Immunol 134:684

Clayberger C, Dekruyff RH, Cantor H (1984) Immunoregulatory activities of autoreactive T-cells: An I-A-specific T cell clone mediates both help and suppression of antibody responses. J Immunol 132:2237

Clayberger C, Dekruyff RH, Cantor H (1985) T cell regulation of antibody responses: an I-A-specific, autoreactive T cell collaborates with antigen-specific helper T cells to promote IgG responses. 134:691

DosReis GA, Shevach EM (1981) The syngeneic mixed leukocyte reaction represents polyclonal activation of antigen-specific T-lymphocytes with receptors for self-Ia antigens. J Immunol 127:2456

Ellis TM, Mokanakumar T (1983) Dissociation of autologous and allogeneic mixed lymphocyte reactivity by using a monoclonal antibody specific for human T helper cells. J Immunol 131:2323

Endres RO, Marrack P, Kappler JW (1983) An IL-2-secreting T cell hybridoma that respond to a self class I histocompatibility antigen in the H-2D region. J Immunol 131:1656

Finnegan A, Needleman B, Hodes RT (1984) Activation of B-cells by autoreactive T cells: cloned autoreactive T cells activate B cells by two distinct pathways. J Immunol 133:78

Folks TM, Sell KW (1984) An autoreactive T hybridoma expressing nonspecific helper acitivity. Cell Immunol 86:183

Gatenby PA, Kotzin BZ, Engleman EG (1981) Induction of immunoglobulin secreting cells in the human autologous mixed leukocyte reaction: regulation by helper and suppressor lymphocyte subsets defined with monoclonal antibodies. J Immunol 127:2130

Glimcher LH, Shevach EM (1982) Production of autoreactive I region restricted T cell hybridomas. J Exp Med 156:640

Glimcher LH, Steinberg AD, House SB, Green I (1980) The autologous mixed lymphocyte reaction in strains of mice with autoimmune disease. J Immunol 125:1832

Glimcher LH, Longo DL, Green I, Schwartz RH (1981) Murine syngeneic mixed lymphocyte response. I. Target antigens are self Ia molecules. J Exp Med 154:1652

Glimcher LH, Schwartz RH, Longo DL, Singer A (1982) The specificity of the syngeneic mixed leukocyte response, a primary anti-I region T-cell proliferative response, is determined intrathymically. J Immunol 129:987

Glimcher LH, Serog B, McKean DJ, Beck BN (1985) Evidence that autoreactive T hybridomas recognize multiple epitopes on the I-Ak molecule. J Immunol 134:1780

Good MF, Boyd AW, Nossal GTV (1983) Analysis of true anti-hapten cytotoxic clones in limiting dilution microcultures after correction for "anti-self" activity: precursor frequencies, Ly-2 and Thy-1 phenotype, specificity, and statistical methods. J Immunol 130:2046

Goto M, Zwaifler NJ (1983) Characterization of the killer cell generated in the autologous mixed leukocyte reaction. J Exp Med 157:1309

Greenberg SJ, Olanow CW, Dawson DV, Crane B, Roses AD (1984) Autologous mixed lymphocyte reaction in patients with myasthenia gravis: correlation with disease activity. J Immunol 132:1229

T-Cell Reactivity to Polymorphic MHC Determinants. II   273

Hausman PB, Raff HV, Gilbert RC, Picker LJ, Stobo JD (1980) T-cells and macrophages involved in the autologous mixed lymphocyte reaction are required for the response to conventional antigen. J Immunol 125:1374

Hausman PB, Stites DB, Stobo JD (1981) Antigen-reactive T-cells can be activated by autologous macrophages in the absence of added antigen. J Exp Med 153:476

Hausman PB, Moody ChE, Innes JB, Gibbons JJ, Wecksler ME (1983) Studies on the syngeneic mixed lymphocyte reaction. III. Development of a monoclonal antibody with high specificity for autoreactive T cells. J Exp Med 158:1307

Hayward AR, Mori M (1984) Human newborn autologous mixed lymphocyte response: Frequency and phenotype of responders and xenoantigen specificity. J Immunol 133:719

Heeg K, Wagner H (1985) Analysis of immunological tolerance to major histocompatibility complex antigens. I. High frequencies of tolerogen-specific cytotoxic T lymphocyte precursors in mice neonatally tolerized to class I major histocompatibility complex antigens. Eur J Immunol 15:25

Heeg K, Zielinski I, Kabelitz D, Wagner H, Reimann J (1985) Anti-MHC-reactive T-cells. II. Clonal specificity analysis of mitogen-activated murine T lymphoblasts. (submitted)

Huber C, Merkenschlager M, Gattringer C, Royston I, Fink V, Braunsteiner H (1982) Human autologous mixed lymphocyte reactivity is primarily specific for xenoprotein determinants absorbed to antigen presenting cells during rosette formation with sheep erythrocytes. J Exp Med 155:1222

James SP, Yenokida GG, Graeff AS, Elson CO, Strober W (1981) Immunoregulatory function of T-cells activated in the autologous mixed lymphocyte reaction. J Immunol 127:2605

Jerne NK (1984) Idiotypic networks and other preconceived ideas. Immunol Rev 79:5

Kagan J, Choi YS (1983) Failure of the human autologous mixed lymphocyte reaction in the absence of foreign antigen. Eur J Immunol 13:1031

Kimoto M, Yoshikubo T, Kishimoto S, Yamamura Y, Kishimoto T (1984) Polyclonal activation of xid B-cells by auto-Ia-reactive T cell clones. J Immunol 132:1663

Lattime EC, Golub SH, Stutman O (1980) Lyt 1 cells respond to Ia bearing macrophages in the murine syngeneic mixed lymphocyte reaction. Eur J Immunol 10:723

Malkovsky M, Medawar PB, Thatcher DR, Toy J, Hunt R, Rayfield LS, Dore C (1985) Acquired immunological tolerance of foreign cells is impaired by recombinant interleukin 2 or vitamin A acetate. Proc Natl Acad Sci USA 82:536

Miller RA, Kaplan HS (1978) Generation of cytotoxic lymphocytes in the autologous mixed lymphocyte culture. J Immunol 212:2165

Nussenzweig MC, Steinman RN (198) Contribution of dendritic cells to stimulation of the murine syngeneic mixed leukocyte reaction. J Exp Med 151:1196

Opelz G, Kiuchi M, Takasugi M, Terasaki PI (1975) Autologous stimulation of human lymphocyte subpopulations. J Exp Med 142:1327

Peck AB, Wigzell H, Janeway C Jr, Andersson LC (1977) Environmental and genetic control of T cell activation in vitro: a study using isolated alloantigen-activated T-cell clones Immunol Rev 35:146

Pfizenmaier K, Trostmann H, Röllinghoff M, Wagner H (1975) Temporary presence of self-reactive cytotoxic T-lymphocytes during murine lymphocytic choriomeningitis. Nature 258:238

Reimann J, Miller RG (1983a) Differentiation from precursors in athymic nude mouse bone marrow of unusual spontaneously cytolytic cells showing anti-self H-2 specificity and bearing T-cell markers. J Exp Med 158:1672

Reimann J, Miller RG (1983b) Generation of autoreactive cytotoxic T lymphocyte under limiting dilution conditions. J Immunol 131:2128

Reimann J, Kabelitz D, Heeg K, Wagner H (1985a) Allorestricted cytotoxic T-cells. Large numbers of allo-H-2Kb-restricted anti-hapten and anti-viral cytotoxic T-cell populations clonally develop in vitro from murine splenic precursor T-cells. J Exp Med 162:592

Rock KL, Benacerraf B (1983) MHC-restricted T cell activation: analysis with T cell hybridomas. Immunol REV 76:29

Rock KL, Benacerraf B (1984a) Thymic T-cells are driven to expand upon interaction with self-class II major histocompatibility complex gene products on accessory cells. Proc Natl Acad Sci USA 81:1221

Rock KL, Benacerraf B (1984b) The role of Ia molecules in the activation of T-lymphocytes. IV. The basis of the thymocyte IL 1 response and its possible role in the generation of the T cell repertoire. J Immunol 132:1654

Smolen JS, Luger TA, Chused TM, Steinberg AD (1981) Responder cells in the human autologous mixed lymphocyte reaction. J Clin Invest 68:1601

Sopori ML, Cohen DA, Cherian S, Roszman TL, Kaplan AM (1984) T-lymphocytes heterogeneity in the rat: separation of distinct rat T-lymphocyte populations which respond in syngeneic and allogeneic mixed lymphocyte reactions. Cell Immunol 87:295

Stockinger B (1984) Cytotoxic T-cell precursors revealed in neonatally tolerant mice. Proc Natl Acad Sci USA 81:220

Stout RD (1984) Inhibition of IL 2 responsiveness of mitogen-stimulated lymphocytes by SMLR-generated plastic adherent suppressor cells. Cell Immunol 85:168

Streilein JW (1979) Neonatal tolerance: Towards a immunogenetic definition of self. Immunol Rev 46:125

Tomonari K (1980) Cytotoxic T cells generated in the autologous mixed lymphocyte reaction. I. Primary autologous mixed lymphocyte reaction. J Immunol 124:1111

Wecksler ME, Kozak RW (1977) Lymphocyte transformation induced by autologous cells. V. Generation of immunologic memory and specificity during the autologous mixed lymphocyte reaction. J Exp Med 146:1833

Wecksler ME, Moody CE, Kozak RW (1981) The autologous mixed lymphocyte reaction. Adv Immunol 31:271

Wolos JA, Smith JB (1982) Helper cells in the autologous mixed lymphocyte reaction. III. Production of helper factor(s) distinct from interleukin 2. J Exp Med 156:1807

Wolos JA, Smith JB (1984) Helper cells in the autologous mixed lymphocyte reaction (AMLR). IV. H-2 restriction and specificity of cytotoxic cells induced by AMLR helper factors. Cell Immunol 87:714

Yamashita U, Shevach EM (1980) The syngeneic mixed leukocyte reaction: the genetic requirements for the recognition of self resembles the requirements for the recognition of antigen in association with self. J Immunol 124:1773

Zanetti M, Altman A, Evans K, Rogers J (1984) Autoreactive rat T-cell lines: establishment and cellular characteristics. Cell Immunol 84:341

Zauderer M, Campbell H, Johnson DR, Seman M (1984) Helper functions of antigen-induced specific and autoreactive T-cell colonies. J Mol Cell Immunol 1:55

Zuberi RI, Altman A (1982) Helper factor production in murine secondary syngeneic mixed leukocyte reactions. J Immunol 128:817

Zuberi RI, Katz DH (1984) Spontaneous proliferation in unfractionated spleen cell culture: autologous mixed lymphocyte reaction (AMLR) which can be differentially regulated by prostaglandins and lymphokines. Cell Immunol 84:299

T-Cell Reactivity to Polymorphic MHC Determinants
III. Alloreactive and Allorestricted T Cells

D. Kabelitz, K. Heeg, H. Wagner, and J. Reimann

1 Current Concepts on Alloreactivity 275
2 The Repertoire of the Unprimed Murine T-Cell Population 277
3 Alloreactive and Allorestricted T-Cell Recognition 279
4 Function and MHC Recognition of T Cells 287
References 288

1 Current Concepts on Alloreactivity

Alloreactive T cells recognize polymorphic nonself MHC determinants that are expressed by different members of the same species. They are detected in specifically stimulated cytotoxic/proliferative responses in vitro (allogeneic mixed leukocyte reaction, allo MLR), and in the graft-versus-host (GvH) or host-versus-graft (HvG) reactions of various transplantation systems in vivo. These primary cell-mediated immune responses are easier to induce and are apparently of a different nature than MHC-restricted T-cell-mediated immune responses to conventional antigens or pathogens. This has always intrigued immunologists (and frustrated transplantation activists). Attempts to explain this preponderance of the T-cell reactivity to allogeneic MHC determinants focused either on a particular "antigenic nature" of MHC-encoded glycoproteins, or assumed a large pool of precursor T cells in normal individuals that specifically recognized allogeneic MHC antigens.

We would like to discuss the phenomenon of T-cell-mediated alloreactivity in the context of three currently proposed interpretations.

1. Alloreactivity represents the allorestricted recognition of allogeneic MHC determinants by T cells.

2. Alloreactivity represents the allorestricted recognition of nonidentified minor histocompatibility antigens by T cells.

3. Alloreactivity results from frequent cross-reactivities of self-MHC-restricted antigen-specific T-cell clones with polymorphic nonself MHC determinants.

The following discussion is an attempt to delineate the genesis and the implications of these three different views on alloreactivity.

T cells might recognize allogeneic MHC determinants in an unrestricted manner (hypothesis 1). T-cell recognition of restricting self-MHC determinants

Institute of Medical Microbiology and Immunology, University of Ulm, D-7900 Ulm

Current Topics in Microbiology and Immunology, Vol. 126
© Springer-Verlag Berlin · Heidelberg 1986

or of allogeneic MHC determinants is allele-specific. If no somatic process instructs the precursor T cell as to which determinants on the alleles of the MHC molecules are shared (monomorphic) and which are allele-specific (polymorphic), these recognition specificities of T cells must be germ-line encoded. There are different versions of this idea (e.g., JERNE 1971; VON BOEHMER et al. 1978; COHN 1983). As a common underlying theme, they conceive alloreactivity and restricted recognition of T cells as the consequence of the phylogenetic and/or ontogenetic path that was followed in generating from a limited pool of germ-line encoded variable region genes, a large repertoire of MHC-restricted receptor specifities in T cells. According to this view, a large pool of T cells with allo-reactive receptor phenotypes would be expected in the unprimed peripheral T-cell pool which would be nonfunctional in a syngeneic environment. In contrast, allorestricted T cells should not be represented in the unprimed peripheral T-cell pool.

Many T-cell clones might recognize undefined nonpolymorphic or (syngeneic/allogeneic) polymorphic minor histocompatibility (H) antigens in an allo-restricted way and thus may seem to constitute an apparently alloreactive T-cell pool (hypothesis 2). This was proposed by proponents of the one-receptor view of T-cell behavior (MATZINGER and BEVAN 1977; MATZINGER 1981). A T-cell repertoire randomly generated during ontogenetic development and/or randomly expanded by somatic diversification would express many allorestricted receptor phenotypes (see paper I, by Reimann et al.). If involvement of MHC determinant recognition is necessary to trigger a functional response in the specific interaction of effector T cells with target cells, only MHC-restricted receptor phenotypes would be detectable by current assay techniques. Following this view, it would be expected that alloreactive T cells are rare and allorestricted minor H-specific T cells are frequent in the peripheral T-cell pool (although technical problems arise in detecting most allorestricted T-cell receptor specificities).

Alloreactivity might result from a particular "immunogenicity" of MHC determinants (hypothesis 3). MHC-encoded molecules are integral membrane glycoproteins (reviewed in STROMINGER 1980). They are antigens because distinct epitopes of these molecules are specifically recognized by T cells and antibodies. „The surface of a protein consists of a complex array of overlapping potential antigenic determinants, in aggregate these approach a continuum" (BENJAMIN et al. 1984). For T cells, the antigenic determinants of autologous/allogeneic MHC molecules are restricted to a limited number of polymorphic epitopes encoded in allelic form within the first and second external domains of MHC genes (HOOD et al. 1983). What is the particular immunogenicity of these few privileged sites on MHC molecules for T cells? "Those [epitopes] to which an individual responds are dictated by the structural differences between the antigen and the host's self-proteins and by host regulatory mechanisms, and are not necessarily an inherent property of the protein molecule reflecting restricted antigenicity or limited antigenic sites" (BENJAMIN et al. 1984). The paradox with MHC molecules is that the polymorphic determinants specifically recognized by T cells are in fact a set of autologous epitopes and its allelic variants. Furthermore, this allele-specific recognition of autologous/allogeneic MHC determinants interferes in a decisive way with the generation of functional phenotypes as well as the receptor repertoire diversity of developing T-cell populations. This indicated a dual role of polymorphic MHC determinants: as antigens that bind to T-cell receptors, and as membrane-associated glycoproteins that mediate an unknown key event in the functional cell-to-cell interaction process. It is questionable if, even in interpretations, these two aspects of T-cell-mediated anti-MHC reactivity should be dissociated.

It has been proposed that alloreactivity results from chance cross-reactions of T cells actually immunized with environmental antigens recognized in the context of self-MHC molecules (PFIZENMAIER et al. 1980; PAUL et al. 1981; KAYE et al. 1984). Alloreactivity would thus represent a low affinity reaction of T-cell receptors with a ligand expressed on the cell surface at high multiplicity. This is supported by the frequently observed cross-reactions of self-restricted antigen-specific T-cell clones with allogeneic MHC determinants. In this view, alloreactive T-cell clones would, of course, be functional in a syngeneic environment. This interpretation gained its main support from the analysis of specific reactivity patterns of cloned T-cell lines. Similar views were proposed earlier in a different experimental system: repeated antigenic stimulation of T cells in vivo resulted in memory T-cell populations that showed specific reactivity to allogeneic MHC determinants (BURAKOFF et al. 1978; FINBERG et al. 1978). This indicated that "alloreactivity reflects a high degree of cross stimulation betwen physiologically relevant antigens associated with self MHC gene products and biologically irrelevant allelic variants of MHC antigens." These interpretations restricted the view of alloreactivity: MHC determinants are neither shaping the repertoire of antigen receptors and functional phenotypes of the T-cell system (hypothesis 1), nor necessarily involved in the transmission of an essential intercellular activation signal (hypothesis 2). They are just considered to be potent immunogens presented at high local concentrations.

It has proved exceedingly difficult to obtain informative experimental data, at either the cellular or the molecular level, to support or exclude any of the hypotheses described above on the nature of alloreactivity.

2 The Repertoire of the Unprimed Murine T-Cell Population

Frequent interactions between cells bearing a certain membrane-associated determinant with cells bearing different membrane receptors for this determinant might indicate either (a) that the determinant "looks" extremely (cross) reactive to many different, clonally distributed receptors, or (b) that many identical/similar receptor specificities with reactivity for the respective determinant are present. Thus, finding a high frequency of alloreactive T cells in unprimed peripheral T-cell populations could indicate either a potent immunogenicity of allogeneic MHC determinants (hypothesis 3), or a high frequency representation of specifically alloreactive T cells (hypothesis 1). The main question therefore is that of demonstrating this exceptionally high frequency of alloreactive T cells in the peripheral unprimed T-cell pool. To approach this question, we have designed a limiting dilution system, in which the repertoire of the splenic cytotoxic T-cell population of young adult mice, raised either under standard-pathogen-free conditions or under germ-free conditions, could be probed (HEEG et al. 1985). The experimental design involved polyclonal induction of splenic T cells (to bypass selective activation requirements of specifically reactive cytotoxic T-lymphocytes [CTL]) and the clonal expansion of the generated T-blasts under limiting dilution conditions (without mitogen, in the presence of growth factor(s) plus filler cells). An exceptionally high cloning efficiency was obtained in this system, as one out of two Lyt-2$^+$ T-blasts gave rise to a cytolytic T-cell clone. The experimental data can thus be considered representative for the murine splenic T-cell pool. As described above, we expected to find a bias of the T-cell repertoire for alloreactive receptor specificities (in support of hypotheses 1 and 3). The data obtained were unexpected as well as incompatible with any of the briefly outlined hypotheses on alloreactivity.

The limiting dilution analysis revealed the following three key findings:

1. The expression of MHC molecules on the cell surface was necessary to enable a functional T-cell recognition. Target cells devoid of MHC determinants on the cell surface were not lysed by any of the hundreds of CTL clones tested. The analyzed T-cell responses were thus reactive to or restricted by MHC determinants.

2. About one out of hundred tested CTL clones specifically lysed a given target cell tested. The T-cell repertoire is thus comprised of at least 10^2 different receptor specificities.

3. There was no bias in the repertoire of unprimed T cells for alloreactive/allorestricted or self-reactive/self-restricted lytic specificities, i.e., every type of MHC-bearing target cell tested had an equal and high chance to be recognized by a CTL clone.

Comparable preliminary data were obtained in the limiting dilution analysis of anti-T3 activated human peripheral blood T-lymphocytes (D. KABELITZ, unpublished).

Unprimed CTL clones thus do not seem to be preferentially reactive to major H antigens, as compared to minor H or conventional antigens, which appears incompatible with any of the currently proposed hypotheses of alloreactivity. We have to consider two alternative interpretations to conceptualize this specificity analysis of T-cell populations. (1) Our limiting dilution system reads out the T-cell receptor diversity as it exists in the unprimed splenic T-cell pool, i.e., as it was generated in an antigen-independent way during the ontogeny of the T-cell system. The unprimed T-cell pool would then contain no bias for self-restricted and alloreactive receptor phenotypes, in contrast to the primed T-cell pool; and it is during the process following immunization that the selective expansion of self-restricted antigen-specific receptor phenotypes would lead to an unequal representation of one type of receptor specificities in the repertoire of primed T-cell populations (although the concomitant appearance of alloreactive receptor phenotypes would remain unexplained). (2) Alternatively, our limiting dilution system might have supported random intraclonal diversification of the receptor repertoire of in vitro developing T-cell populations (REIMANN and MILLER 1985). The absence of an antigen-mediated specific "regulation" of this diversification process under our in vitro conditions would have resulted in the expression of a random sample of a clonal population of diversified receptor specificities, while the bias of the primed T-cell receptor repertoire for self-restricted (and alloreactive) specificities would be introduced into the (more physiological) process of antigen-stimulated T-cell receptor diversification in the syngeneic in vivo environment. To approach this problem, we have focused our interest on a comparative analysis of clonal specificities expressed by mitogen-activated T-lymphoblast populations and by antigen-activated T-lymphoblast populations.

3 Alloreactive and Allorestriced T-Cell Recognition

In the preceding paper (by Heeg et al.) we have presented evidence that self-reactive receptor phenotypes may predominate early in ontogeny as well as early in the course of an antigen-stimulated T-cell response in a syngeneic environment. We have speculated that self-restricted receptor phenotypes may be derived from self-reactive receptor phenotypes. This generated the idea that allorestricted receptor phenotypes might develop from alloreactive receptor phenotypes in the course of a T-cell response in an allogeneic environment. This idea was at the origin of an extensive series of experiments, in which the generation of allorestricted receptor specificities was analyzed under limiting dilution conditions in mitogen-driven and in antigen-stimulated cytotoxic T-cell responses in vitro. Although it remains to be formally demonstrated that allorestricted specificity patterns originate from alloreactive specificities, we have found surprisingly high frequencies of cytotoxic lymphocyte precursors that generate in vitro CTL clones with exquisitely specific allorestricted lytic reactivity.

Previous attempts to demonstrate the existence of allorestricted antigen-specific murine T cells have used the opposite approach, i.e., they have eliminated the respective alloreactive T cells through negative selection procedures in vitro (STOCKINGER et al. 1980, 1981; NAGY et al. 1981), or in vivo (WILSON et al. 1976; DOHERTY and BENNINK 1979), or through neonatal tolerization protocols (VON BOEHMER and HAAS 1976; PFIZENMAIER et al 1976; ZINKERNAGEL 1976) prior to the in vitro induction of T cells with antigen presented on allogeneic accessory cells. The thus generated specific allorestricted T-cell reactivity was usually low, considerably lower than the reactivity towards the respective antigen presented by syngeneic accessory cells. Our approach to study allorestricted T-cell reactivity patterns did not rely on any of these selection procedures. We detected allorestricted reactivity patterns in unselected T-cell populations comprising the full repertoire of alloreactive receptor phenotypes. Data from comparable systems have been published (TEH 1979; GOOD and NOSSAL 1983). Our limiting dilution analysis involved different antigens (hapten, viral determinants, minor histocompatibility antigens) and different allogeneic MHC combinations of human and murine responder T cells/stimulator cells. The experimental data generated up to now are described in the following.

1. Coculture of CBA ($H-2^k$), BALB/c ($H-2^d$), or C57Bl/6 ($H-2^b$) splenic or thymic responder T cells with trinitrophenyl (TNP)-modified allogeneic stimulator cells resulted in high frequencies of CTL clones (1/30–1/300) that lysed the relevant TNP-modified allogeneic target cells (REIMANN et al. 1985a). This

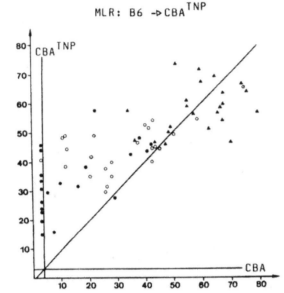

Fig. 1. Allorestricted lytic patterns are generated predominantly when low numbers of responder cells per culture are seeded. Limiting numbers of B6 responder cells were cocultured with TNP-modified CBA stimulator cells. The lytic response was read out at day 8 of incubation against CBA or CBA^{TNP} target cells. There were 500 (▲), 250 (○) and 125.62 (●) splenic responder cells per microculture

was found for all six allogeneic strain combinations tested. The majority of clonally developing CTL populations were specific for the stimulating allogeneic H-2 determinant(s) in that they did not lyse TNP-modified syngeneic or third party allogeneic target cells. The responder cell number plated per microwell critically influenced the cytolytic reactivity patterns. As shown in Fig. 1, allorestricted TNP-specific CTL clones were primarily detected in microcultures set up with low responder cell numbers (which thus had a high probability of clonality), whereas alloreactive cytotoxic patterns predominated in microcultures set up with high responder cell numbers. As TNP might modify surface MHC molecules in such a way as to mimick "neo" MHC antigens (LEVY et al. 1984), we used other antigens for the induction of allorestricted CTL populations. High frequencies of allorestricted virus-specific CTL clones were found when, for example, B6 splenic responder cells were cocultured with herpes simplex virus (HSV)-infected CBA stimulator cells. A representative experiment is shown in Fig. 2, which further illustrates that the appearance of allorestricted lytic patterns in this system was always dependent on the culture period: while alloreactive lytic patterns predominated at day 7 of culture, allorestricted HSV-specific reactivity patterns were more frequent at day 11 of culture. As further evident from Fig. 2, the large majority of cytotoxic lymphocyte precursors that developed into allorestricted CTL clones under our in vitro conditions expressed the Lyt-1$^+$, 2$^+$ surface phenotype. The results obtained with TNP and HSV antigens were not reproducible with minor H antigens. In various combinations tested, we did not observe minor H-specific allorestricted lytic patterns (e.g., B10 stimulated with CBA, read out against CBA and B10.BR; B10 stimulated with BALB/c, read out against BALB/c and B10.D2; Fig. 3). This is in contrast to the

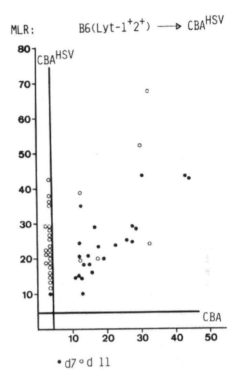

Fig. 2. Allorestricted lytic patterns predominate at late time points of culture. Cell sorter separated Lyt-1$^+$, 2$^+$ splenic responder cells from B6 mice were cocultured under limiting dilution conditions with herpes simplex virus (HSV)-infected CBA stimulator cells. Lytic responses were read out against HSV-infected or noninfected CBA Con A blast target cells at day 7 (●) and at day 11 (○) of in vitro culture

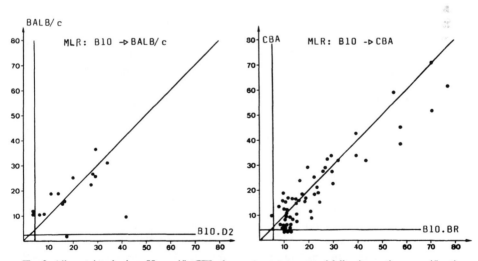

Fig. 3. Allorestricted minor H-specific CTL clones are not generated following antigen-specific stimulation under limiting dilution conditions. Splenic B10 responder cells were cocultured with CBA stimulator cells (*right*) or BALB/c stimulator cells (*left*). The cytolytic response was tested against CBA and B10.BR target cells (*right*) or against BALB/c and B10.D2 target cells (*left*)

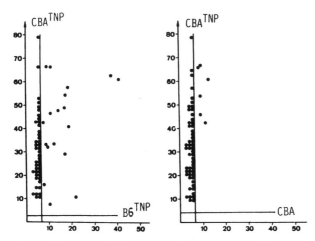

Fig. 4. Allorestricted CTL receptor phenotypes are stabile for extended culture periods. B6 splenic responder cells were cocultured with TNP-modified CBA stimulator cells under limiting dilution conditions. At day 10, individual microcultures were tested for cytolytic activity against CBA, CBA^{TNP}, and syngeneic B6^{TNP} target cells. Cells were cloned by micromanipulation from microcultures displaying allorestricted lytic patterns and cultured for an additional 12 days in the presence of interleukin-2 and CBA^{TNP} stimulator cells. The cytolytic readout was then repeated against CBA, CBA^{TNP}, and B6^{TNP} target cells

mitogen-stimulated (antigen-independent) induction protocol where large numbers of minor H-specific allorestricted CTL clones were detected (Fig. 6). Allorestricted receptor phenotypes were furthermore "spontaneously" generated at low frequency in limiting dilution cultures stimulated with unmodified allogeneic cells (REIMANN et al. 1985a), which led us to speculate that anti-(syngeneic/allogeneic) MHC reactivity may be at the origin, from where (self/allo)-restricted T-cell receptor phenotypes develop. The specificity pattern of allorestricted CTL clones generated in limiting dilution cultures was maintained for extended periods of time as shown by single cell cloning experiments (Fig. 4). B6 splenic responder cells were cocultured under limiting dilution conditions with TNP-modified CBA stimulator cells. At day 10, individual microcultures were read out against CBA, CBA^{TNP} and syngeneic B6^{TNP} targets. Cells were cloned by micromanipulation from microcultures displaying allorestricted lytic patterns (i.e., that lysed CBA^{TNP} targets exclusively) and cultured for additional 12–14 days in the presence of CBA^{TNP} stimulator cells and conditioned medium. The repeated cytolytic readout demonstrated that the vast majority of cloned CTL populations retained their TNP-specific allorestricted receptor phenotype over a 20 day in vitro culture period (Fig. 4). We have been unable to induce allorestricted CTL clones using lymph node cells as responder cells, whereas self-restricted TNP-specific CTL clones were readily induced in high frequency (1/100–1/200) from such lymph node cells (J. Reimann, unpublished).

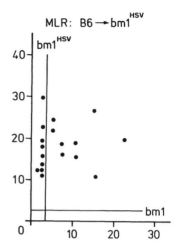

Fig. 5. Allogeneic H-2K molecules are restriction elements for allorestricted HSV-specific CTL clones. B6 (H-2K^b) splenic responder cells were cocultured with HSV-infected bm1 (H-2K^{bm1}) stimulator cells under limiting dilution conditions. The lytic response was read out against HSV-infected and noninfected bm1 target cells

2. Normal C57Bl/6 (B6) (H-2^b) responder cells were cocultured with HSV-infected mutant bm1 (H-2K^{bm1}) stimulator cells (and vice versa). The estimated frequencies of CTL clones that lysed HSV-infected bm1 targets ranged from 1/70 to 1/300 (REIMANN et al. 1985b). The estimated frequencies of CTL clones that lysed the respective noninfected allogeneic (bm1) targets, were 3–5 fold lower. The specificity of the lytic response was assessed by split well analysis using allogeneic bm1 targets, either HSV-infected or noninfected, and HSV-infected syngeneic B6 targets. As shown in Fig. 5, allorestricted HSV-specific cytolytic patterns were clearly discernible. Similar results were obtained using the hapten TNP as antigen (REIMANN et al. 1985b). This system allowed us to define the restricting element as a mutant allogeneic H-2K^b molecule.

3. We have employed limiting dilution analyses to quantitate the frequencies of alloreactive and allorestricted CLP in populations of mitogen-activated T-blasts (HEEG et al. 1985). Two key observations were made: (a) allorestricted antigen-specific lytic patterns could be clearly distinguished from the equally frequent alloreactive lytic patterns (frequencies 1/50–1/200); and (b) allorestricted lytic patterns were only seen with low numbers of responder cells seeded per well while at high responder cell numbers per well alloreactive lytic patterns predominated (als already observed in the antigen-specific induction protocol). When the lytic response of cultures set up with low numbers of responder T-blasts was read out against TNP-modified and nonmodified allogeneic targets, about half of the positive cultures displayed an allorestricted lytic pattern in the combination H-2^b anti-H-2^k-TNP, about 65% in the combination H-2^k anti-H-2^b-TNP, and roughly 25% in the combination H-2^k anti-H-2^d-TNP. Even more striking was the allorestricted H-Y-specific readout: about 40% of the microcultures with female CBA responder cells lysed only allogeneic male BALB/c targets, but not female BALB/c targets (Fig. 6a). In another minor H system, CBA T-blasts (H-2^k) were assayed against DBA/2 (H-2^d) and B10.D2 (H-2^d) targets, and three lytic patterns were observed; almost half of the positive cultures lysed

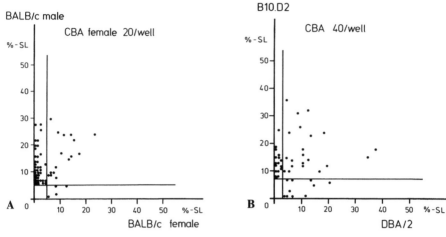

Fig 6A, B. Allorestricted lytic reactivity is generated in CTL populations developing from mitogen-activated T-cell blasts. T-blasts of the indicated mouse strain were seeded at 20 or 40 cells/well. After 5 days, individual microcultures were split and tested for cytolytic activity against the indicated target cells. **A** Responder: female CBA (20/well); targets: male BALB/c or female BALB/c. **B** Responder: CBA (H-2^k) (40/well); targets: DBA/2 (H-2^d) or B10.D2 (H-2^d)

both targets equally well (alloreactive pattern), about 35% lysed only DBA/2 but not B10.D2 targets, while about 20% of positive cultures lysed only B10.D2 but not DBA/2 targets (allorestricted minor H-specific patterns) (Fig. 6b). The frequencies calculated for minor H-specific allorestricted CTL clones were again in the range of 1/40 to 1/80 (HEEG et al. 1985).

4. In preliminary experiments (K. Heeg, unpublished), we have been able to generate allorestricted HSV-specific CTL in vivo. Lethally irradiated CBA (H-2^k) mice were infected with HSV and reconstituted 24 h later with B10 (H-2^b) thymocytes. Spleen cells were taken from these mice after additional 4 days and cultured under limiting dilution conditions with B10 peritoneal exudate filler cells. These splenic T cells gave rise in high frequencies (1/400–1/800) to allo(H-2^k)restricted HSV-specific CTL clones (Fig. 7).

5. Peripheral blood human T cells were cocultured with allogeneic Epstein-Barr virus (EBV)-transformed lymphoblastoid cell lines (LCL) in a modified limiting dilution culture system (KABELITZ et al. 1985a). The estimated frequencies of CTL clones that lysed the stimulating allogeneic LCL target ranged from 1/70 to 1/200, while frequencies of CTL clones that lysed the respective non-transformed Con A blast target were 3–40 fold lower (KABELITZ et al. 1985b). This discrepancy was not due to differences in susceptibility to lysis between LCL and Con A blast targets, as Con A blast targets were efficiently lysed by allo-LCL-stimulated CTL clones in a lectin-facilitated readout that bypassed antigen-specific CTL/target recognition (Fig. 8). The calculated frequencies of CTL clones generated in allo-LCL-stimulated limiting dilution cultures that lysed HLA-mismatched third party LCL or responder-derived autologous LCL targets were again 3–10 fold lower than those measured against the stimulating

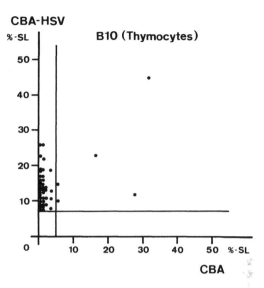

Fig. 7. Allorestricted HSV-specific CTL are generated in vivo. CBA mice were lethally irradiated and subsequently infected with HSV. After 24 h, the mice were reconstituted with 10^8 B10 thymocytes. The mice were killed 4 days later, and splenocytes were cultured under limiting dilution conditions together with B10 peritoneal exudate filler cells. After 6 days, the cultures were split and tested for cytotoxic reactivity against HSV-infected or noninfected CBA target cells. Specific lysis values of individual microcultures are plotted

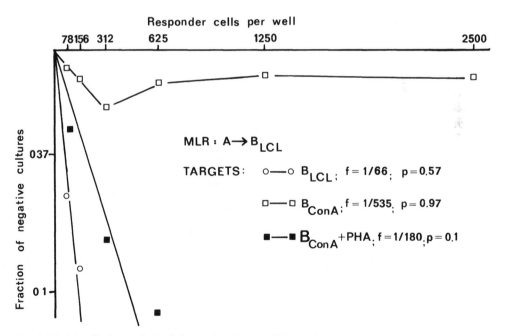

Fig. 8. Limiting dilution analysis of allorestricted human CTL. T cells from donor A were cocultured with irradiated cells from an allogeneic EBV-transformed lymphoblastoid cell line (B_{LCL}) under modified LD conditions. Individual wells were split and tested for cytolytic activity against the stimulating LCL target (B_{LCL}; O–O) as well as against Con A blast targets derived from the allogeneic LCL cell donor in the absence (□–□) or presence (■–■) of PHA. The logarithm of the fraction of negative cultures is plotted against the number of responder cells per well. The CTL precursor frequency against Con A blast target cells was calculated from the linear part of the curve

Table 1. A large fraction of peripheral blood T cells is induced to clonal development by stimulation with allogeneic EBV-transformed lymphoblastoid cell lines (LCL)

MLR[a]			Estimated CTL precursor frequency		
Responder	Stimulator	Target	Expt 1	Expt 2	Expt 3
A	B_{LCL}	B_{LCL}	1/66	1/71	1/203
		C_{LCL}	1/405	1/222	nd[b]
		A_{LCL}	nd	nd	1/560

[a] E-rosette purified T cells were cocultured under modified limiting dilution conditions with irradiated allogeneic LCL stimulator cells in the presence of interleukin-2. After 10–12 days, individual microcultures were split into 2–3 aliquots and tested against various LCL target cells as indicated. A, B, C refer to HLA-mismatched individuals.
[b] nd = not done

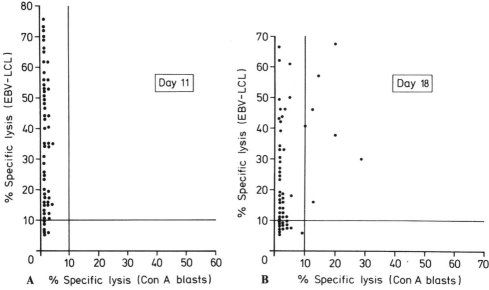

Fig. 9A, B. Allorestricted human CTL receptor phenotypes are stabile upon restimulation. Responder T-cells (78 to 312 per well) were cocultured with allogeneic LCL stimulator cells. At day 11, all microcultures were split and tested for cytolytic activity against the stimulating LCL and the respective Con A blasts. **A** Individual microcultures showing allorestricted cytolytic patterns were selected and restimulated in the presence of interleukin-2. **B** The cytolytic readout was then repeated after 7 days against the same target cells

allogenic LCL (Table 1). A detailed split well analysis indicated that a large fraction of CTL clones induced in this system showed exquisitely specific allorestricted reactivity to LCL membrane antigens (KABELITZ et al. 1985b). As shown for murine allorestricted TNP-specific CTL clones, LCL-specific allorestricted human CTL clones also maintained their specific pattern of lysis for prolonged culture periods. Individual microcultures selected at day 11 for allorestricted lytic reactivity were restimulated for additional 7 days in the presence of interleukin-2. The repeated lytic readout at day 18 of culture showed that the majority of microcultures had retained their allorestricted lytic pattern (Fig. 9).

Our results obtained in various experimental systems using both human and murine primary CTL clones thus indicated that allorestricted T-cell recognition can be induced in unselected mature T-cell populations.

4 Function and MHC Recognition of T Cells

Allogeneic MHC molecules might "function" (by an unknown mechanism) in a way similar or identical to that of autologous MHC molecules that are involved in physiological lymphocyte interactions. This was originally proposed by D. Katz in working on the "allogeneic effect" (reviewed in KATZ 1977). Phenomenologically, the allogeneic effect is indistinguishable from the autologous effect, suggesting that parallel mechanisms underlie the allogeneic interactions he observed in vivo and the physiological regulatory phenomena occurring in syngeneic lymphocyte populations. He concluded: „It is conceivable that the allogeneic effect is a true reflection of the basic regulatory mechanisms controlling the immune system, in the sense that a form of autoreactivity may underlie many (or all) of the cellular interactions concerned with such regulation" (p. 528). We have discussed this idea in the context of self-reactivity and alloreactivity. A major difference lies in the fact that we have described the problem of self-reactivity and alloreactivity exclusively under the aspect of T-cell repertoire development, while D. Katz views it exclusively under the aspect "MHC mediated functional regulatory control mechanism(s)". We have to search for a way to bridge the gap in our understanding of the influence of MHC molecules on the expression of a particular functional phenotype by a T-cell population, and the role of MHC molecules in directing the diversification of recognition specificities of T-cell receptors.

We have described a comparative clonal specificity analysis of primary self- and allorestricted cytotoxic T-cell responses under limiting dilution conditions in vitro, either specifically induced by different antigenic stimulations or polyclonally induced by mitogen activation. The observed lytic patterns were compared between the two alternative systems, between microwells containing CTL populations with a high probability of monoclonality, and between wells containing CTL populations of multiclonal origin. From this type of analysis the following picture emerged: In the antigen-driven limiting dilution system, self-restricted lytic patterns were almost exclusively found in monoclonal CTL populations, while polyclonal CTL populations displayed self-restricted and self-reactive lytic patterns (Fig. 4 in paper II, by Heeg et al., this volume). In the mitogen-driven limiting dilution system, equal numbers of self-restricted and self-reactive lytic patterns were found in monoclonal CTL populations (generated from the unprimed murine splenic T-cell pool), while self-reactive lytic patterns were notably absent in polyclonal CTL populations (HEEG et al. 1985). In the antigen-driven limiting dilution system, allorestricted lytic patterns were frequently expres-

288   D. Kabelitz et al.

sed by monoclonal CTL populations, while polyclonal CTL populations were exclusively alloreactive (see Fig. 1). Experimental data generated in the mitogen-driven limiting system were similar; almost equal numbers of allorestricted and alloreactive lytic patterns were found in monoclonal CTL populations, while exclusively alloreactive patterns were seen with polyclonal CTL populations.

In the attempt to interpret these data along the lines proposed above, we would have to distinguish between the generation of anti-MHC reactivity (i.e., the recruitment of T cells into the response), and the development of restricted T-cell receptor phenotypes out of these recruited anti-MHC-reactive T-cell receptor phenotypes. In antigen-driven CTL responses, this transition from self-reactive to self-restricted receptor phenotypes is rapid and not detectable by current assay techniques under monoclonal conditions, but becomes manifest in mitogen-driven CTL responses (which are not subjected to antigen-driven selection). Self-reactivity becomes apparent in antigen-stimulated polyclonal responses, in which many CTL are recruited into "self-reactivity." Some "safety mechanism" prevents excessive accumulation of self-reactive CTL under polyclonal conditions, as is evident from the mitogen-driven limiting dilution system in which self-reactive CTL are not detectable under polyclonal conditions. Under antigen-driven monoclonal conditions, this repertoire development functions "normally" for alloreactive $\rightarrow$ allorestricted CTL populations. But under polyclonal antigen- or mitogen-driven conditions, alloreactive T cells accumulate, as they are not able to further develop into the respective allorestricted T cells. Hence, this presumably MHC allele-specific regulation of recruitment and of intraclonal generation of restricted recognition displays different phenomenologies in syngeneic and allogeneic environments. This might possibly offer a chance to understand some aspects of autoreactivity and alloreactivity.

Acknowledgements. The expert technical assistance of Astrid Bellan, Anja Otterbein, Christiane Steeg and Claudia Zanker is gratefully acknowledged.

References

Benjamin DC, Berzofsky JA, East IJ, Gurd FRN, Hannum C, Leach SJ, Margoliash E, Michael JG, Miller A, Prager EM, Reichlin M, Sercarz EE, Smith JS, Todd PE, Wilson AC (1984) The antigenic structure of proteins: a reappraisal. Ann Rev Immunol 2:67

Burakoff SJ, Finberg R, Glimcher L, Lemonnier F, Benacerraf B, Cantor H (1978) The biological significance of alloreactivity. The ontogeny of T-cell sets specific for alloantigens or modified self antigens. J Exp Med 148:1414

Cohn M (1983) The T-cell receptor mediating restrictive recognition of antigen. Cell 33:657

Doherty PC, Bennink JR (1979) Vaccinia-specific cytotoxic T-cell responses in the context of H-2 antigens not encountered in thymus may reflect aberrant recognition of a virus-H-2 complex. J Exp Med 149:150

Finberg R, Burakoff SJ, Cantor H, Benacerraf B (1978) Biological significance of alloreactivity: T cells stimulated by Sendai virus-coated syngeneic cells specifically lyse allogeneic target cells. Proc Natl Acad Sci USA 75:5145

Good MF, Nossal GJV (1983) Clones of cytotoxic T-lymphocytes reactive to haptenated allogeneic cells: precursor frequency and characteristics as determined by split culture approach. Proc Natl Acad Sci USA 80:1693

Heeg K, Zielinski I, Kabelitz D, Wagner H, Reimann J (1985) Anti-MHC reactive T-cells. II. Clonal specificity of mitogen activated cytotoxic T-lymphoblasts. (submitted)

Hood L, Steinmetz M, Malissen B (1983) Genes of the major histocompatibility complex of the mouse. Ann Rev Immunol 1:529

Jerne NK (1971) The somatic generation of immune recognition. Eur J Immunol 1:1

Kabelitz D, Herzog WR, Zanker B, Wagner H (1985a) Human cytotoxic T-lymphocytes. I. Limiting dilution analysis of alloreactive cytotoxic T-lymphocyte precursor frequencies. Scand J Immunol 22:329

Kabelitz D, Reimann J, Herzog WR, Heeg K, Wagner H (1985b) Allorestricted cytotoxic T-cells. Large numbers of human peripheral blood precursor T-cells clonally develop into allorestricted antiviral cytotoxic T-cell populations in vitro. (submitted)

Katz DH (1977) Lymphocyte differentiation, recognition, and regulation. Academic, New York

Kaye J, Jones B, Janeway CA (1984) The structure and function of T cell receptor complexes. Immunol Rev 81:39

Levy RB, Dower SK, Shearer GM, Segal DM (1984) Trinitrophenyl modification of H-2k and H-2b spleen cells results in enhanced serological detection of K^k-like determinants. J Exp Med 159:1464

Matzinger P (1981) A one-receptor view of T-cell behavior. Nature 292:497

Matzinger P, Bevan MJ (1977) Hypothesis. Why do so many lymphocytes respond to major histocompatibility antigens? Cell Immunol 29:1

Nagy ZA, Baxevanis CN, Ishii N, Klein J (1981) Ia antigens as restriction molecules in Ir-gene controlled T-cell proliferation. Immunol Rev 60:59

Paul WE, Sredni B, Schwartz RH (1981) Long-term growth and cloning of non-transformed lymphocytes. Nature 294:697

Pfizenmaier K, Starzinski-Powitz A, Rodt H, Röllinghoff M, Wagner H (1976) Virus and trinitrophenyl hapten-specific T-cell-mediated cytotoxicity against H-2 incompatible target cells. J Exp Med 143:999

Pfizenmaier K, Stockinger H, Röllinghoff M, Wagner H (1980) Herpes simplex virus specific $H-2D^k$ restricted T lymphocytes bear receptors for $H-2D^d$ alloantigen. Immunogenetics 11:169

Reimann J, Miller RG (1985) Rapid changes in specificity within single clones of cytolytic effector cells. Cell 40:571

Reimann J, Heeg K, Miller RG, Wagner H (1985a) Alloreactive T-cells. I. Alloreactive and allorestricted cytotoxic T-cells. Eur J Immunol 15:387

Reimann J, Kabelitz D, Heeg K, Wagner H (1985b) Allorestricted cytotoxic T-cells. Large numbers of allo-$H-2K^b$-restricted anti-hapten and anti-viral cytotoxic T-cell populations clonally develop in vitro from murine splenic precursor T-cells. J Exp Med 162:592

Stockinger H, Pfizenmaier K, Hardt C, Röllinghoff M, Wagner H (1980) H-2 restriction as a consequence of intentional priming: T-cells of fully allogeneic chimeric mice as well as normal mice respond to foreign antigens in the context of H-2 determinants not encountered on thymic epithelial cells. Proc Natl Acad Sci USA 77:7390

Stockinger H, Bartlett R, Pfizenmaier K, Röllinghoff M, Wagner H (1981) H-2 restriction as a consequence of intentional priming. Frequency analysis of alloantigen-restricted, trinitrophenyl-specific cytotoxic T lymphocyte precursors within thymocytes of normal mice. J Exp Med 153:1629

Strominger JL (1980) Structure of products of the major histocompatibility complex in man and mouse. In: Fougereau M, Dausset J (eds) Progress in Immunology IV. Academic, New York, p 541

Teh HS (1979) Frequency estimates of cytotoxic precursors to trinitrophenyl-modified alloantigens and determination of the degree of crossreactivity between allodeterminants and trinitrophenyl-modified self determinants. Immunogenetics 8:99

von Boehmer H, Haas W (1976) Cytotoxic T lymphocytes recognize allogeneic tolerated TNP-conjugated cells. Nature 261:141

von Boehmer H, Haas W, Jerne NK (1978) Major histocompatibility complex-linked immune responsiveness is acquired by lymphocytes of low responder mice differentiating in the thymus of high responder mice. Proc Natl Acad Sci USA 75:2439

Wilson DB, Fischer-Lindahl K, Wilson DH, Sprent J (1976) The generation of killer cells to trinitrophenyl-modified allogeneic targets by lymphocyte populations negatively selected to strong alloantigens. J Exp Med 146:361

Zinkernagel RM (1976) H-2 restriction of virus-specific cytotoxicity across the H-2 barrier. Separate effector T-cell specificities are associated with self-H-2 and with the tolerated allogeneic H-2 in chimeras. J Exp Med 144:933

Appearance of New Specificities in Lectin-Induced T-Cell Clones Obtained from Limiting Dilution T-Cell Cultures*

P. Benveniste and R.G. Miller

1 Introduction 291

2 Material and Methods 292

3 Results 293
3.1 Con A Induced Cultures Seeded at Limiting Dilution Can Lyse More Than One Target Cell by Day 9 293
3.2 Cold Target Inhibition Analysis of Day 9 Cultures 294
3.3 Cold Target Inhibition Analysis of Day 9 Cultures in the Presence of Con A 296

4 Discussion 297

References 298

1 Introduction

Clones of cytotoxic T lymphocytes (CTL), from either short term, limiting dilution cultures or long term lines, have been widely used to study the T-cell specificity repertoire. These studies have been largely premised on the assumptions that all the CTL within a clone have the same specificity, that this specificity is stable in time, and that the CTL developed from a precursor which was already committed to the specificity expressed by the CTL in the clone. All three of these assumptions have been brought into question by recent reports (Brooks 1983; Brooks et al. 1982, 1983; Claesson and Miller 1984, 1985; Shortman et al. 1983, 1984; Reimann and Miller 1985; Teh et al. 1982; Wilson and Shortman 1984).

Many long term CTL lines can, when cultured with appropriate growth factors, develop an NK-like lytic capacity (Brooks 1983; Brooks et al. 1982). Some long term CTL lines, when cultured without their appropriate stimulator cells, can develop an additional lytic activity specific for self MHC (Claesson and Miller 1985). In both instances, the specificity of the CTL lines has changed. These types of specificity changes can be classified as "late" changes in the sense that they occur within an established population of apparently mature cells that can be clearly demonstrated as being CTL on the basis of both cell surface markers and function. However, it can also be argued that CTL lines are not cell lines in the usual sense but instead represent a continuously differentiating cell popula-

---

Ontario Cancer Institute and Department of Immunology, University of Toronto, 500 Sherbourne St., Toronto, Ontario M4X 1K9, Canada
* Supported by MRC of Canada (MT-3017) and the National Cancer Institute of Canada

tion whose specificity is maintained only in the presence of the appropriate factors and cells (CLAESSON and MILLER 1984, 1985).

Specificity changes can also be seen in short term limiting dilution cultures. Shortman and colleagues (SHORTMAN et al. 1983, 84) have made extensive studies of "specificity degradation" to an NK-like phenotype in lectin-activated short term limiting dilution cultures. At early culture times specific cytolytic effector cells can be identified, but at late times only nonspecific NK-like effector cells having the morphology of large granular lymphocytes can be seen. REIMANN and MILLER (1985) have also showed specificity changes in short term limiting dilution microcultures, but used specific stimulator cells rather than lectin to initiate the response. They found "early" changes within a developing clone of CTL: when limiting dilution microcultures are tested at different times after culture initiation for their ability to lyse different members of an appropriate panel of target cells, specificity changes are seen within a single clone. Some possible patterns of lysis are seen at all culture times (favored) whereas others are seen only early (unfavored), with the clone switching to a favored lytic pattern at later times. The effector cells appear to be highly specific CTL. However, when maintained for an even longer period of time, some cultures could change to an NK-like lytic phenotype similar to that reported by SHORTMAN et al. (1983, 1984), and the cells would acquire the morphology of large granular lymphocytes (REIMANN and MILLER unpublished). The above results suggest that in the lectin-driven system of SHORTMAN et al. (1983, 1984), it might be possible that the developing clones of effector cells display multiple specificities before becoming nonspecific. In the study reported here, we have used a lectin-driven limiting dilution culture system similar to that of SHORTMAN et al. (1983), and present evidence that single clones of effector cells at late times contain more than one specificity.

2 Material and Methods

Strains of Mice. C3H/HeJ (H-2^k), DBA/2J (H-2^d) and C57BL/10J (H-2^b) mice were purchased from Jackson Laboratories. Mice were used at 8–12 weeks of age.

Factors. Mouse Con A supernatant (SN), rat Con A SN: 5×10^6 spleen cells/ml were incubated for 48 h in culture medium containing 5 μg/ml Con A. Supernatants were harvested and used at concentrations previously found to be optimal for CTL induction. EL4-PMA: Murine EL4 thymona cells (10^6/ml) were incubated for 48 h with 10 ng/ml phorbol myristyl acetate (PMA) as described previously (REIMANN and MILLER 1985). 2MLR SN: Supernatants of 2° MLR were obtained as previously described (CLAESSON and MILLER 1984).

Culture Conditions. Spleen cells, 50–300 cells/microwell (60 replicates/cell concentration) were cultured in flat bottom plates (Nunclon). Each well also contained 0.4 μg/well of Con A, 0.5×10^6 irradiated (1500 rads) syngeneic feeder cells, and an optimal concentration of one of four factors – Con A mouse SN (25%), rat Con A SN (10%), EL4-PMA (6%), or 2MLR SN (25%) – in a final volume of 0.2 ml of αMEM medium supplemented with 10% FCS, 2ME, and

Appearance of New Specificities in Lectin-Induced T-Cell Clones 293

Hepes buffer. Cultures were incubated at 37°C for either 6 or 9 days in a humidified atmosphere of 5% CO_2 in air.

Cytotoxicity Assay. Day 2 Con A blasts from either C57BL/10 (H-2^b) or DBA/2 (H-2^d) spleen cells were labelled with ^{51}Cr for 2 h and washed 3 times in medium containing α-methyl-D-mannoside as described previously (REIMANN and MILLER 1985). Cultures were then split into two equal aliquots which were tested for their ability to lyse DBA/2 or C57BL/10 target cells in a 4-h ^{51}Cr release assay. Cultures were scored positive if ^{51}Cr release was superior to two standard deviations above spontaneous release.

Cold Target Inhibition Experiments. Identical trays, at least 6 trays per experiment, each tray containing 60 cultures seeded with 50 cells per culture were all split into four aliquots on day 9. Unlabelled and labelled target cells were added in ratios of 30:1, 20:1, or 10:1 cold H-2^b or H-2^d to hot H-2^d or H-2^b and vice versa. Hot targets (1000/well) were added 20–30 min after addition of cold targets. After 4 h incubation, 0.1 ml was removed from each culture and counted on a gamma counter. Analysis was restricted to cultures lysing both targets. Percent inhibition was calculated as 100 − (mean % lysis of double positives in the presence of cold target × 100/mean % lysis of double positives in the absence of cold target).

3 Results

3.1 Con A Induced Cultures Seeded at Limiting Dilution Can Lyse More Than One Target Cell by Day 9

C3H (H-2^k) spleen cells were cultured at concentrations ranging from 50 to 300 cells per microwell, 60 replicates per cell concentration, in the presence of an optimal concentration of one of four different factors: mouse and rat Con A SN, EL4-PMA SN, or 2°MLR SN. All cultures also included 5×10^5 irradiated syngeneic spleen cells (C3H) and Con A (0.4 μg/well). After 6 and 9 days of incubation, two equal aliquots were removed from each culture and assayed for cytotoxic activity against two different allogeneic target cells (day 2 Con A blasts) derived from C57BL/10 (H-2^b) and DBA/2 (H-2^d), in a 4-h ^{51}Cr release assay. Limiting dilution theory was used to calculate the frequencies of the lectin-induced cytotoxic effector cells and a detailed analysis was made of the patterns of lysis in those groups of cultures seeded well below (at least four fold) limiting dilution concentration of one precursor cell per well.

On day 6, some cultures could lyse H-2^b targets and others could lyse H-2^d targets. For each target, the fraction of positive cultures as a function of the number of cells per culture fit one hit limiting dilution theory for all four factors tested. The fraction of cultures lysing one target which could also lyse the other (i.e., the fraction of double positives) was consistent with independent precursors of each specificity happening to be in the same well by chance alone as assessed by χ^2 analysis. Table 1 gives results of a representative experiment.

By day 9, the situation was different. Some cultures could still lyse H-2^b targets and other could lyse H-2^d targets. Again, for each target, the fraction of po-

Table 1. Frequencies of alloreactive effector cells at day 6 of culture in the presence of four different factors

	Precursor frequency		
	H-2^d	H-2^b	χ^2 (Double positives)
Mouse Con A SN (25%)	1/555	1/159	2.32
Rat Con A SN (10%)	1/735	1/643	1.02
EL4-PMA (6%)	1/827	1/486	0
2 MLR SN (25%)	1/1187	1/1123	0.25

C3H spleen cells were cultured at concentrations ranging from 50 to 300 cells/culture in the presence of 5×10^5 irradiated syngeneic feeder cells, 0.4 μg/well Con A, and different factors as indicated for 6 days. Cultures were then split and assayed against both H-2^b and H-2^d day 2 Con A blast in a 4-h ^{51}Cr release assay.
Entries are precursor frequencies calculated according to the limiting dilution analysis of PORTER and BERRY (1963). χ^2 analysis of wells lysing both targets is consistent with a precursor of each specificity being independently present in the double positive wells

Table 2. Frequencies of alloreactive effector cells at day 9 of culture in the presence of four different factors

	Precursor frequency		
	H-2^d	H-2^b	χ^2 (Double positives)
Mouse Con A SN (25%)	1/202	1/240	3
Rat Con A SN (10%)	1/331	1/297	8.96
EL4-PMA (6%)	1/138	1/150	6.13
2 MLR SN (25%)	1/550	1/525	0.07

Cultures were performed as in Table 1. Assay was on day 9. χ^2 analysis of wells lysing both targets suggests that a single precursor can give rise to effector cells lysing both targets

sitive cultures as a function of the number of cells per culture fit one hit limiting dilution theory for all four factors tested, the only difference being that the frequencies were two- to three fold higher. However, the fraction of cultures lysing one target which could also lyse the other was very much increased to the point ($\chi^2 > 3$), where it was no longer consistent with independent precursors of each specificity happening to be by chance alone in the same well. Table 2 gives results of a representative experiment.

3.2 Cold Target Inhibition Analysis of Day 9 Cultures

The high frequency of double positive cultures observed on day 9 coupled with the observation that good fits to one hit limiting dilution theory were still obtained implied that either the effector cells had become nonspecific, or that new

Appearance of New Specificities in Lectin-Induced T-Cell Clones 295

Table 3. Frequencies of double positive cultures obtained at day 9

H-2^d	H-2^b	H-2^d+H-2^b
1/331	1/297	1/372
1/98	1/93	1/111
1/193	1/129	1/212
1/230	1/109	1/230
1/616	1/411	1/579
1/142	1/157	1/193
1/342	1/215	1/446
1/320	1/267	1/492

C3H spleen cells were cultured for 9 days with irradiated syngeneic feeder cells, Con A, and rat Con A SN as above, split and assayed against H-2^b and H-2^d target cells. A limiting dilution fit was obtained for each target and for the cultures lysing both targets

specificities were developing as the clone expanded. Since the highest frequency of double positives was found using the rat Con A SN (Table 2), cultures grown using this factor were selected for further analysis. Table 3 lists results from 8 independent experiments. It is clear that most cultures are double positives. In order to assess the specificity of the effector cells in these cultures, cold target inhibition experiments were performed.

In all experiments, a complete limiting dilution curve was measured for each target and those groups of cultures seeded at least four fold below the limiting dilution concentration of one precursor per well were assayed by cold target inhibition. There is thus a high probability that the cultures analysed were mounting a clonal response. If the effector cells by day 9 are no longer specific, then one would expect the lysis of a given labelled target to be equally well inhibited either by identical unlabelled targets or by unrelated unlabelled targets. Conversely, if the clones contain specific effector cells of several different specificities then unlabelled targets identical to the labelled target cells should be the most effective competitors.

A minimum of 60 cultures containing 50 responder cells/well were set up as above, incubated 9 days, and split into 4 equal aliquots. These were tested against labelled target A (e.g., DBA/2, H-2^d), labelled target A plus unlabelled target A, labelled target A plus unlabelled target B (e.g., C57BL10, H-2^b), and labelled target B. A second group of 60 cultures or more was tested against labelled B, labelled B plus unlabelled B, labelled B plus unlabelled A, and labelled A. Both groups were measured at cold to hot target ratios of 10 to 1, 20 to 1, and 30 to 1. Thus a single experiment involved analysis of a minimun of 360 cultures split into four groups. All cultures included 25 mM α-methyl-D-mannoside (αMM) to block any residual Con A remaining in the cultures. Figure 1 shows results of one such experiment. Although both cold targets provided competition, the cold target identical to the hot target was usually a statistically significantly better competitor. Thus using the Wilcoxon rank pair test for the data at a cold:hot ratio of 10:1, one finds values of $p = 0.0314$ (Fig. 1a) and $p = 0.0197$ (Fig. 1b). Similar results were obtained in four other independent experiments.

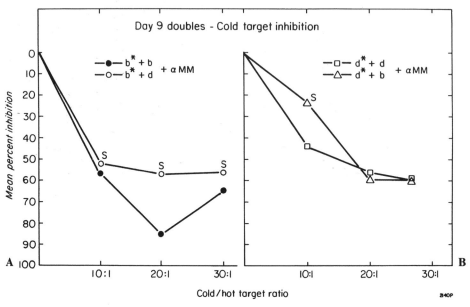

Fig. 1A, B. Cold target inhibition of day 9 cultures showing double specificity in the presence of αMM. Day 9 cultures of 50 C3H spleen cells were split into four aliquots and assayed agains H-2^b and H-2^d targets. Half of the trays were cold target inhibited with H-2^b and H-2^d at the ratios of cold to hot targets shown and assayed either on H-2^b hot (**A**) or H-2^d hot (**B**). Significant % inhibition was obtained at all three ratios with H-2^d cold and assayed on H-2^b, and at a 10:1 ratio with H-2^b cold assayed on H-2^d hot targets

Although the relatively high level of nonspecific competition seen suggests there may be nonspecific effector cells, additional specific competition was also always seen. This suggests that the cultures contain effector cells of different specificities. Since these cultures were originally seeded well below the limiting dilution point, there is a high probability that these different specificities developed within a single clone of effector cells.

3.3 Cold Target Inhibition Analysis of Day 9 Cultures in the Presence of Con A

Since the phenomenon of dual specificity (or nonspecificity) in day 9 Con A induced cultures was originally described (SHORTMAN et al. 1983) using a lectin-dependent cytotoxicity assay, we performed cold target experiments as described above, except that αMM was not added and any remaining Con A in the cultures could contribute to the effects seen. To our surprise, the apparent specificity of the cold target inhibition was greatly augmented (Fig. 2), and the data are strongly suggestive of two different populations of allospecific effector cells in the cultures.

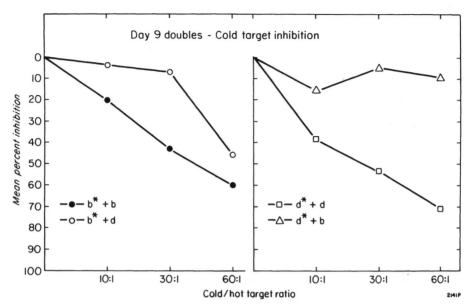

Fig. 2. Cold target inhibition of day 9 cultures showing double specificity in the absence of αMM. Day 9 cultures of 50 C3H spleen cells were split into four aliquots and assayed against H-2^b and H-2^d targets. Half of the trays were cold target inhibited with cold H-2^b and H-2^d at the ratios shown. When assayed on hot H-2^b, cold H-2^b target inhibited significantly more than cold H-2^d; similarly when assayed on hot H-2^d, cold H-2^d inhibition was more pronounced than with cold H-2^b. This experiment was performed in the absence of αMM in the assay media

4 Discussion

The phenomenon of "degradation of specificity" or aquisition of an NK-like pattern of lysis has been well documented by SHORTMAN et al. (1983, 1984). Using the same limiting dilution approach, we asked whether there could be a stage preceding the loss of specificity in which multiple specificities could be seen, i.e., could we be looking at the development of new specificities within a single clone? We reproduced the anomalous day 9 patterns of lysis found in Con A induced cultures containing low numbers of spleen cells, i.e., cultures that on day 6 were monospecific, by day 9 were capable of lysing at least two targets. We showed that this dual specificity is linked to the source of the factor used, rat Con A SN being the optimal inducer of double positive cultures. Reasoning that if only NK-like cells were present in day 9 cultures, cold inhibition would be nonspecific, we inhibited the double positive cultures with unlabelled competitors. According to limiting dilution theory, the cultures on which cold target competition were performed had a high probability of clonality. Cold target inhibition experiments were statistically consistent with the presence of two distinct specificities, albeit superimposed on a polyspecific NK-like type of cell. Statistical analysis reproducibly showed the presence of a new specificity which was not present at early stages of the cultures and which could not be completely inhibited by the specific cold target.

Surprisingly, the presence of at least two specific effector cells was most obvious when αMM was not included in the final assay, i.e., Con A remaining from the initial culture period or added externally (data not shown) allowed distinction by cold target inhibition betwen two specific effector cells present on day 9 in much clearer fashion than in its absence. The mechanism of action of Con A in both activation of a lectin-dependent CTL and its effect on specific CTL is still controversial. As SITKOVSKY et al. (1982, 1984) have described, an inhibition of monospecificity by a direct effect on the effector cell and an enhancement of the lectin-dependent cytotoxicity by an effect on the target cells are found with doses of the lectin similar to the ones used here. However, our results are difficult to explain on this basis since if this were the case, both specificities should be affected in the same way.

On the other hand, KANE and CLARCK (1984) have described an MHC restricted pattern of activation of lectin induction of CTL, i.e., in order to polyclonally activate a CTL precursor by a lectin, the precursor has to recognize the lectin in the context of MHC on an MHC-bearing cell, making the mitogen activation requirements similar to those for antigen-specific activation. One possible explanation for our observation of a specific inhibition of a double positive culture would be that the inhibited CTL is recognizing Con A in association with the appropriate MHC so that targets of the inappropriate MHC could not compete. In the absence of Con A, the effect is less evident, perhaps due to the background of NK-like cells induced after 9 days of incubation.

We conclude that the day 9 double positive cultures contain CTL of at least two different specificities that have both developed within a single clone and that a stage of polyspecificity appears to precede the stage of NK-like nonspecificity in these cultures. Thus it appears that generation of T-cell diversity can occur in a lectin-activated culture in a manner similar to that previously reported for a conventional mixed lymphocyte reaction (REIMANN and MILLER 1985).

References

Brooks CG (1983) Reversible induction of natural killer cell activity in cloned murine cytotoxic lymphocytes. Nature 305:155–158

Brooks CG, Kuribayashi K, Sale GE, Henney CS (1982) Characterization of five cloned murine cell lines showing high cytolytic activity against Yac-1 cells. J Immunol 128:2326–2336

Brooks CG, Urdal D, Henney CS (1983) Lymphokine driven 'differentiation' cytotoxic T cell clones into cells with NK-like specificity: correlations with display of membrane macromolecules. Immunol Rev 72:43–72

Claësson MH, Miller RG (1984) Functional heterogeneity in allospecific cytotoxic T lymphocyte clones. I. CTL clone express strong anti-self suppressive activity. J Exp Med 160:1702–1716

Claësson MH, Miller RG (1985) Functional heterogeneity in allospecific cytotoxic T lymphocyte clones. II. Development of syngeneic cytotoxicity in the absence of specific antigenic stimulation. J Immunol 134:684–690

Kane K, Clark WR (1984) The role of class I MHC products in polyclonal activation of CTL function. J Immunol 133:2857–2863

Appearance of New Specificities in Lectin-Induced T-Cell Clones 299

Porter EH, Berry RJ (1963) The efficient design of transplantable tumor assays. Br J Cancer 17:583–595

Reimann J, Miller RG (1985) Rapid changes in specificity within a single clone of cytotoxic effector cells. Cell 40:571–581

Shortman K, Wilson A, Scollay R, Chen WF (1983) Development of large granular lymphocytes with anomalous nonspecific cytotoxicity in clones derived from Ly-2$^+$ T cells. Proc Natl Acad Sci USA 80:2728–2732

Shortman K, Wilson A, Scollay R (1984) Loss of specificity in cytolytic T lymphocyte clones obtained by limit dilution culture of Ly-2$^+$ T cells. J Immunol 132:584–593

Sitkovsky MM, Pasternack MS, Eisen HN (1982) Inhibition of cytotoxic T lymphocyte activity by concanavalin-A. J Immunol 129:1372–1376

Sitkovsky MV, Pasternack MS, Lugo JF, Klein JR, Eisen HN (1984) Isolation and partial characterization of Con-A receptors on cloned cytotoxic T lymphocytes. Proc Natl Acad Sci USA 81:1519–1523

Teh HS, Bennink J, Von Boehmer H (1982) Selection of the T cell repertoire during ontogeny: limiting dilution analysis. Eur J Immunol 12:887

Wilson A, Shortman K (1984) Degradation of specificity in cytotoxic T lymphocyte clones: mouse strain dependence and interstrain transfer of nonspecific cytolysis. Eur J Immunol 14:951–956

Syngeneic Cytotoxicity and
Veto Activity in Thymic Lymphoid Colonies and
Their Expanded Progeny

M.H. Claësson and C. Röpke

1 Introduction 301
2 Materials and Methods 301
3 Results 302
3.1 Characteristics of Thymic Lymphoid Colonies 302
3.2 Cytotoxic Activity 304
4 Discussion 306
5 Summary 308
References 308

1 Introduction

MHC restriction and self-tolerance of the mature T lymphocyte are acquired during the ontogeny of the cells (Zinkernagel 1978; Zinkernagel and Doherty 1979). The thymus appears to be essential in this process, probably by selection and regulation of self-reactive early T-cell precursors from which the mature phenotype may arise by positive selection through somatic mutation (Zinkernagel 1978; von Boehmer et al. 1978). Self-reactivity, however, potentially carries the possibility of autoaggression leading to tissue and organ destruction. However, the mechanisms by which the various degrees of self-reactivity are regulated during T-cell differentiation in the thymus are poorly understood.

In the present work we demonstrate the existence of specific syngeneic cytotoxic reactivity in lymphocyte clones from short-term expansion cultures derived from thymus cortex and medulla. We also show that such newly established lymphocyte clones possess antiself suppressor activity of the veto type (Miller 1980; Muraoka and Miller 1980), an activity which may be of importance for down-regulation of autoaggression and the maintenance of self-tolerance in the normal thymus environment.

2 Materials and Methods

Animals. Mice of the strains BALB/c, C3H, and C57Bl/6 were obtained from the Panum Institute stock. SJL mice were purchased at Gl. Bomholtgård, Laven, Denmark. Animals were used at the age of 8–10 weeks.

Institute of Medical Anatomy, Dept. A, University of Copenhagen, The Panum Institute, 3 Blegdamsvej, DK-2200 Copenhagen N

302   M.H. Claësson and C. Röpke

Colony Assay and Cell Culture. Thymocytes were obtained by standard procedures and separated into PNA$^+$ and PNA$^-$ cells according to the method of EISENTHAL et al. (1982). The cells were then suspended in methylcellulose (MC) culture medium in the presence of FCS, horse serum, supernatant from 2 days Con A activated rat spleen cells, 2% α-methyl mannoside (Sigma), PHA, and 2-ME according to methods described in detail elsewhere (RÖPKE and CLAËSSON 1985; RÖPKE 1984). Cells were seeded into 33-mm plastic culture dishes at cell densities from 1×10^4–2×10^5/ml. For expansion culture, individual colonies were picked from the MC at day 7 of culture and transferred to 96 round bottom well microculture plates (Nunc, Roskilde, Denmark) containing 200 μl RPMI culture medium with 10% FCS, 2-ME, 10% rat Con A-supernatant (SN), and 10^5 syngeneic, mictomycin-treated spleen cells.

Cytotoxic Assay. After expansion for 7 days, 100 μl were removed from each well and replaced with 1000–2000 ^{51}Cr labelled target cells in 100 μl RPMI medium. After 4 h, 100 μl supernatant were recovered from each well and counted for radioactivity in a gamma counter. Spontaneous release was calculated from at least 30 individual feeder cell cultures without added colony cells. Cytotoxic activity greater than the spontaneous release counts plus $2 \times$ SD was considered to reflect specific killing.

To study the influence of colony cells on cytotoxic activity directed against the haplotype of the colony cells (veto activity), individual or mass collected day 7 colonies or expanded day 14 colonies were added to 200 μl MLC cultures in which the stimulator cells shared haplotype with the colony cells. Cell numbers were 10^5 responder and 3×10^5 stimulator spleen cells, and 20% rat Con A-SN was added to all MLC cultures. In experiments assaying specificity in this system a third party type stimulator cell was included in the MLC. Cytotoxicity tests were performed as mentioned above, the controls in these experiments being MLC cultures without added colony cells. Cytotoxic activity lower or higher than the mean control value plus $2 \times$ SD was considered suppressed and stimulated, respectively. All assay cultures contained in addition 2% α-methylmannoside to block any effect of Con A and PHA.

Target Cells. Tumor cell lines RBL-5 (H-2^b), P-815 (H-2^d) and L cells (H-2^k) were kept as continous cultures in vitro. In addition we used 2–3 days Con A stimulated normal spleen cells of the appropriate haplotype. Targets were labelled with 150 μCi ^{51}Cr in PBS, containing 5% FCS, for at least 60 min and washed four times prior to assay.

Antibodies and Fluorescence Microscopy. Monoclonal fluorescein labelled antibodies against Lyt-1 and Lyt-2 antigens were purchased from Becton Dickinton, California, USA. For enumeration of Lyt-1 and Lyt-2 positive cells in colonies, 500 to 1000 antibody-labelled cells were counted in a Leitz Ortholux II epifluorescence microscope.

3   Results

3.1   Characteristics of Thymic Lymphoid Colonies

The most important data regarding our culture system are summarized in Table 1. From these data it appears that thymic colonies are derived from relatively

Table 1. Characteristics of thymic lymphoid colonies

	Nonseparated thymocytes	PNA$^+$ thymocytes	PNA$^-$ thymocytes	Reference
Cloning efficiency	0.017%	0.014%	0.051%	RÖPKE (1984)
Colony cells:				
% Lyt-1$^+$	74 ± 5[a]	85 ± 10	93 ± 4	RÖPKE and CLAËSSON (1986)
% Lyt-2$^+$	91 ± 2	96 ± 1	98 ± 1	
Numbers at day 10	nd	8 × 10^3	12 × 10^3	
Cortisol IC$_{50}$[b]	nd	2 × 10^{-8}M	2 × 10^{-6}M	CLAËSSON and RÖPKE (1983)
Colony-forming cells:	Thy-1 dull	H-2 bright	Lyt-1 medium Lyt-2 bright	TL dull	RÖPKE (1984)

[a] Mean value of 10 individual colonies ± SEM
[b] Cortisol was added to the culture dish at day 1 of culture

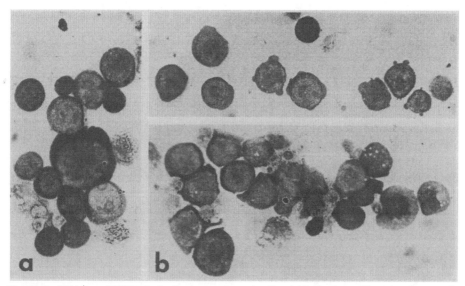

Fig. 1a, b. PNA$^+$- and PNA$^-$-derived colony cells at day 7 and 14 of culture. Note the absence of granulated cells

mature cell subsets and are composed of lymphocytes belonging to the cytotoxic/suppressor cell lineages. Furthermore, it appears that colonies derived from PNA$^+$ and PNA$^-$ subsets respectively exhibit different growth kinetics and sensitivity to growth inhibition induced by cortisol.

Figure 1 shows the morphology of C3H mouse colony cells at days 7 and 14 of culture. The vast majority of cells are typical small and medium sized lymphocytes without any cytoplasmatic granulation.

3.2 Cytotoxic Activity

Cytotoxic activity against both syngeneic and allogeneic targets (see below) was demonstrated in individual colonies as early as day 7 of culture, but the activity was lower than that of expanded colonies (data not included).

Seven-day expanded colonies (see above) were assayed in a 4-h ^{51}Cr release assay against Cr-labelled syngeneic (L cell fibroblasts or Con A blasts) or allogeneic (P815 mastocytoma cells or Con A blasts) cells of the H-2^k or and H-2^d haplotypes respectively. Table 2 summarizes the results of six separate experiments. Approximately 30% of the PNA$^+$-derived colonies and 15% of the PNA$^-$-derived colonies exhibited significant cytotoxic activity against syngeneic target cells ($p<0.05$) when compared to the activity of equal numbers of microcultures containing mitomycin-treated feeder cells only (see Sect. 2). In comparison, only 7% and 8% of the two colony types, respectively, killed allogeneic H-2^d target cells. Table 2 also shows that colony-mediated killing of YAC cells was low. Cytotoxic activity of C3H thymus colonies against the haplotypes H-2^b and H-2^s was much lower than the activity against H-2^d cells (data not included).

We asked the question whether the same individual colony is capable of killing both syngeneic and allogeneic target cells. Individual 7-day expanded colonies were split and the same colony assayed against syngeneic L cells and allogeneic P815 cells. Figure 2 shows the results from such an experiment. It is obvious that an individual colony kills either syngeneic or allogeneic targets. Thus, only 2 out of 160 colonies killed both target cells.

The development of MHC restriction in thymocytes is believed to be based on positive selection within the thymus of lymphoid precursors with an intermediate affinity for self molecules exposed to their antigen receptors by thymic epithelial cells (ZINKERNAGEL 1978; VON BOEHMER et al. 1978; CHIEN et al. 1984). The risk of autoaggression in cytotoxic T-cell precursors with strong affinities for self-structures appears possible during the selection process. However, autoagression is never observed in normal uncultured thymic cell preparations, although easily demonstrable in expanded thymus lymphocyte clones as shown above. This discrepancy might suggest that the development of autoaggression

Table 2. Cytotoxicity in 7 day expanded C3H mouse thymic colonies. Number of cytotoxic colonies/total colonies. Results from six separate experiments

Colonies obtained from	Target cell H-2	Experiment[a]					
		1	2	3	4	5	6
PNA$^+$ cells	H-2^k	28/60	27/60	9/30	10/30	13/60[b]	10/102[b]
	H-2^d	5/60	n.t.	3/30	2/30	3/60[b]	5/60[c]
PNA$^-$ cells	H-2^k	5/60	9/60	1/30	4/30	20/60[b]	13/102[b]
	H-2^d	8/60	n.t.	3/27	3/30	4/60[b]	1/60[c]

[a] Experiments 1–4 assayed on L cells (H-2^k) and P815 cells (H-2^d) respectively
[b] Target cells were 2 day Con A activated blast cells
[c] Target cells were YAC tumor cells

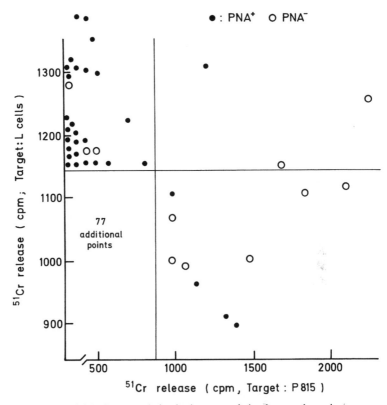

Fig. 2. Cytotoxic activity of individually expanded colonies assayed simultaneously against syngeneic (L cells) and allogeneic (P815) target cells. The *horizontal* and *vertical lines* represent the mean ^{51}Cr release of 60 microcultures containing feeder cells only + 2×SD. *Open symbols* and *closed symbols* represent cytotoxic activity of PNA⁻- and PNA⁺-derived colonies respectively

in the normal thymus is under a strong negative regulation. Antiself suppressor activity of the veto type (MILLER 1980; MURAOKA and MILLER 1980) has been claimed, but has actually never been proved to exist in the thymic environment. In light of our and others' recent work (CLAËSSON and MILLER 1984; FINK et al. 1984), demonstrating powerful veto activity within individual cytotoxic T-cell clones, we have looked for such activity in the thymic cell colonies. Figure 3 shows the results. Six and 11 out of 21 PNA⁺- and PNA⁻-derived C3H thymic colonies, respectively, added to individual micro MLC (H-2^d anti-H-2^k), significantly ($p<0.05$) inhibited the development of anti-H-2^k reactivity. On expansion the colonies lost this activity and even appeared to enhance development of cytotoxicity in the assay MLC. In order to study the specificity of this antiself suppressor activity, PNA⁺- and PNA⁻-derived colony cells (H-2^k) were mass harvested and added to an H-2^b anti-(H-2^k + H-2^d) MLC. Cytotoxic activity was assayed at day 5 of culture. Only the anti-H-2^k reactivity was inhibited indicating the veto nature of this suppression (Fig. 4).

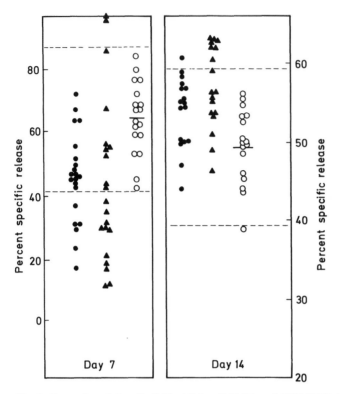

Fig. 3. Cytotoxic activity of individual 5 days BALB/c anti-C3H MLC. Individual day 7 colonies or 7 day expanded colonies from C3H mouse thymus were added to a total of 78 MLC cultures. The *open symbols* represent cytotoxic activity of individual control MLC without addition of colony cells. *Stippled lines* represent cytotoxic activity of control MLC ± 2×SD. Target cells were C3H activated blast cells. Spontaneous ^{51}Cr release was less than 25% of total release. ●, addition of PNA$^+$ cell derived colonies; ▲, addition of PNA$^-$ cell derived colonies

4 Discussion

The two major observations of the present work are that day 7 thymic lymphoid colonies of the Lyt-1$^+$2$^+$ phenotype possess antiself suppressor activity of the veto type (MILLER 1980; MURAOKA and MILLER 1980) and that, on expansion, the colonies loose their suppressor activity and a significant proportion develop syngeneic cytotoxic reactivity.

Thymocytes are known to possess proliferative reactivity when exposed to irradiated syngeneic spleen cells (WU and THOMAS 1985), the target structure for recognition being associated with class II antigens encoded by Ia, I region genes of the MHC. Such reactivity is believed to be essential for the proliferation and selection of MHC restricted and self-tolerant mature T cells within the thymus of the helper/inducer lineages (CHIEN et al. 1984; ROCK and BENACERRAF 1984). Similarly, the syngeneic cytotoxic reactivity of the cloned Lyt-2$^+$ thymic lymphocytes shown in the present work may in some way reflect a selection mechanism

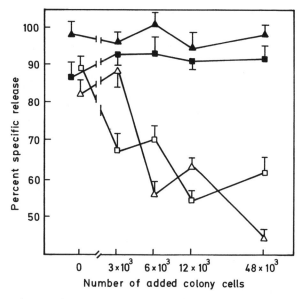

Fig. 4. Cytotoxic activity of 5 day C57B1/6 anti-(C3H+BALB/c) MLC cultures (1 ml volumes) after addition of various numbers of day 7 mass harvested PNA$^+$ (□ ■) and PNA$^-$ (△ ▲) cell derived C3H thymic lymphoid colony cells. *Bars* represent SD of six replicate assay cultures. Target cells were C3H Con A activated blast cells (□ △) and P815 tumor cells (■ ▲)

for the cytotoxic T-cell lineages. Under bulk culture conditions self-directed cytotoxicity may be impossible to demonstrate due to the presence of strong suppressor activity which downregulates autoaggression. Our results suggest this possibility by showing that antiself suppression precedes the development of syngeneic cytotoxicity within individual clones, although we have not yet formally proven that the two activities exist in the same clone at different time intervals. Support for this hypothesis comes from recent work showing strong veto activity in normal allospecific CTL clones (CLAËSSON and MILLER 1984; FINK et al. 1984) and the finding that such CTL clones may express high levels of syngeneic cytotoxic reactivity (CLAËSSON and MILLER 1985). We thus believe that antiself suppression of the veto type is a basic and necessary property of all T-cell clones with a cytotoxic potential. This idea goes also well with a hypothesis where MHC class II self antigens on thymic stromal cells are stimulatory whereas class I self antigens are inhibitory to intrathymic lymphocyte proliferation.

It was shown recently that self-reactive T-cell clones or T-cell hybridomas on subcloning and expansion may undergo somatic mutation in their genes encoding the antigen specific receptor molecules, loose self-reactivity and become semiallo or totally alloreactive (REIMANN and MILLER 1985; AUGUSTIN and SIM 1984). This process is not dependent on antigenic stimulation, but occurs at random at a low but significant rate. In the present study, we only identified very few clones which exhibited both syngeneic and allogeneic reactivity, so we were unable to demonstrate directly that alloreactive T-cell clones are derived from precursor cells with syngeneic reactivity. Our data, showing that the majority of syngeneic reactive clones are derived from cells in the thymic cortex (PNA$^+$ cells), which is the site of production for the vast majority of thymocytes, are in line with this possibility.

Although it was recently shown that allospecific cytotoxic T-cell clones on expansion may undergo degradation of specificity and exhibit NK-like activity (BROOKS et al. 1983; SHORTMAN et al. 1983), we do not think that the syngeneic reactivity observed in the present work bears any relationship to NK activity. First, YAC cells, known to be sensitive to NK killing, were only killed by few PNA$^+$-derived colonies, which might have reacted with the K^k haplotype (syngeneic reactivity) of the YAC cells. More convincingly, the killing of allogeneic blast cell targets other than those of H-2^d haplotype was very low although such target cells are easily killed by T cells with NK-like activity (BROOKS et al. 1982). Finally, the morphology of colony cells was typical of that of activated cytotoxic T lymphocytes without occurrence of cytoplasmatic granulation.

5 Summary

T-cell colonies of Lyt-1$^+$2$^+$ phenotype were generated from PNA$^+$ and PNA$^-$ C3H thymus cells. Individual colonies expanded for 7 days in subculture were assayed for cytotoxic activity against syngeneic and allogeneic target cells in a 4-h ^{51}Cr-release assay. Approximately 30% of PNA$^+$ and 15% of PNA$^-$ cell derived colonies exhibited significant syngeneic cytotoxic activity, whereas less than 10% of the colonies expressed allogeneic cytotoxic activity. Only very few colonies simultaneously expressed cytotoxic activity against both syngeneic and allogeneic target cells.

Individual and mass collected colonies were assayed for antiself suppressor (veto) activity in a MLC system where the stimulator and the colony cells were of identical haplotype. Both day 7 individual and mass collected colonies inhibited generation of cytotoxic cells in the MLC, whereas 7 day expanded colonies lost their activity. Our data suggest that self-aggression in individual cytotoxic thymic lymphocyte clones is downregulated by cells with veto activity within the clones.

Acknowledgement. This work was supported by grants from the Danish Medical Research Council and the Danish Cancer Foundation.

References

Augustin AA, Sim GK (1984) T-cell receptors generated via mutations are specific for various major histocompatibility antigens. Cell 39:5–12

Brooks CG, Kuribayashi K, Sale GE, Henney CS (1982) Characterization of five cloned murine cell lines sharing high cytolytic activity against YAC-1 cells. J Immunol 128:2326–2335

Brooks CG, Urdal DL, Henney CS (1983) Lymphokinedriven "differentiation" of cytotoxic T-cell clones into cells with NK-like specificity: Correlation with display of membrane macromolecules. Immunol Rev 72:43–87

Syngeneic Cytotoxicity and Veto Activity in Thymic Lymphoid Colonies   309

Chien Y, Gascoigne NR, Kavaler J, Lee NE, Davis MM (1984) Somatic recombination in murine T cell receptor gene. Nature 309:322–326

Claësson MH, Miller RG (1984) Functional heterogeneity in allospecific cytotoxic T cell clones. I. CTL clones express strong anti-self suppressive activity. J Exp Med 160:1702–1716

Claësson MH, Miller RG (1985) Functional heterogeneity in allospecific cytotoxic T lymphocyte clones. II. Development of syngeneic cytotoxicity in the absence of specific antigenic stimulation. J Immunol 134:684–690

Claësson MH, Röpke C (1983) Colony formation by subpopulations of T lymphocytes. IV. Inhibitory effect of hydrocortisone as human and murine T cell subsets. Clin Exp Immunol 54:554–560

Eisenthal A, Nachtigal D, Feldman M (1982) The in vitro generation of suppressor lymphocytes involves interactions between PNA$^+$ and PNA$^-$ thymocyte populations. Immunology 46:697–704

Fink PJ, Rammensee HG, Bevan MJ (1984) Cloned cytolytic T cells can suppress primary cytotoxic responses directed against them. J Immunol 133:1775–1781

Miller RG (1980) An immunological suppressor cell inactivating cytotoxic T lymphocyte precursor cells recognizing it. Nature 287:544–546

Muraoka S, Miller RG (1980) Cells in bone marrow and in T cell colonies grown from bone marrow can suppress generation of cytotoxic T lymphocytes directed against their self antigens. J Exp Med 152:54–71

Reimann J, Miller RG (1985) Rapid changes in specificity within single clones of cytolytic effector cells. Cell (to be published)

Rock K, Benacerraf B (1984) The role of Ia molecules in the activation of T lymphocytes. IV. The basis of the thymocyte IL 1 response and its possible role in the generation of the T cell repertoire. J Immunol 132:1654–1662

Röpke C (1984) Characterization of T lymphocyte colony-forming cells in the mouse. The colony-forming cells is confined to Lyt1, 2, 3$^+$ cell subsets in the thymus and the lymph nodes. J Immunol 132:1625–1631

Röpke C, Claësson MH (1985) T-lymphocyte colony formation by thymic and peripheral lymphocytes in methylcellulose culture. Thymus 7:49–63

Röpke C, Claësson MH (1986) Proliferative kinetics, phenotype and cytotoxic function of thymic and peripheral T cell colonies. Scand J Immunol 23:243–250

Shortman K, Wilson A, Scollay R, Chen W-F (1983) Development of large granular lymphocytes with anomalous, nonspecific cytotoxicity in clones derived from Lyt-2$^+$ T cells. Proc Natl Acad Sci USA 80:2728–2732

von Boehmer H, Haas W, Jerne NK (1978) Major histocompatibility complex-linked immune responsiveness is acquired by lymphocytes of low-responder mice differentiating in thymus of high-responder mice. Proc Natl Acad Sci USA 75:2439–2442

Wu S, Thomas DW (1985) Syngeneic responses by murine thymocytes: A role for non-MHC and non-MLS genes. J Immunol 134:10–15

Zinkernagel RM (1978) Thymus and lymphohemopoietic cells: their role in T cell maturation in selection of T cells, H-2 restriction specificity and in H-2 linked Ir gene control. Immunol Rev 42:202–270

Zinkernagel RM, Doherty PG (1979) MHC-restricted cytotoxic T cells: studies on the biological role of polymorphic major transplantation antigens determining T-cell restriction specificity, function and responsiveness. Adv Immunol 27:51–177

Functional Analysis of a Self-I-A Reactive T-Cell Clone Which Preferentially Stimulates Activated B Cells

T. Saito and K. Rajewsky

1 Introduction 311
2 Derivation of a Self-I-A Reactive T-Cell Clone, D11-22 312
3 D11-22 Directly Stimulates B Cells in the Absence of Added Antigen 312
4 D11-22 Helps Antigen-Specific Responses in the Presence of Antigen 313
5 Discussion 315
6 Summary 315
References 316

1 Introduction

Autoreactive T cells have been isolated in the form of continuously growing lines (Zauderer et al. 1984; Clayberger et al. 1984; Kimoto et al. 1984; Finnegan et al. 1984) or hybridomas (Glimcher and Shevach 1982; Rock and Benacerraf 1983, Endres et al. 1983; Nagase et al. 1984). Such T cells may participate in syngeneic mixed lymphocyte reaction (reviewed by Battisto and Ponzio 1981). However, it is not clear whether they play a regulatory role under physiological conditions (Hausman and Stobo 1979; Smith and Knowlton 1979; Lattime et al. 1981; Goto and Zvaifler 1983).

In an attempt to isolate immunoglobulin idiotype-specific T-cell lines, which is one category of autoreactive T cells, we isolated a T-cell clone which directly stimulates syngeneic B cells in a MHC-restricted way in the absence of exogeneous antigens. Functional analysis of the clone failed to reveal an idiotypic specificity but showed that the cells stimulate every hundredth B cell into proliferation and antibody formation and also help antigen-specific responses in the presence of antigen, suggesting that the clone may preferentially stimulate "activated" B cells.

Most of the results concerning the characterization of the clone have been described in a previous paper (Saito and Rajewsky 1985). In this article, we summarize the previous evidence, add some information, and discuss the possible physiological role of self-I-A reactive T cells.

Institute for Genetics, University of Cologne, D-5000 Cologne

312   T. Saito and K. Rajewsky

Table 1. Proliferation of D11-22 cells

Feeder cells							Serum in medium	Proliferation[b]
Mouse strain	Cell source	H-2						
		K	A	E	D			
A. C57BL/6	SC	b	b	b	b		FCS	+
B10.A(4R)	SC	k	k	b	b			−
B10.A(5R)	SC	b	b	k	d			+
B10.MBR	SC	b	k	k	q			−
B. C57BL/6	SC						FCS	+
	LPS-last							+
	Thymocyte							−
	SAC [a]							+
C. C57BL/6	SC						MS	+
	LPS-blast						MS	+

[a] T-cell and B-cell depleted splenic adherent cells (SAC): Glass-adherent cells were prepared from B-cell depleted SC by panning on goat antimouse Ig coated dishes. Adherent cells were further treated with anti-Thy1 and Lyt-2 plus complement
[b] Proliferation was measured by ^{3}H-thymidine uptake. Cultures giving a stimulation index ≥ 20 were scored as "+". For details see SAITO and RAJEWSKY (1985)

2 Derivation of a Self-I-A Reactive T-Cell Clone, D11-22

Since we intended to establish idiotype-specific T-cell clones, C57BL/6 mice were immunized with the monoclonal anti-NP antibody B1-8 (IgM, λ1) (RETH et al. 1978), and lymph node T cells were cultivated in the presence of B1-8 and irradiated spleen cells (SC). Vigorous growth was observed but turned out later to be independent of the presence of antibody B1-8. The cells were cloned and one clone, named D11-22, was analyzed in detail. Approximately one third of the total collection of clones ($\cong 20$) seemed to be similar to D11-22 in functional terms.

The phenotype of clone D11-22 is Thy1$^+$, Ly1$^+$, Lyt2$^-$, and sIg$^-$. The cells proliferate in the presence of syngeneic SC in the culture. Proliferation of D11-22 is I-A restricted (A in Table 1) and also occurs in the medium supplemented with mouse serum (MS) instead of FCS (C in Table 1). Irradiated SC, LPS-blasts and splenic adherent cells as feeder cells induce a proliferative response of D11-22 cells (B in Table 1). The response was inhibited by addition of monoclonal anti-I-A^b antibody. These results suggest that D11-22 cells recognize the I-A^b molecule as such or a self-antigen in association with I-A^b.

3 D11-22 Directly Stimulates B Cells in the Absence of Added Antigen

D11-22 cells stimulate syngeneic B cells into proliferation (Table 2) and into antibody formation. The PFC response was also I-A restricted. The I-A restriction

Functional Analysis of a Self-I-A Reactive T-Cell Clone   313

Table 2. B-cell proliferation in response to D11-22 cells[a]

B cells	T cells		(^{3}H)-TdR uptake (cpm)
B	–	–	414
B	–	LPS	29230
B[b]	–	LPS	94
–	D11-22	–	52
–	⚡ D11-22	–	72
B	D11-22	–	15686
B	⚡ D11-22	–	4951
B	D11-22	–	2870

[a] 1×10^4 T cells were seeded with either 1×10^5 nonirradiated or 5×10^5 irradiated T-cell depleted SC ("B") in 0.2 ml culture.
[b] ⚡ = irradiated

in the PFC response does not only apply to the activation of D11-22 cells but also to their collaboration with B cells because monoclonal anti-I-A[b] antibody completely inhibited PFC induction even when it was added after the D11-22 cells had been activated. This result suggests that B-cell stimulation by D11-22 is due to a direct interaction between T and B cells. This was further substantiated using two different protocols. In the first, D11-22 cells were shown to stimulate only syngeneic but not allogeneic B cells even in the presence of irradiated syngeneic feeder cells. A similar result was obtained in another type of experiment in which a mixture of syngeneic and allogeneic B cells were cocultured with D11-22 and after 4 days B cell blasts were treated with anti-H-2 antibody plus complement to determine which type of B cells was stimulated. From these experiments we concluded that D11-22 directly stimulated B cells in a MHC-restricted way.

In order to characterize the B-cell population responding to D11-22, we analyzed the frequency of the responding B cells and their polyclonality. The frequency of B cells responding to D11-22 is approximately 1/100 at a saturating dose of T cells in a limiting dilution analysis. It is unlikely that the low frequency simply reflects the restriction of responsiveness to blast cells because D11-22 cells stimulate small B cells separated on a Percoll density gradient or by a cell sorter as well as unfractionated cells. B-cell stimulation by D11-22 was polyclonal since the frequency of PFC of various specificities among the Ig-secreting cells are indistinguishable among the blast cells stimulated by LPS or D11-22 (SAITO and RAJEWSKY 1985).

4 D11-22 Helps Antigen-Specific Responses in the Presence of Antigen

D11-22 cells also affect antigen-specific antibody responses. In an in vivo transfer experiment in which cloned T cells and naive B cells were transferred into ir-

314   T. Saito and K. Rajewsky

Table 3. Helper function of D11-22 cells in an antigen-induced in vivo response[a]

T cell	B cell	Antigen	IgG1 anti-NP antibody (ug/ml)
D11-22	B	–	<0.1
–	B	NP-CG	<0.1
	SC	NP-CG	940
E3[b]	B	NP-CG	95
D11-22	B	NP-CG	26

[a] Data from SAITO and RAJEWSKY (1985). In primary adoptive cell transfer experiments, irradiated C57BL/6 mice were reconstituted with 1×10^7 T-cell depleted SC ("B") and 3×10^6 T cells. Control groups were injected with whole SC or B cells alone. Mice were bled on day 13 and titer of anti-NP antibodies were determined by RIA
[b] NP-CG-specific helper T-cell clone

Table 4. Helper function of D11-22 cells in antigen-induced in vitro responses[a]

Stimulating antigen [b]	Anti-TNP IgG1 antibody (ng/ml) induced by	
	–	D11-22
–	36	91
TNP- KLH	51	865
NP- KLH	58	86
KLH	48	94
TNP- OVA	25	895
OVA	15	80
NP- CG	31	110

[a] 4×10^5 T-cell depleted SC from TNP-KLH primed C57BL/6 mice were seeded together with 1×10^4 T-cell clones in 0.2 ml culture. Titers of IgG1 anti-TNP antibody in culture supernatants of 8 days culture were determined by RIA
[b] 30 ng/ml

radiated recipients, D11-22 helps (4-hydroxy-3-nitrophenyl)acetyl (NP)-specific responses to a NP-chicken gamma globulin (CG) conjugate (Table 3). No response was observed in the absence of antigen. The helper function for the antigen-specific response was also observed in vitro in the primary response to (4-hydroxy-5-iodo-3-nitrophenyl)acetyl-polymerized flagellin (NIP-POL) (a TI-II antigen) or in the secondary T cell-dependent (TD) antitrinitrophenyl (TNP) response. In the latter case, as shown in Table 4, D11-22 helps specific antibody formation only in the presence of the relevant antigen in the culture. In the case of the primary anti-NP response to NIP-POL, D11-22 induces IgG1 anti-NP antibodies, which is not observed in the presence of control T cells such as normal splenic T cells and keyhole limpet hemocyanin (KLH) or NP-CG-specific T-cell clones. Since KLH-specific T cells support a specific IgG1 response in the presence of NP-KLH, D11-22 mimics MHC-restricted, antigen-specific T cells in the presence of a TI-II antigen. However, the induction of IgG1 by D11-22 was not observed in the presence of splenic T cells, suggesting that self-I-A reactive T cells like D11-22 are generally inactive in the system (SAITO and RAJEWSKY 1985).

5 Discussion

The evidence that the T-cell clone described here is autoreactive is as follows: 1. The cells proliferate in the presence of syngeneic spleen cells in mouse serum. 2. The clone helps antigen-specific responses in vivo. 3. B-cell stimulation by D11-22 cells is polyclonal and MHC-restricted. If the cells were specific for a minor antigen present at a concentration in the nanogram range per ml in FCS, B-cell stimulation should be antigen-specific. If the cells are specific for a major antigen present in FCS in microgram concentrations, B-cell stimulation should be MHC-nonrestricted as seen when B cells are mixed with KLH-specific cloned T cells in the presence of a high dose of KLH.

D11-22 cells appear to recognize I-A^b as such or some other self antigen in association with I-A^b. The fact that the T cells stimulate only every hundredth B cell polyclonally is compatible with both possibilities since it could reflect quantitative heterogeneity of I-A expression as well as heterogeneity with respect to the expression of some other antigen. In our attempts to identify a second antigen in addition to I-A^b we failed to obtain evidence for an idiotypic specificity of D11-22 cells or the involvement of some other differentiation antigen expressed in the B-cell lineage (SAITO and RAJEWSKY 1985).

Increased reactivity of antigen-specific B cells to respond to D11-22 in the presence of antigen in vivo and in vitro may reflect the increased expression of I-A molecules on B cells after cross-linking of sIg (MOND et al. 1981). Thus, D11-22 cells would preferentially stimulate "activated" B cells. B cells responding to direct stimulation by D11-22 may consist of large activated B cells and small "excited" B cells expressing high amounts of I-A molecules on the surface (ROEM et al. 1984). The frequency of D11-22 responsive B cells (1/100) might reflect the frequency of these types of B cells in the mouse.

As the main point of the present analysis, self-I-A reactive T cells like D11-22 apparently have the capacity to specifically help the induction of antibody responses by antigens for which they are not specific. Such cells might also be involved in idiotypic regulation in that they may enhance idiotype expression in concert with anti-idiotypic antibody. Thus, considering also that autoreactive T cells like D11-22 can be easily isolated from the mouse, this cell type, generally inactive in the system, may play a physiological role in the amplification of various kinds of B-cell responses.

6 Summary

A self-I-A reactive T-cell clone has been isolated that proliferates in the presence of irradiated syngeneic spleen cells in mouse serum. The cells directly stimulate every hundredth B cell into proliferation and antibody formation. The cells may recognize self-I-A as such. The clone also augments antigen-specific antibody responses in vivo and in vitro in the presence of antigen, suggesting that the cells preferentially stimulate "activated" B cells. The results suggest that self-Ia reactive T cells, generally inactive in the system, may locally help B cell responses to antigens which the T cells do not themselves recognize.

Acknowledgements. We wish to thank Ms. C. Uthoff-Hachenberg for excellent technical help. T.S. was supported by an Alexander von Humboldt Foundation Fellowship. This work was supported by the Deutsche Forschungsgemeinschaft through SFB 74.

References

Battisto JR, Ponzio NM (1981) Autologous and syngeneic mixed lymphocyte reactions and their immunological significance. Prog Allergy 28:160

Clayberger C, Dekruyff RH, Cantor H (1984) Immunoregulatory activities of autoreactive T cells: an I-A-specific T cell clone mediates both help and suppression of antibody responses. J Immunol 132:2273

Endres RO, Marrack P, Kappler JW (1983) An IL2-secreting T cell hybridoma that responds to a self class I histocompatibility antigen in the H-2D region. J Immunol 131:1656

Finnegan A, Needleman B, Hodes RJ (1984) Activation of B cells by autoreactive T cells: cloned autoreactive T cells activate B cells by two distinct pathways. J Immunol 133:78

Glimcher LH, Shevach EM (1982) Production of autoreactive I region-restricted T cell hybridomas. J Exp Med 156:640

Goto M, Zvaifler NJ (1983) Characterization of the killer cell generated in the autologous mixed lymphocyte reaction. J Exp Med 157:1309

Hausman PB, Stobo JD (1979) Specificity and function of a human autologous reactive T cell. J Exp Med 149:1537

Kimoto M, Yoshikubo T, Kishimoto S, Yamamura Y, Kishimoto T (1984) Polyclonal activation of xid B cells by auto-Ia-reactive T cell clones. J Immunol 132:1663

Lattime EC, Gilles S, David C, Stutman O (1981) Interleukin 2 production in the syngeneic mixed lymphocyte reaction. Eur J Immunol 11:67

Mond JJ, Seghal E, Kung J, Finkelman FD (1981) Increased expression of I-region-associated antigen (Ia) on B cells after cross-linking of surface immunoglobulin. J Immunol 127:881

Nagase F, Walter SJ, Thorebecke GJ, Bona CA (1984) Characterization of a (BALB/c × C57BL/6) F1 T cell hybridoma with double specificity: recognition of antigen in context of I-A^d and autoreactivity to I-A^b. Eur J Immunol 14:625

Reth M, Hämmerling GJ, Rajewsky K (1978) Analysis of the repertoire of anti-NP antibodies in C57BL/6 mice by cell fusion. I. Characterization of antibody families in the primary and hyperimmune response. Eur J Immunol 8:393

Rock KL, Benacerraf B (1983) The role of Ia molecule in the activation of T lymphocytes III. Antigen-specific, Ia-restricted, interleukin 2-producing T cell hybridomas with detectable affinity for the restricting I-A molecule. J Exp Med 157:359

Roem NW, Leibson HJ, Zlotnik A, Kappler J, Marrack P, Cambier JC (1984) Interleukin-induced increase in Ia expression by normal mouse B cells. J Exp Med 160:679

Saito T, Rajewsky K (1985) A self-I-A reactive T cell clone directly stimulates every hundredth B cells and helps antigen-specific B cell responses. Eur J Immunol 15:927

Smith JB, Knowlton P (1979) Activation of suppressor T cells in human autologous mixed lymphocyte culture. J Immunol 123:419

Zauderer M, Campbell H, Johnson DR, Seman M (1984) Helper function of antigen-induced specific and autoreactive T cell clones. J Mol Cell Immunol 1:65

Printed by Publishers' Graphics LLC USA
MO20120905-313